Principles and Foundations of
Health Promotion and Education

SEVENTH EDITION

Principles and Foundations of Health Promotion and Education

SEVENTH EDITION

Randall R. Cottrell, D.ED., MCHES
Professor, University of North Carolina Wilmington & Professor Emeritus, University of Cincinnati

James T. Girvan, Ph.D., M.P.H.
Professor Emeritus, Boise State University

Denise M. Seabert, Ph.D., MCHES
Professor & Associate Dean, Ball State University

Caile Spear, Ph.D., MCHES
Professor, Boise State University

James F. McKenzie, Ph.D., M.P.H., MCHES
Professor Emeritus, Ball State University

330 Hudson Street, NY, NY 10013

Senior Portfolio Manager: *Michelle Yglecias*
Content Producer: *Susan Malloy*
Portfolio Management Assistant: *Nicole Constantine*
Managing Producer, Science: *Nancy Tabor*
Full-service Vendor and Compositor: *Cenveo® Publisher Services*
Project Manager: *Norine Strang*
Copyeditor: *Michael Rossa*
Cover Designer: *Tamara Newnam*
Rights & Permissions Project Manager: *Laura Murray*
Rights & Permissions Management: *Ben Ferrini*
Manufacturing Buyer, Higher Ed.: *Stacey Weinberger*
Executive Product Marketing Manager: *Neena Bali*
Cover Photo Credit: *Rawpixel/Alamy*

Acknowledgements of third party content appear on page 367, which constitutes an extension of this copyright page.

Library of Congress Cataloging-in-Publication Data

Names: Cottrell, Randall R., author. | Girvan, James T., author. | Seabert, Denise, author. | Spear, Caile, author. | McKenzie, James F., author.

Title: Principles and foundations of health promotion and education / Randall R. Cottrell, James T. Girvan, Denise M. Seabert, Caile Spear, James F. McKenzie.

Description: Seventh edition. | Glenview, IL : Pearson Education, Inc., [2018] | Includes bibliographical references and index.

Identifiers: LCCN 2016038665| ISBN 9780134517650 (alk. paper) | ISBN 0134517652 (alk. paper)

Subjects: | MESH: Health Education | Health Promotion | Models, Educational | United States

Classification: LCC RA440.5 | NLM WA 590 | DDC 613--dc23 LC record available at https://lccn.loc.gov/2016038665

2   17

www.pearsonhighered.com

ISBN 10: 0-134-51765-2
ISBN 13: 978-0-134-51765-0

CONTENTS

Chapter 5 Ethics and Health Education/Promotion 136

Chapter 6 The Health Education Specialist: Roles, Responsibilities, Certifications, and Advanced Study 163

This is an exciting time to be studying and/or entering the field of health education/ promotion. There continues to be unparalleled interest in health as evidenced by the growing numbers of students entering training programs, numerous new products and services designed to address health issues, and the dramatic growth in information and information-seeking behaviors of those interested in knowing about their health. Yet we are facing problems that are dramatic with the aging of the population, the shifting demographics of populations, the continuing challenges that come from new biological and social threats to health, and the explosive growth of social media and apps that are related to health issues. In Burke's preface to the second edition of *Connections*, he refers to "the radical changes that lay ahead, caused by developments in communications and information technology, and of the urgent need to understand the process of scientific and technological change, the better to manage its increasingly unexpected ripple effects" (Burke, 2007).

Therein lies the challenge to crafting a book to serve as the foundational introduction to the field of health education/promotion. Most would agree that change is the only constant in our world today—and that change is happening more rapidly and with greater consequence with each passing year. How then do Cottrell et al. provide a foundation for a profession as complex and changing as health education/promotion? Let me give you two illustrations of that challenge. First, in my lifetime there have been incredible changes in our thinking about subjects such as nutrition. In that time we've gone from a basic seven, to a basic four, to a daily food guide with five groups, then a food wheel providing a platter for daily food choices, then a food guide pyramid followed by MyPyramid, and now MyPlate (U.S. Department of Agriculture, 2013). Certainly, nutrition is not the only health-related content that changes so rapidly with changes in science and technology.

Second, as I look back one decade to 2006, no one then knew what the Zika virus was, Facebook and Twitter had barely come into use, the Human Genome Project had just been completed, iPhones and iPads had not yet been introduced, and this country had not yet had an African American president. Think about the implications of this kind of rapid change in the field of health education/promotion. Those responsible for the training of health education specialists/ promoters must train our students to be able to practice 10 years from now, in a world that does not yet exist, to address problems that are as yet unknown and to be able to use tools that do not yet exist.

The best definition of education I've ever heard has been attributed to Albert Einstein, but its origin is unclear. However, I believe that "education is what's left over after you forget everything you've been taught." If you agree, you realize that we need to put into place not content related to fields of study such as health education/promotion, but the building blocks that let aspiring professionals and others continue to grow in their understanding and professional practice. Cottrell and colleagues come as close as I've seen among the "foundations" books to achieving this.

Here's what the seventh edition of *Principles and Foundations of Health Promotion and Education* does to address the theme of change. The authors provide foundational history and philosophical guidelines allowing for consideration, thought, application, and adaptation. They don't prescribe, they provide building blocks. They do this in the context of applying multiple pedagogies in their chapters. I am particularly appreciative of their Practitioner's Perspective, A Day in the Career, Case Studies, and Critical Thinking Questions and Activities. These worked so well in the sixth edition and have been significantly updated and improved.

I am especially pleased to say that consistent with the theme of change, Chapter 10 on future trends in health education/promotion captures the essence of the forces driving these changes, and it is an interesting look at the implications for the profession and practice of health education/promotion. Because of the overall tenor of the book and each of the elements I've discussed, it is critically important that a book such as this is available to those beginning their study of the field of health education/promotion.

Welcome to the future.

Robert S. Gold, Ph.D, DrPH, FASHA, FAAHB
University of Maryland

References

Burke, James (2012-02-21). *Connections* (Kindle Locations 93–95). Simon & Schuster. Kindle Edition.
U.S. Department of Agriculture. A brief history of USDA food guides. Retrieved September 1, 2013, from http://www.choosemyplate.gov/food-groups/downloads/MyPlate/ABriefHistoryOfUSDAFoodGuides.pdf.

Many students enter the profession of health education/promotion knowing only that they are interested in health and wish to help others improve their health status. Typically, students' interest in health education/promotion is derived from their own desire to live a healthy lifestyle and not from an in-depth understanding of the historical, theoretical, and philosophical foundations of this profession. Other than perhaps a high school health education teacher, many students do not know any health education specialists. In fact, most beginning students are unaware of employment opportunities, the skills needed to practice health education/promotion, and what it would be like to work in a given health education/promotion setting.

This text is written for such students. The contents will be of value to students who are undecided as to whether health education/promotion is the major they want to pursue, as well as for new health education/promotion majors who need information about what health education/promotion is and where health education specialists can be employed. The text is designed for use in an entry-level health education/promotion course in which the major goal is to introduce students to health education/promotion. In addition, it may have value in introducing new health education graduate students, who have undergraduate degrees in fields other than health education/promotion, to the health education/promotion profession.

▷ New to the Seventh Edition

- Significant rewrites to make information in the chapters flow better in sequence for students.
- All chapters have been updated for currency including tables, figures, references, terminology, end-of-chapter materials, Weblinks, and appendices.
- Additional within-chapter application scenarios.
- Many of the Practitioner's Perspective boxes have been replaced, offering fresh insights from current practitioners addressing such areas as health education certification (CHES), Eta Sigma Gamma, professional associations, internships, and careers in healthcare settings and university wellness centers among others.

Important new issues and trends covered include

- the impact of healthcare reform on health education/promotion;
- Whole School, Whole Community, Whole Child Model;

- Health Education Specialist Practice Analysis 2015 (HESPA);
- *Healthy People 2020*;
- updated responsibilities, competencies, and sub-competencies of a health education specialist;
- program accreditation for freestanding undergraduate public/community health programs; and
- The Patient Protection and Affordable Care Act's implications for public/community health education.

▷ Chapter Overview

Chapter 1, "A Background for the Profession," provides an overview of health education/promotion and sets the stage for the remaining chapters. Chapter 2, "The History of Health and Health Education/Promotion," examines the history of health and health care, as well as the history of health education/promotion. This chapter was written to help students understand the tremendous advances that have been made in keeping people healthy, and it provides perspective on the role of health education/promotion in that effort. One cannot appreciate the present without understanding the past. The chapter will bring students up to date with the most recent happenings in the profession, such as the new Patient Protection and Affordable Care Act and the Whole School, Whole Community, Whole Child Model. Chapters 3, 4, and 5 provide what might best be called the basic foundations. All professions, such as law, medicine, business, and teacher education, must provide students with information related to the philosophy, theory, and ethics inherent in the field.

Chapter 6, "The Health Education Specialist: Roles, Responsibilities, Certifications, and Advanced Study," is designed to acquaint new students with the skills that are needed to practice in the field of health education/promotion. It also explains the certification process to students and encourages them to begin thinking of graduate study early in their undergraduate programs. New information related to changes in the competencies and sub-competencies of a health education specialist based on the 2015 Health Education Specialist Practice Analysis (HESPA) study is incorporated into this chapter. Chapter 7, "The Settings for Health Education/Promotion," introduces students to the job responsibilities inherent in different types of health education/promotion positions and provides a discussion of the pros and cons of working in various health education/promotion settings. With its "A Day in the Career of . . ." sections and the "Practitioner's Perspective" boxes, this chapter is unique among introductory texts. An important warning is provided to students to be careful what they post to social networking Web sites, and information is included on landing one's first job and how to excel in a health education/promotion career. This chapter truly provides students with important insights into the various health education/promotion settings and the overall practice of health education/promotion.

Chapter 8, "Agencies, Associations, and Organizations Associated with Health Education/Promotion," introduces students to the many professional agencies, associations, and organizations that support health education/promotion. This is an extremely important chapter because all health education specialists need to know of these resources and allies. All introductory students are encouraged to join one or more of the professional associations described in this chapter. For that reason, contact information for all of the professional associations discussed is included in the chapter. Chapter 9, "The Literature of Health Education/Promotion," directs students to the information and resources necessary to work in the field. Included in this chapter is basic information related to the Internet and the World Wide Web that should be especially helpful to new students. With the explosion of knowledge related to health, being able to locate needed resources is a critical skill for health education specialists. Finally, health education/promotion students need to consider what future changes in health knowledge, policy, and funding may mean to those working in health education/promotion. They must learn to project into the future and prepare themselves to meet these challenges. Chapter 10, "Future Trends in Health Education/Promotion," is an attempt to provide a window into the future for today's health education/promotion students.

As one reads the text, it will be apparent that certain standard features exist in all chapters. These are designed to help the student identify important information, guide the student's learning, and extend the student's understanding beyond the basic content information. Each chapter begins by identifying objectives. Before reading a chapter, students should carefully read the objectives because they will guide the student's learning of the information contained in that chapter. After reading a chapter, it may also be helpful to review the objectives again to be certain major points were understood. Being able to respond to each objective and define each highlighted term in a chapter is typically of great value in understanding the material and preparing for examinations.

Throughout the text take note of the "Practitioner's Perspective" boxes. These are boxes written by health education/promotion professionals who are currently working in the field. Some of the boxes relate to working in a particular setting, while others focus on such areas as ethics, certification, internships, hiring, Eta Sigma Gamma, and graduate study. There is a total of 18 "Practitioner's Perspective" boxes, 9 of them new to this edition.

At the end of each chapter, the student will find a brief summary of the information contained in that chapter. Following the summary are review questions. Students are encouraged to answer these questions because they provide an additional method for targeting learning and reviewing the chapter's contents. A case study follows the review questions. Case studies allow readers to project themselves into realistic health education situations and problem solve how to handle such situations. Next, readers will find critical thinking questions designed to extend readers' learning beyond what is presented in the chapter. They require readers to apply what they have learned, contemplate major events, and project their learning into the future. A list of activities, designed to extend readers' knowledge beyond what can be obtained by reading the chapter, follows the critical thinking questions. In some activities students are asked to apply or synthesize the chapter's information. In others, students are encouraged to get actively involved with experiences that will help integrate learning from the text with a practical, real-world setting. By completing these activities, students should have a better understanding of health education/promotion. The activities are followed by Weblinks, which have been updated and expanded for this edition. Weblinks are sites that students can access to read more about a topic, extend their learning, or obtain interesting and important resource materials. Each chapter ends with a list of references the authors used to develop the chapter. All references are cited in the chapter, and students can use the references to obtain more detailed information on a topic from an original source when they desire to do so.

▷ Supplements

The following instructor supplements are available with the seventh edition:

- An Instructor's Manual that includes a synopsis, an outline, teaching ideas, Web site activities, and video resources for each chapter.
- A Test Bank that includes multiple-choice, true/false, and essay questions for each chapter. A computerized Test Bank is also available.
- PowerPoint presentations that feature chapter outlines and key points from the text.

Many thanks to Michelle LaClair, Pennsylvania State College of Medicine, for her careful revision of these resources. All of the supplements are available in electronic format only; they can be downloaded by signing in at Pearson's Instructor Resource Center at http://www .pearsonhighered.com/educator.

We authors readily acknowledge that the information contained in this text represents our bias regarding what material should be taught in an introductory course. There may be important introductory information we have not included, or we may have included information that may not be considered introductory by all users. We welcome and encourage comments and feedback, both positive and negative, from all users of this text. Only with such feedback can we make improvements and include the most appropriate information in future editions.

Randall R. Cottrell
James T. Girvan
Denise M. Seabert
Caile Spear
James F. McKenzie

ACKNOWLEDGMENTS

First, we would like to thank all of the health education faculty who have adopted each new edition of our text and all of the students who have used the text. The response we have received has been truly gratifying. Without you, we would not be writing the seventh edition of our text.

We would also like to thank Pearson for producing the book. We would especially like to thank Michelle Yglecias and Susan Malloy for their editorial guidance as well as Norine Strang for her hard work on this project.

We would like to express our sincere appreciation to those health education/promotion professionals who served as reviewers for the seventh edition. They had many good ideas that we tried to incorporate whenever possible. The reviewers were Becky Corran, New Mexico State University, Doña Ana Community College; Stephen Firsing, Coastal Carolina University; Katie Darby Hein, University of Georgia; Jennifer H. Herman, Simmons College; Pamela Hoalt, Malone University; Stephanie Malinenko, Daemen College; Keely Rees, University of Wisconsin, La Crosse; Brenda Simonson, Niagara County Community College; Jennifer Tripken, Marymount University; and Ashley Wennerstrom, Tulane University.

We would also like to thank the reviewers of previous editions: Jerome Kotecki, Ball State University; Erin Largo-Wight, University of North Florida; Sarah Rush, University of Alabama; Erica Sosa, University of Texas at San Antonio; Lori Turner, University of Alabama; Linda Wray, Pennsylvania State University; John Batacan, Idaho State University; Holly Harring, University of South Carolina; Joanna Hayden, William Paterson University; Adriana Rascon-Lopez, University of Texas at El Paso; Manoj Sharma, University of Cincinnati; Erica Sosa, University of Texas at San Antonio; Georgia Polacek, University of Texas, San Antonio; Kathleen Allison, Lock Haven University; Gregg Kirchofer, Canisius College; Dawn Larsen, Minnesota State University, Mankato; Sharon Thompson, the University of Texas, El Paso; M. Allison Ford, Florida Atlantic University; Mike Perko, University of North Carolina Greensboro; Georgia Johnston, the University of Texas, San Antonio; Craig Huddy, Concord College; Whitney Boling, University of Houston; Virginia Noland, University of Florida; R. Morgan Pigg, Jr., University of Florida; Marilyn Morrow, Illinois State University; Steve Nagy, Western Kentucky University; Emily Tyler, University of North Carolina at Greensboro (with additional helpful feedback from Julie Orta, MPH student); and Marianne Frauenknecht, Western Michigan University. Special thanks to Steven Crowley at Boise State University for his assistance with the Philosophy chapter.

Finally, we would like to dedicate this book to the people in our lives who mean the most to us: our spouses, Karen, Georgia, Bonnie, Matt, and Glen; our children, Kyle, Lisa, Kory, Nollis, Jennifer, Erik, Becky, Erik, Anne, Greg, Clark, Nathan, Elias, and Devin; our grandchildren, Kaylee, Anna, Emily, Jonah, Rose, Aevan, Olin, Mitchell, Julia, and Ansley; and our parents, Russell and Edith Cottrell, Terry and Margaret Girvan, Gordon and Betty McKenzie, Paul and Judy Seabert, and Ellen and Robert Spear.

Chapter 1

A Background for the Profession

Chapter Objectives

After reading this chapter and answering the questions at the end,
you should be able to:

- Define the terms *health, health education, health promotion, disease prevention, public health, community health, global health, population health,* and *wellness.*
- Describe the current status of health education/promotion.
- Define *epidemiology.*
- Explain the means by which health or health status can be measured.
- List and explain the goals and objectives of health education/promotion.
- Identify the practice of health education/promotion.
- Explain the following concepts and principles:

  a. health field concept
  b. levels of prevention
  c. risk factors
  d. health risk reduction
  e. chain of infection
  f. communicable disease model
  g. multicausation disease model
  h. selected principles of health education/promotion—*participation, empowerment, advocacy, social media,* and *cultural competence*

Health education/promotion has come a long way since its early beginnings. Health education/promotion as we know it today dates back only about 80 years, but the progress in development has accelerated most rapidly in the past 35 years (Glanz & Rimer, 2008). As the profession has grown and changed, so have the roles and responsibilities of health education specialists. The purpose of this book is to provide those new to this profession with a sense of the past—how the profession was born and on what principles it was developed; a complete understanding of the present—what it is that health education specialists are expected to do, how they should do it, and what guides their work; and a look at the future—where the profession is headed, and how health education specialists can keep pace with the changes to be responsive to those whom they serve.

This chapter provides a background in the terminology, concepts, and principles of the profession. It defines many of the key words and terms used in the profession, briefly discusses why health education/promotion is referred to as an emerging profession, looks at the current state of the profession, shows how health and health status have been measured, outlines the goals and objectives of the profession, identifies the practice of health education/promotion, and discusses some of the basic, underlying concepts and principles of the profession.

▷ Key Words, Terms, and Definitions

Each chapter introduces new terminology that is either important to the specific content presented in the chapter or used frequently in the profession. This chapter discusses the more common terms that will be used throughout this text. Like the profession, these words and definitions have evolved over the years. The most recent effort occurred in 2011 (Joint Committee on Health Education and Promotion Terminology [Joint Committee], 2012). The 2011 Joint Committee was convened by the American Association for Health Education (AAHE) of the American Alliance for Health, Physical Education, Recreation, and Dance (AAH-PERD) (see Chapter 8 for information on professional associations). The Joint Committee is charged with reviewing and updating the terminology of the profession. The members of the 2011 Joint Committee were composed of representatives from the member organizations in the Coalition of National Health Education Organizations (see Chapter 8), the National Commission for Health Education Credentialing, Inc. (see Chapter 6), and governmental agencies (Joint Committee, 2012). Before this meeting, there had been seven major terminology reports developed for the profession over the past 80 years with the first dating back to 1927 (Johns, 1973; Joint Committee on Health Education Terminology, 1991a, 1991b; Joint Committee, 2001; Moss, 1950; Rugen, 1972; Williams, 1934; Yoho, 1962).

Before presenting some of the key terms used in the profession, an in-depth discussion of the word *health* may be helpful. Health is a difficult concept to put into words, but it is one that most people intuitively understand. The World Health Organization (WHO) has defined health as "the state of complete mental, physical and social well being not merely the absence of disease or infirmity" (WHO, 1947, p. 1). This classic definition is important because it identifies the vital components of health and further implies that health is a holistic concept involving an interaction and interdependence among these various components. A number of years after the writing of the WHO definition, Hanlon (1974) defined health as "a functional state which makes possible the achievement of other goals and activities. Comfort, well-being, and the distinction between physical and mental health differ in social classes, cultures, and religious groups" (p. 73). And more recently, the WHO (1986) has stated that "To reach a state of complete physical, mental, and social well-being, an individual or group must be able to identify and to realize aspirations, to satisfy needs, and to change or cope with the environment. Health is, therefore, seen as a resource for everyday life, not the object of living. Health is a positive concept emphasizing social and personal resources, as well as physical capacities" (p. 5). In other words, good health should not be the goal of life but rather a vehicle to reaching one's goals of life. We feel that these major concepts of health are captured in the definition that states that **health** "is a *dynamic* state or condition that is multidimensional (i.e., physical, emotional, social, intellectual, spiritual, and occupational) a resource for living, and results from a person's interactions with and adaptation to the environment"

(Joint Committee, 2012, p. 10). As such, health can exist in varying degrees—ranging from good to poor and everywhere in between—and depends on each person's individual circumstances. "For example, a person can be healthy while dying, or a person who is quadriplegic can be healthy in the sense that his or her mental and social well-being is high and physical health is as good as it can be" (Hancock & Minkler, 2005, p. 144).

In addition to the word *health*, it is also important to have an understanding of the following key terms and definitions:

community health—"the health status of a defined group of people and the actions and conditions to promote, protect and preserve their health" (Joint Committee, 2012, p. 15)

health education—"any combination of planned learning experiences using evidence based practices and/or sound theories that provide the opportunity to acquire knowledge, attitudes, and skills needed [to] adopt and maintain healthy behaviors" (Joint Committee, 2012, p. 17)

health promotion—"any planned combination of educational, political, environmental, regulatory, or organizational mechanisms that support actions and conditions of living conducive to the health of individuals, groups, and communities" (Joint Committee, 2012, p. 18) (See **Figure 1.1** for the relationship between health education and health promotion.)

disease prevention—"the process of reducing risks and alleviating disease to promote, preserve, and restore health and minimize suffering and distress" (Joint Committee, 2001, p. 99)

public health—"an organized effort by society, primarily through its public institutions, to improve, promote, protect and restore the health of the population through collective action. It includes services such as health situation analysis, health surveillance, health promotion, prevention, infectious disease control, environmental protection and sanitation, disaster and health emergency preparedness and response, and occupational health, among others" (WHO, 2016a)

▶ **Figure 1.1** Relationship between health education and health promotion

Source: From J. F. McKenzie, B. L. Neiger, and R. Thackeray, *Planning, Implementing and Evaluating Health Promotion Programs: A Primer*. 6th ed., p. 5, Fig 1.1 © 2013 Reproduced by permission of Pearson Education, Inc., Upper Saddle River, NJ.

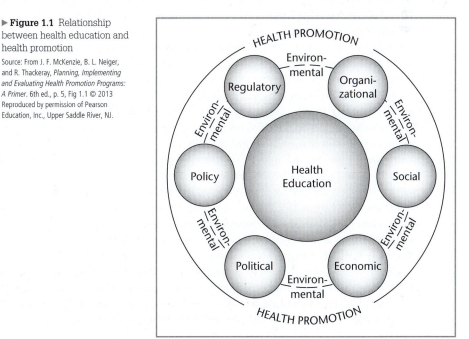

global health—"health problems, issues, and concerns that transcend national boundaries and are beyond the control of individual nations, and are best addressed by cooperative actions and solutions" (Joint Committee, 2012, p. 17)

population health—"a cohesive, integrated, and comprehensive approach to health care that considers the distribution of health outcomes within a population, the health determinants that influence distribution of care, and the policies and interventions that affect and are affected by the determinants" (Nash, Fabius, Skoufalos, Clarke, & Horowitz, 2016, p. 448)

wellness—"an approach to health that focuses on balancing the many aspects, or dimensions, of a person's life through increasing the adoption of health enhancing conditions and behaviors rather than attempting to minimize conditions of illness" (Joint Committee, 2012, p. 10)

Before we leave the discussion about key words and terms of the profession, it should be noted that there is not complete agreement on terminology. We could easily have found another definition for each of the terms presented here written by either a respected scholar in health education/promotion or a legitimate professional or governmental health agency.

▷ The Health Education/Promotion Profession

Historically, there have been a number of occasions that can be pointed to as "critical" to the development of health education/promotion. (See Chapter 2 for an in-depth presentation of the history.) But there has been no time in which the status of the profession has been more visible to the average person or as widely accepted by other health professionals as it is today. Much of this notoriety can be attributed to the health promotion era of public health history that began about 1974 in the United States.

The United States' first public health revolution spanned the late 19th century through the mid-20th century and was aimed at controlling the harm (morbidity and mortality) that came from infectious diseases. By the mid-1950s, many of the infectious diseases in the United States were pretty much under control. This was evidenced by the improved infant mortality rates, the reduction in the number of children who were contracting childhood diseases, the reduction in the overall death rates in the country, and the increase in life expectancy (see **Table 1.1**). With the control of many communicable diseases, the focus moved to the major chronic diseases such as heart disease, cancer, and strokes—diseases that were, in large part, the result of the way people lived.

It became clear, by the mid-1970s, that the greatest potential for reducing morbidity, saving lives, and reducing healthcare costs in the United States was to be achieved through health promotion and disease prevention. At the core of this approach was health education/promotion. In 1980, the U.S. Department of Health, Education, and Welfare (USDHEW) presented a blueprint of the health promotion and disease prevention strategy in its first set of health objectives in the document called *Promoting Health/Preventing Disease: Objectives for a Nation* (USDHEW, 1980). This document proposed a total of 226 objectives divided into three main areas—preventive services, health protection, and health promotion. This was the first time a comprehensive national agenda for prevention had been developed, with specific goals and objectives for anticipated gains (McGinnis, 1985). In 1985, it was apparent that only about one half of the objectives established in 1980 would be reached by 1990, another

TABLE 1.1 **Life expectancy at birth, at 65 years of age, and at 75 years of age, according to sex: United States, selected years 1900–2010**

Year	At Birth			At 65 Years			At 75 Years		
	Both Sexes	Male	Female	Both Sexes	Male	Female	Both Sexes	Male	Female
1900	47.3	46.3	48.3	11.9	11.5	12.2	*	*	*
1950	68.2	65.6	71.1	13.9	12.8	15.0	*	*	*
1980	73.7	70.7	77.4	16.4	14.1	18.3	10.4	8.8	11.5
2010	78.7	76.2	81.0	19.1	17.7	20.3	12.1	11.0	12.9

* = Data not available

Source: Data from U.S. Department of Health and Human Services, National Center for Health Statistics (NCHS). (2015). *Health, United States, 2014: With Special Feature on Adults Aged 55-64.* Hyattsville, MD: Author

one fourth would not be reached, and progress on the others could not be judged because of the lack of data (Mason & McGinnis, 1990). Even though not all objectives were reached, the planning process involved in the 1980 report demonstrated the value of setting goals and listing specific objectives as a means of measuring progress in the nation's health and healthcare services. These goals and objectives published by the U.S. Department of Health and Human Services (USDHHS), now in their fourth generation as *Healthy People 2020*, have defined the nation's health agenda and guided its health policy since their inception. (See Chapter 2 for more on *Healthy People 2020*.)

Now more than 10 years into the 21st century, the health of the people in the United States is better than any time in the past. "By every measure, we are healthier, live longer, and enjoy lives that are less likely to be marked by injuries, ill health, or premature death" (Institute of Medicine [IOM], 2003, p. 2). Yet, we could do better. Four modifiable health risk behaviors— "lack of exercise or physical activity, poor nutrition, tobacco use, and drinking too much alcohol—cause much of the illness, suffering, and early death related to chronic diseases and conditions" (Centers for Disease Control and Prevention [CDC], 2016a, ¶2). Thus, "behavior patterns represent the single most prominent domain of influence over health prospects in the United States" (McGinnis, Williams-Russo, & Knickman, 2002, p. 82).

As the health agenda has become more clearly defined, so has the health education/ promotion profession. In 1998, the U.S. Department of Commerce and Labor formally recognized "health educator" as a distinct occupation, thus demonstrating that the health education/promotion profession is moving in the right direction. More recently a study titled "Marketing the Health Education Profession: Knowledge, Attitudes, and Hiring Practices of Employers" conducted by Hezel Associates (2007) was conducted. Through this study the term *health education specialist* has gained favor over the use of the term *health educator*. A **health education specialist** has been defined as "an individual who has met, at a minimum, baccalaureate-level required health education academic preparation qualifications, who serves in a variety of settings, and is able to use appropriate educational strategies and methods to facilitate the development of policies, procedures, interventions, and systems conducive to the health of individuals, groups, and communities" (Joint Committee, 2012, p. 18). Thus the term *health education specialist* will be used throughout the remainder of this book.

Clearly, there is a need for health education/promotion interventions provided by health education specialists in the United States both today and in the future.

▷ Measuring Health or Health Status

Though the definition of health is easy to state, trying to quantify the amount of health an individual or a population possesses is not easy. Most measures of health are expressed using health statistics based on the traditional medical model of describing ill health (injury, disease, and death) instead of well health. Thus, the higher the presence of injury, disease, and death indicators, the lower the level of health; the lower the presence of injury, disease, and death indicators, the higher the level of health. Out of necessity we have defined the level of health with just the opposite—ill health (McKenzie, Pinger, & Kotecki, 2012).

The information gathered when measuring health is referred to as **epidemiological data**. These data are gathered at the local, state, and national levels to assist with the prevention of disease outbreaks or control those in progress and to plan and assess health education/promotion programs. Epidemiology is one of those disciplines that helps provide the foundation for the health education/promotion profession. **Epidemiology** is defined as "the study of the distribution and determinants of health-related states or events (including disease), and the application of this study to the control of diseases and other health problems" (World Health Organization, 2016b). In the following sections, several of the more common epidemiological means by which health, or lack thereof, are described and quantified.

Rates

A **rate** "is a measure of some event, disease, or condition in relation to a unit of population, along with some specification of time" (National Center for Health Statistics [NCHS], 2015, p. 442). Rates are important because they provide an opportunity for comparison of events, diseases, or conditions that occur at different times or places. Some of the more commonly used rates are death rates, birth rates, and morbidity rates. **Death rates** (the number of deaths per 100,000 resident population), sometimes referred to as *mortality* or *fatality rates*, are probably the most frequently used means of quantifying the seriousness of injury or disease. (See **Table 1.2** for death rates and **Table 1.3** for an example of a formula used to tabulate rates.) "The transition from wellness to ill health is often gradual and poorly defined. Because death, in

TABLE 1.2 **Crude death rates for all causes and selected causes of death: United States, 2014**

Cause	Deaths per 100,000 Population
All causes	823.7
Diseases of the heart	192.7
Malignant neoplasms (cancer)	185.6
Cerebrovascular diseases (stroke)	41.7
Suicide	13.4
Motor vehicle-related injuries	11.1
Homicide	5.0

Source: Data from U.S. Department of Health and Human Services, National Center for Health Statistics (NCHS). (2015). *Health, United States, 2014: With Special Feature on Adults Aged 55-64.* Hyattsville, MD: Author.

EPIDEMIOLOGY Jaime Harding

CURRENT POSITION: Health Promotion Program Manager

EMPLOYER: Central District Health Department, Boise, Idaho

DEGREE/INSTITUTION/YEAR: Master of Health Science, Boise State University, August 2006; Bachelor of Science, Athletic Training and Bachelor of Science, Health Promotion, Boise State University, May 2001.

MAJOR: Health Science—Health Policy emphasis (graduate); Athletic Training (undergraduate); Health Promotion (undergraduate)

Describe your past and current professional positions and how you came to hold the job you now hold (How did you obtain the position?): During my senior year of undergraduate work, I interned at Saint Alphonsus Regional Medical Center in the Marketing Department. Upon my graduation, the internship position led into a full-time employment opportunity within the same department. I worked in this capacity for approximately one year when I obtained a promotional opportunity to work for the Idaho Department of Health and Welfare (IDHW). I worked in several capacities for the IDHW for ten years. Specifically, my positions were in the Division of Medicaid in the Regional Medicaid Services office as a Health Resources Coordinator in Medicaid's managed care program, Healthy Connections; in the Diabetes Prevention and Control Program; in the Physical Activity and Nutrition Program as a Health Program Specialist and finally as a Physical Activity and Nutrition Program Manager. These experiences honed my skills in grant writing to agencies such as the CDC and the U.S. Administration of Aging, negotiating and managing contracts, supervising employees, facilitating statewide networks for prevention activities, and creating and overseeing program budgets. Having these skills helped me obtain the Health Promotion Program Manager position at Central District Health Department in April 2012, where I helped guide the local health department's shift away from working on individual behavior change activities to that of broad-based population impact to increase access to physical activity and healthy eating opportunities.

Describe the duties of your current position: Within the Office of Health Promotion, my staff and I primarily focus on increasing access to physical activity and healthy eating along with reducing tobacco initiation and use. I also oversee the implementation of a senior fall prevention program and an agency worksite wellness program. Additionally, I conduct semiannual and annual performance reviews along with providing regular coaching and mentoring to staff. I lead staff in strategic and policy agenda planning utilizing a policy, systems, and environmental change approach to influence broad-based population impact, and negotiate and manage contracts with multiple agencies such as IDHW and non-profit organizations. These are my major position duties. I'm also involved with staff in providing technical assistance and training to community partners, participating on state and local coalitions, alliances, and advisory boards with a physical activity, nutrition, tobacco prevention, and healthy aging emphasis.

Describe what you like most about this position: After working for ten years at a state agency, I've enjoyed gaining local-level experience. I appreciate the opportunity to work in each community to spend time developing and fostering relationships while gaining an understanding of the specific needs of that community. I have noticed I spend more time fostering partnerships through face-to-face meetings and phone calls than through email communication.

Describe what you like least about this position: Stable and ongoing funding for primary prevention has been problematic for public health. In the past, most funding opportunities came to us in a categorical manner or with a disease-specific focus. Recently, we are starting to see a shift to funding primary prevention work that is

BOX

1.1

continued

focused on mitigating chronic disease risk factors through broad-based population work. Public health funding continues to be inadequate and inconsistently funded so this is an ongoing challenge. Because we are often underfunded, we are limited on available human resources, which results in a challenge to have adequate staff to meet the workload demands.

In addition, we often have problems with programmatic silos in public health resulting in duplication of effort. Programs tend to work independently of each other, often using the same community-based partners. Unfortunately, in a small state like Idaho, many community-based partners are serving on multiple coalitions and alliances. It is not uncommon for me to attend two different coalition meetings within a short period of time and usually the same core group of people is in attendance. We talk about integration and streamlining efforts among programs and community partners, but it is difficult to put this into practice.

How do you use health data/epidemiology in your current position? We use health data to inform us on the current and changed state of our communities. These data help us determine the priority needs in each community for addressing access to physical activity, healthy eating, and tobacco use prevention. Within our four-county jurisdiction, we are working with several communities to implement the CDC-developed Community Health Assessment and Group Evaluation (CHANGE) Tool. The CHANGE Tool community health assessment affords us an opportunity to assess community strengths, identify areas for improvement, and assist the community with prioritizing community needs related to population-based strategies. Currently, we rely on state-collected data such as the CDC's Behavioral Risk Factor Surveillance

System (BRFSS) and Youth Risk Behavior Surveillance System (YRBSS) to assess health behaviors, but we recognize there are health data gaps in Idaho. There are efforts underway to address these data gaps and develop a clearinghouse to store chronic disease risk factor data. We use best practice or evidence-based practices in our community-based work to create lasting, sustainable change. Our goal is to create an environment where the healthy choice is the default choice for all individuals.

What recommendations/advice do you have for current health education students desiring to become community health educators? I work with interns on a regular basis and am often interviewed by students seeking guidance for entering the public health field. I recommend developing skills to become a strong written and oral communicator. Much of our work is done through written documents and via oral presentations. I'm often asked to present to the Central District Health Department Board of Health or other groups within the community so being organized and comfortable with public speaking is key. Additionally, I write grant applications, reports, contracts, and communicate via email so strong written skills are a necessity. I recommend that students be nimble and flexible in their careers. Students need to know that an entry-level position may not be their dream job but it serves as an opportunity to develop skills and relationships with other individuals working in the field. It is a way to gain experience so when promotional opportunities are available, they can apply for them. It's also critical that students connect with working professionals through local, state, and national societies and associations. Oftentimes, networking opens the door for employment opportunities.

TABLE 1.3 **Selected mortality rates and their formulas**

Rate	Definition	Example (U.S. 2014)
Crude death rate $= \dfrac{\text{Number of deaths (all cause)}}{\text{Estimated midyear population}} \times 100{,}000$		799.5/100,000
Age-specific death rate $= \dfrac{\text{Number of deaths, } 45-54}{\text{Estimated midyear population, } 45-54} \times 100{,}000$		407.1/100,000
Cause-specific mortality $= \dfrac{\text{Number of deaths, (HIV)}}{\text{Estimated midyear population}} \times 100{,}000$		2.7/100,000

Source: Data from U.S. Department of Health and Human Services, National Center for Health Statistics (NCHS). (2015). *Health, United States, 2014: With Special Feature on Adults Ages 55-64.* Hyattsville, MD: Author.

contrast, is a clearly defined event, it has continued to be the most reliable single indicator of health status of a population. Mortality statistics, however, describe only a part of the health status of a population, and often only the endpoint of an illness process" (USDHHS, 1991, p. 15). Rates can be expressed in three forms: (1) crude, (2) adjusted, and (3) specific. A **crude rate** is the rate expressed for a total population. An **adjusted rate** is also expressed for a total population but is statistically adjusted for a certain characteristic, such as age. A **specific rate** is a rate for a particular population subgroup such as for a particular disease (i.e., disease-specific) or for a particular age of people (i.e., age-specific). Examples include calculating the death rate for heart disease in the United States or the age-specific death rate for 45- to 54-year-olds.

There are three other epidemiological terms that are used to describe the magnitude of a rate of some event, disease, or condition in a unit of population. They are (1) **endemic**—occurs regularly in a population as a matter of course, such as heart disease in the United States; (2) **epidemic**—an unexpectedly large number of cases of an illness, specific health-related behavior, or other health-related event in a population, like the recent Ebola outbreak in West Africa; and (3) **pandemic**—an outbreak over a wide geographical area, such as a continent. An example of a recent pandemic was the H1N1 flu outbreak in the United States. As you continue your preparation to become a health education specialist, you will be introduced to more and more epidemiological principles and terms.

Life Expectancy

Life expectancy is another means by which health or health status has been measured. However, it is also based on mortality. Even with this limitation, life expectancy has been described as "the most comprehensive indicator of patterns of health and disease, as well as living standards and social development" (CDC, 1994, pp. 2–8). **Life expectancy** "is the average number of years of life remaining to a person at a particular age and is based on a given set of age-specific death rates—generally the mortality conditions existing in the period mentioned. Life expectancy may be determined by sex, race and Hispanic origin, or other characteristics using age-specific death rates for the population with that characteristic" (NCHS, 2015, p. 424). The most frequently used times to state life expectancy are at birth, at the age of 65, and more recently at age 75 (see Table 1.1). It must be remembered that life expectancy is an average for an entire cohort (usually a single birth year) and is not necessarily a useful predictor for any one individual. In terms of evaluating the effect of chronic disease on a population, life expectancies calculated *after* birth have been found to be more useful measures than life expectancy *at* birth because life expectancy at birth reflects infant mortality rates.

Years of Potential Life Lost

A third method by which health or health status has been measured is **years of potential life lost (YPLL)**. YPLL "is a measure of premature mortality" (NCHS, 2015, p. 446) (see **Table 1.4**) and is calculated by subtracting a person's age at death from 75 years. For example, for a person who dies at age 30, the YPLL are 45. Until 1996, the U.S. government used age 65 in calculating YPLL, but because life expectancy in the United States has continued to increase and is greater than 75 years, that age is now used (NCHS, 2015).

Disability-Adjusted Life Years

The three measures of health and health status noted previously are commonly used in the United States and other developed countries. However, because mortality does not express the burden of living with disability (for example, the resulting paralysis from an automobile crash or the depression that often follows a stroke), the WHO and the World Bank developed a measure called **disability-adjusted life years (DALYs)**. One DALY can be thought of as one lost year of "healthy" life as a result of being in states of poor health or disability (Murray & Lopez, 1996; WHO, 2008).

To calculate total DALYs for a given condition in a population, years of life lost (YLL) and years lived with disability (YLD) of known severity and duration for that condition must each be estimated, then the total summed. For example, to calculate DALYs incurred through road accidents in India in 1990, add the total years of life lost in fatal road accidents and the total years of life lived with disabilities by survivors of such accidents (Murray & Lopez, 1996, p. 7).

Figure 1.2 presents the DALYs for selected regions of the world. As noted, "DALYs in Africa are at least two times higher than in any other region" (WHO, 2008, p. 40).

TABLE 1.4 **Age-adjusted years of potential life lost (per 100,000 population) before age 75 for selected leading causes of death: United States, 1990 and 2013**

Cause	1990	2013
Malignant neoplasms	2,003.8	1,328.6
Diseases of the heart	1,617.7	952.3
Unintentional injuries (accidents)	1,162.1	1,051.2
Suicide	393.1	401.6
Homicide	417.4	229.8
Cerebrovascular diseases (stroke)	259.6	158.1
Chronic lower respiratory diseases	187.4	176.6
Diabetes mellitus	155.9	168.3
HIV	383.8	58.1
Chronic liver disease and cirrhosis	196.9	176.9
Influenza and pneumonia	141.5	82.3

Source: Data from U.S. Department of Health and Human Services, National Center for Health Statistics (NCHS). (2015). *Health, United States, 2014 with Special Feature on Adults Aged 55-64.* Hyattsville, MD: Author, p. 93.

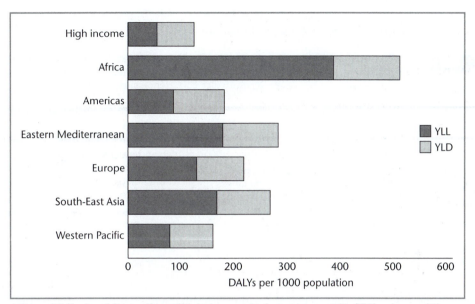

▲ **Figure 1.2** Burden of disease: Years of life lost as a result of premature mortality (YLL) and years of life lived with a disability (YLD) per thousand by region, 2004

Source: From "Burden of Disease: DALYs" in *The Global Burden of Disease: 2004 Update*. © World Health Organization, 2008. Reproduced by permission of the World Health Organization. http://www.who.int/healthinfo/global_burden_disease/GBD_report_2004update_part4.pdf DALYs, disability-adjusted life years

Health-Related Quality of Life

Even though DALYs go beyond measuring health in terms of just mortality, they really do not get at the quality of life (QOL). Although QOL refers to a person or group's general well-being, **health-related quality of life (HRQOL)** encompasses "those aspects of overall quality of life that can be clearly shown to affect health—either physical or mental" (CDC, 2011a, ¶3). Healthcare providers have often used HRQOL to measure the effects of chronic disease in their patients to better understand how a disease interferes with a person's daily life. Similarly, public health professionals have used HRQOL to measure the effects of numerous disorders, short- and long-term disabilities, and diseases in different populations. Tracking HRQOL in different populations can identify subgroups with poor physical or mental health and can help guide policies or other interventions to improve their health (CDC, 2011a).

Increasingly, health professionals have been using the concept of HRQOL to quantify and track the health status of people. Measures of HRQOL are now included on a number of different health surveys, including the Behavioral Risk Factor Surveillance Survey (BRFSS) and the National Health and Nutrition Examination Survey (NHANES) (see next section for discussion of these surveys). Both the BRFSS and the NHANES use the standard four-item "Healthy Days" core questions (CDC HRQOL-4) created by the Centers for Disease Control and Prevention (CDC) and presented in Box 1.2.

Health Surveys

Data collected through surveys conducted by governmental agencies are other means by which health or health status has been measured in the United States. Six examples are

"Healthy Days" Core Questions (CDC HRQOL-4)

1. Would you say that in general your health is:
   a. Excellent
   b. Very good
   c. Good
   d. Fair
   e. Poor

2. Now thinking about your physical health, which includes physical illness and injury, for how many days during the past 30 days was your physical health not good?

3. Now thinking about your mental health, which includes stress, depression, and problems with emotions, for how many days during the past 30 days was your mental health not good?

4. During the past 30 days, approximately about how many days did poor physical or mental health keep you from doing your usual activities, such as self-care, work, or recreation?

Source: Centers for Disease Control and Prevention (CDC). (2011a). *Health-related Quality of Life.* Available from http://www.cdc.gov/hrqol/methods.htm.

presented here. The first two, the National Health Interview Survey (NHIS) and the NHANES, are conducted by the National Center for Health Statistics (NCHS). The NHIS, which has been used for more than 50 years, is a household survey in which respondents are asked a number of questions about their health and health behavior. One of the questions, for example, asks the respondents to describe their health status using one of five categories: excellent, very good, good, fair, or poor.

The NHANES data are collected using a mobile examination center. Through personal interviews, physical examinations, and clinical and laboratory testing, data are collected on a representative group of Americans. These examinations result in the most authoritative source of standardized clinical, physical, and physiological data on the U.S. population. Included in the data are the prevalence of specific conditions and diseases and data on blood pressure, blood cholesterol, body mass index, nutritional status and deficiencies, and exposure to environmental toxins (CDC, 2016b).

The third example of data collected from surveys actually comes from a family of surveys called the National Health Care Surveys. These surveys are designed to "answer key questions of interest to health care policy makers, public health professionals, and researchers" (CDC, 2012a, ¶1). The National Health Care Surveys are used to study resource use, including staffing, quality of care, disparities in health care services, and diffusion of certain healthcare technologies (CDC, 2012a). The fourth example of data collected through a survey is the data collected through the BRFSS. The BRFSS is the nation's premier system of adult health-related data regarding health-related risk behaviors, chronic health conditions, and use of preventive services. Using telephone survey techniques, these data are collected by individual states, territories, and the District of Columbia through cooperative agreements with the CDC (CDC, 2014).

Because of the success of the BRFSS, a similar surveillance system was begun for youth. The Youth Risk Behavior Surveillance System (YRBSS) was developed in 1990 to monitor priority health-risk behaviors that contribute markedly to the leading causes of death, disability, and social problems among youth and adults in the United States. The six categories of priority health-risk behaviors include (1) tobacco use; (2) unhealthy dietary behaviors; (3) inadequate physical activity; (4) alcohol and other drug use; (5) sexual behaviors that contribute to unintended pregnancy and sexually transmitted diseases, including HIV infection; and (6) behaviors that contribute to unintentional injuries and violence (CDC, 2015a).

The final survey presented, the National College Health Assessment (NCHA), collects health data about college students. The NCHA is the only one presented here that is not conducted by a governmental agency. The NCHA is carried out by the professional organization American College Health Association (ACHA) (see Chapter 8 for more on this association). The ACHA developed the NCHA, which can be conducted as either a paper-pencil or online survey, to assist schools in collecting data about students' habits, behaviors, and perceptions about topics such as alcohol, tobacco, and other drug use; mental health; weight, nutrition, and exercise; personal safety and violence; and sexual health. The ACHA charges schools for conducting the NCHA, but the schools have the flexibility to select the surveying method, sample size, priority population, and time it is offered (ACHA, 2016).

▷ Using Health Data in Health Education/Promotion

In this section, we would like to give you an example of how health education specialists may use data. As you will soon learn, a major task of health education specialists is to assist those in the priority population (individuals, groups, and communities) in obtaining, maintaining, and improving their health. Often this means planning some type of health education/promotion program that can be used by those in the priority population. These programs should be based on the needs of the priority population, and the needs are often described using data.

For example, let's say a health education specialist is working for a local (county) health department at a time when the state health department has just made funds available through a competitive grant process to deal with the high rates of cancer in the state. Because of some past concerns about cancer in the county, her supervisor has suggested she seek funding. Though she has heard some residents express concern about possible higher rates of cancer, she is really not sure about the type of cancer or whether there is a specific group of people affected. Therefore, she needs to be able to describe the potential problem and identify a priority population. One approach would be to determine if there are any health disparities associated with cancer in her county. It has long been "recognized that some individuals are healthier than others and that some live longer than others do, and that often these differences are closely associated with social characteristics such as race, ethnicity, gender, location, and socioeconomic status" (King, 2009, p. 339). These gaps between groups have been referred to as *health disparities* (also called health inequalities in some countries). More formally, **health disparity** has been defined as the difference in health between populations often caused by two health inequities—lack of access to care and lack of quality care (McKenzie & Pinger, 2015).

One place to start looking for cancer health disparities would be the cancer mortality rates (i.e., crude and age-adjusted) for the state as a whole compared with the county where the health education specialist works. These data may be available from the NCHS or another center within the CDC, from the state department of health, or from a university research center. Comparisons could also be made based on the mortality rates for various types of cancer. If the health education specialist knew what types of cancers were of greatest concern in the county, she could then examine the data for the county on the basis of certain demographic characteristics that have been associated with certain cancers. So the health education specialist may be using sex-, age-, or race/ethnicity-specific rates to compare various subgroups while looking for disparities. Once the health education specialist identifies a subgroup problem with a type of cancer, she may turn to data from the BRFSS to look for risk behaviors that are known to contribute to or cause the type of cancer identified. Again, the health education specialist may find the needed data in a state or local agency or university as well. Using different sources of data should help the health education specialist find the focus of her program for the priority population and put her in a position to compete for the grant money from the state department of health. Examples of what the health education specialist may have found through this process are higher rates of prostate cancer in African American men between the ages of 45 and 64 years or a higher prevalence of certain types of leukemia in children younger than 15 years of age.

In summary, to get to the point of being able to identify a priority population (i.e., a certain subgroup of people) and program focus (i.e., risk factors associated with a certain type of cancer), several different types of data were used. Initially, the health education specialist used cancer mortality data, then prevalence rates for various types of cancer and different subgroups, and finally risk factor data for various types of cancer.

▷ The Goal and Purpose of the Profession

The ultimate goal of all service professions, including health education/promotion, is to improve the quality of life, even though the quality of life is difficult to quantify (Raphael, Brown, Renwick, & Rootman, 1997). However, many professionals feel that there is a direct relationship between quality of life and health status. Quality of life is usually improved when health status is improved, or, as Ashley Montagu (1968, p. 206) has stated, "The highest goal in life is to die young, at as old an age as possible." To that end, "the goal of health education is to promote, maintain, and improve individual and community health. The teaching-learning process is the hallmark and social agenda that differentiates the practice of health education from that of other helping professions in achieving this goal" (National Commission for Health Education Credentialing, Inc. [NCHEC], 1996, pp. 2–3).

Because quality of life and health status are complex variables, they are not usually changed in a short period of time. To reach these goals, people usually work their way through a number of small steps over a period of time that equip them with all that is necessary to impact both their health status and, in turn, their quality of life. Thus, it is the work of health education specialists to create interventions (programs) that can assist people in working toward better health. This work is reflected in the purpose of health education that "is to positively influence the health behavior of individuals and communities as well as the living and working conditions that influence their health" (Coalition for National Health Education Organizations [CNHEO], 2007, p. 1).

▷ The Practice of Health Education/Promotion

While the practice of health education specialists is outlined in the responsibilities and competencies presented in Chapter 6, as previously noted in our discussion of the use of data, the primary role of health education specialists is to develop appropriate health education/

promotion programs for the people they serve. The practice of health education/promotion is based on the assumption "that beneficial health behavior will result from a combination of planned, consistent, integrated learning opportunities. This assumption rests on the scientific evaluations of health education programs in schools, at worksites, in medical settings, and through mass media" (Green & Ottoson, 1999, pp. 93–94). The results of these *scientific evaluations*, referred to by Green and Ottoson, are one source of data that contribute to a body of data known as evidence. **Evidence** is data that can be used to make decisions about planning. When health education specialists practice in such a way that they systematically find, appraise, and use evidence as the basis for decision making when planning health education/promotion programs it is referred to as **evidence-based practice** (Cottrell & McKenzie, 2011).

Although the practice of health education specialists is easily stated, it is by no means easy to carry out. Much time, effort, practice, and on-the-job training are required to be successful. Even the most experienced health education specialists find program development challenging because of the constant changes in settings, resources, and priority populations (McKenzie, Neiger, & Thackeray, 2013).

The specific steps taken to develop a health education/promotion program vary depending on the planning model used (see Chapter 4); most models include the following steps (McKenzie et al., 2013) (see Figure 4.17):

1. Assessing the needs of the priority population
2. Setting goals and objectives
3. Developing an intervention that considers the peculiarities of the setting
4. Implementing the intervention
5. Evaluating the results

Therefore, it becomes the practice of health education specialists to be able to carry out all that is associated with these tasks.

Over the years, to be educated to serve as a health education specialist, individuals have been trained in three different types of academic programs—community health education, public health education, and school health education. In recent years, mostly because of the profession's movement toward accreditation of all undergraduate programs in health education, there has been a movement to just two preparation tracks as opposed to three in the past. Community health education programs are increasingly switching over to public health education to meet accreditation requirements (see Chapter 6 for more on accreditation).

▷ Basic Underlying Concepts of the Profession

Previously mentioned in this chapter and discussed in greater detail in Chapter 2, the profession of health education/promotion is one that has been built on the principles and concepts of a number of disciplines and professions. Pieces of community development and organizing, education, epidemiology, medicine, psychology, and sociology can be found within health education/promotion. In the sections that follow, we present some of the basic underlying concepts of the profession. Please note that we have not exhausted the discussion of each of these topics but, rather, present sufficient information to allow a basic understanding of each.

The Health Field Concept and the Determinants of Health

Soon after the Canadian government implemented its national health plan that ensured health care for all Canadians, it began to look more closely at the health field as a way of improving Canadians' health. The **health field** is a term the government described as being far more encompassing than the "healthcare system." This term was much broader and included all matters that affected health (Lalonde, 1974). Because the health field was such a broad concept, it was felt that there was a need to develop a framework that would subdivide the concept into principal elements so that the elements could be studied. Such a framework was developed and called the **health field concept** (Laframboise, 1973).

The health field concept divided the health field into four elements: (1) human biology, (2) environment, (3) lifestyle, and (4) healthcare organization. "These four elements were identified through an examination of the causes and underlying factors of sickness and death in Canada, and from an assessment of the parts the elements play in affecting the level of health in Canada" (Lalonde, 1974, p. 31). **Human biology** "includes all those aspects of health, both physical and mental, which are developed within the human body as a consequence of the basic biology of man [sic] and the organic make-up of an individual" (Lalonde, 1974, p. 31). This includes not only the genetic inheritance of an individual but also the processes of maturation and aging and the complex interaction of the various systems of the human body (Lalonde, 1974). The element of **environment** "includes all those matters related to health which are external to the human body and over which the individual has little or no control" (Lalonde, 1974, p. 32). Some examples of things often included in the element of environment are geography, climate, community size, industrial development, economy, and social norms.

The element of **lifestyle** comprises the "aggregation of decisions by individuals which affect their health and over which they more or less have control" (Lalonde, 1974, p. 32). In more recent times, lifestyle has been more commonly referred to as **health behavior** (those behaviors that impact a person's health). The fourth element in the health field concept is healthcare organization. **Healthcare organization** "consists of the quantity, quality, arrangement, nature and relationships of people and resources in the provision of health care" (Lalonde, 1974, p. 32). This fourth element is often referred to as the healthcare system.

The utility of the health field concept has proved to be helpful over the years, both in Canada and the United States. Its greatest importance may have been to bring attention to the concept of health promotion and disease prevention. Before this point in history, the primary focus of health care had been on the cure of disease, not the prevention of disease. In fact, it was stated that the health field concept put human biology, environment, and lifestyle on equal footing with healthcare organization (Lalonde, 1974). Since its development, studies using this concept in both Canada and the United States have provided a greater understanding of what contributes to morbidity and mortality and what health professionals can do to help improve the health of those they serve.

Using a similar framework as that of the elements of the health field concept, it is now believed that the health of populations is shaped by five intersecting domains (i.e., the **determinants of health**): (1) genetics (e.g., sex, age, and individual characteristics), (2) individual behavior (e.g., diet, physical activity, and alcohol use), (3) social circumstances (e.g., education, socioeconomic status, housing, and crime), (4) environmental and physical influences (e.g., safe water, where a person lives, and crowding conditions), and (5) health services (e.g., access to quality health care, cost, and lack of insurance coverage) (CDC, 2015b; IOM, 2001;

McGinnis, 2001; McGovern, Miller, & Hughes-Cromwick, 2014; USDHHS, 2014a) (also see the discussion of Multicausation Disease Model later in this chapter). These domains are dynamic and vary in impact depending on where one is in the life cycle (IOM, 2001).

In addition to understanding the determinants of health as they contribute to a person's current state of health, the **social determinants of health** also play a critical role in the health of people and communities. Social determinants of health are "conditions in the environments in which people are born, live, learn, work, play, worship, and age that affect a wide range of health, functioning, and quality-of-life outcomes and risks. Conditions (e.g., social, economic, and physical) in these various environments and settings (e.g., school, church, workplace, and neighborhood) have been referred to as "place" (USDHHS, 2014b, ¶4). Like the determinants of health, the social determinants of health (see **Figure 1.3**) encompass five areas: (1) economic stability (e.g., poverty, employment, housing stability such as homelessness or foreclosure, and food security); (2) education (e.g., high school graduation rates, enrollment in higher education, language, and literacy); (3) social and community context (e.g., perceptions of discrimination and equity, civic participation, and incarceration); (4) health and health care (e.g., access to health care, access to primary care, and health literacy); and (5) neighborhood and built environment (e.g., quality of housing, environmental conditions, access to healthy foods, and crime and violence) (USDHHS, 2014b). Addressing these social determinants of health can impact the health of large numbers of people in ways that can be sustained over time.

We know that genetics play a big part in late-onset diseases such as diabetes, cancer, and cardiovascular disease, whereas employment and income (social circumstances) have a significant

▶ **Figure 1.3** Social determinants of health

Source: U.S. Department of Health and Human Services (USDHHS). 2014. *Healthy People 2020: Social determinants of health*. Retrieved March 9, 2016, from https://www.healthypeople.gov/2020/topics-objectives/topic/social-determinants-of-health.

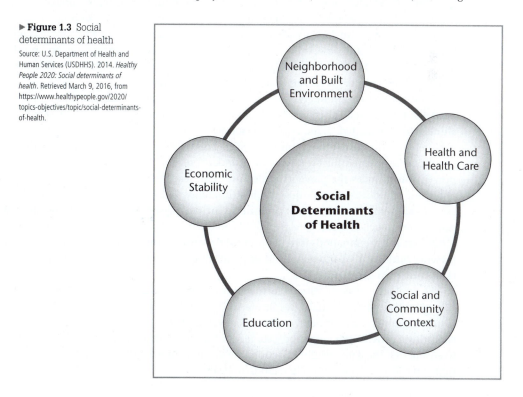

influence on health and health care throughout life. Further, environmental aspects also impact health. For example, families with access to sidewalks and safe neighborhoods (neighborhood and built environment) are more likely to engage in health-enhancing behaviors.

> On a population basis, using the best available estimates, the impacts of various domains on early deaths in the United States distribute roughly as follows: genetic predispositions, about 30%; social circumstances, 15%; environmental exposures, 5%; behavioral patterns, 40%; and shortfalls in medical care about 10%. But more important than these proportions is the nature of the influences in play where the domains intersect. Ultimately, the health fate of each of us is determined by factors acting not mostly in isolation but by our experience where domains interconnect. Whether a gene is expressed can be determined by environmental exposures or behavioral patterns. The nature and consequences of behavioral choices are affected by our social circumstances. Our genetic predispositions affect the health care we need, and our social circumstances affect the health care we receive. (McGinnis et al., 2002, p. 83)

The Levels and Limitations of Prevention

The word *prevention* has already been used several times in this chapter. We now want to formally define the term, present the different levels of prevention, and briefly discuss the limitations of prevention. **Prevention**, as it relates to health, has been defined as the planning for and the measures taken to forestall the onset of a disease or other health problem before the occurrence of undesirable health events. This definition presents three distinct levels of prevention: primary, secondary, and tertiary prevention. **Primary prevention** comprises those preventive measures that forestall the onset of illness or injury during the prepathogenesis period (before the disease process begins) (McKenzie & Pinger, 2015). Examples of primary prevention measures include wearing a safety belt, using rubber gloves when there is potential for the spread of disease, immunizing against specific diseases, exercising, and brushing one's teeth. Any health education/promotion program aimed specifically at averting the onset of illness or injury is also an example of primary prevention.

Illness and injury cannot always be prevented. In fact, many diseases, such as cancer and heart disease, can establish themselves in humans and cause considerable damage before they are detected and treated. In such cases, the sooner a condition is detected and medical personnel intervene, the greater the chances of limiting disability and preventing death. Such identification and intervention are known as secondary prevention. More specifically, **secondary prevention** includes the preventive measures that lead to an early diagnosis and prompt treatment of a disease or an injury to limit disability and prevent more serious pathogenesis. Good examples of secondary prevention include personal and clinical screenings and examinations such as blood pressure, blood cholesterol, and mammograms. The goal of such screenings and examinations is not to prevent the onset of the disease but rather to detect its presence during early pathogenesis, thus permitting early treatment and limiting disability (McKenzie & Pinger, 2015).

The final level of prevention is **tertiary prevention**. It is at this level that health education specialists work to retrain, reeducate, and rehabilitate the individual who has already incurred disability, impairment, or dependency. Examples of some tertiary measures include educating a patient after lung cancer surgery or working with an individual who has diabetes to ensure that the daily insulin injections are taken. **Figure 1.4** provides a visual representation of the levels of prevention in relation to health status.

▶ **Figure 1.4** Levels of prevention

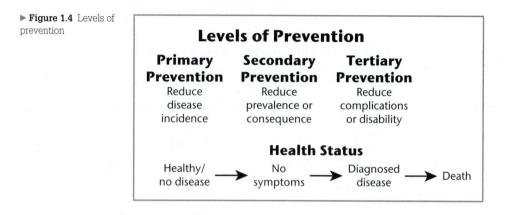

Though health education specialists can intervene at any of the three levels of prevention and can have a great deal of success, it should be obvious from the previous discussion of the health field concept and the determinants of health that prevention is not the "magic bullet" for an endless life. Prevention does have its limits. McGinnis (1985) has noted four major categories of limitations: (1) biological, (2) technological, (3) ethical, and (4) economic. Biological limitations center on life span. How long should individuals expect to live healthy lives or, for that matter, how long should they expect to live at all? Even with the best inputs and a bit of luck, one should not expect to live longer than 80 to 110 years. Body parts will eventually wear out from use.

Technological advances also have their limitations. Today, healthcare workers have a vast array of technical equipment available to help them care for their patients, but technology still has not been able to eradicate AIDS or malaria or to explain the cause of Alzheimer's disease.

Prevention is also limited by ethical concerns (see Chapter 5). Even though helmets would increase the chances of survival in automobile crashes, is it ethical to have a law that says all drivers and passengers in automobiles must wear them? Or is it ethical to penalize people via fines, taxes, or surcharges for acting in unhealthy ways, such as driving an automobile without a safety belt on, buying and using tobacco products, or for not having a smoke detector and fire extinguisher in the home?

Finally, prevention has economic limitations. Prevention is limited by the amount of money that is put into it. Though the exact figures are difficult to determine, it is commonly understood that less than 5 percent of all dollars spent on health in the United States each year are spent on essential public health services, government public health activity, and population-based public health activity (Turnock, 2012). Stated another way, approximately 95 percent of the two trillion plus dollars spent on health in the United States each year is spent on curing ill health, not on health promotion and disease prevention (Sultz & Young, 2011).

Risk Factors

The health field concept, the determinants of health, and the social determinants of health have provided those interested in health issues with a framework from which the health field can be studied. The levels of prevention and their limitations have provided this same group of people with a time frame from which to plan to help forestall the onset of, limit the spread of, and rehabilitate after pathogenesis or another health problem. What none of these concepts fully discloses is the focus at which health promotion and disease prevention programming should be aimed, **risk factors**. A risk factor is "any attribute, characteristic or exposure of an individual that increases the likelihood of developing a disease or injury (WHO, 2016c, ¶1). Risk factors increase the probability of morbidity and premature mortality but do not guarantee that people with a risk factor will suffer the consequences.

Risk factors can be divided into two categories: (1) **modifiable risk factors** (changeable or controllable) and (2) **nonmodifiable risk factors** (nonchangeable or noncontrollable). The former include such factors as sedentary lifestyle, smoking, and poor dietary habits—things that individuals can change or control whereas the latter group includes factors such as age, sex, and inherited genes—things that individuals cannot change or do not have control over. Note that these two categories of risk factors are often interrelated. In fact, the combined potential for harm from a number of risk factors is greater than the sum of their individual potentials. For example, asbestos workers have an increased risk for cancer because of their exposure to this carcinogen. Further, if they smoke, they have a 30 times greater chance of developing lung cancer than do their nonsmoking coworkers and 90 times greater chance of getting lung cancer than do people who neither work with asbestos nor smoke. The risk increases further if they have an inherited respiratory disease.

Knowledge about the impact of risk behaviors has continued to grow. In looking back over the 20th century, we have seen disease prevention change "from focusing on reducing environmental exposures over which the individual had little control, such as providing potable water, to emphasizing behaviors such as avoiding use of tobacco, fatty foods, and a sedentary lifestyle" (Breslow, 1999, p. 1030). As noted previously, approximately 40 percent of the early deaths in the United States each year are caused by behavior patterns that could be modified by preventive interventions (McGinnis et al., 2002). Therefore, much of the focus of the work of health education specialists has been to help individuals identify and control their modifiable risk factors.

Health Risk Reduction

To focus on specific risk factors, health education specialists must have a basic understanding of both communicable (infectious) and noncommunicable (noninfectious) diseases. **Communicable diseases** are those diseases for which biological agents or their products are the cause and that are transmissible from one individual to another (McKenzie & Pinger, 2015), and **noncommunicable diseases** or illnesses are those that cannot be transmitted from an infected person to a susceptible, healthy one (McKenzie & Pinger, 2015). Our intent in this section and the ones that follow is not to present information on all possible diseases and their related risk factors that a health education specialist may have to develop programs for, but rather to provide a general understanding of the spread and cause of disease. (See **Table 1.5** for leading causes of death and their risk factors.)

Before moving on, we would like to make a special note about one of the data presented in **Figure 1.5**. The term *leading causes of death* is used in this figure. That term refers to "the primary pathophysiological conditions identified at the time of death, as opposed to the root

TABLE 1.5 **Leading causes of death and associated risk factors for all ages: United States, 2010**

Rank	Cause	Risk Factors
1	Diseases of the heart	Tobacco use, high blood pressure, elevated serum cholesterol, diet, diabetes, obesity, lack of exercise, alcohol abuse, genetics
2	Malignant neoplasms (cancer)	Tobacco use, alcohol misuse, diet, solar radiation, ionizing radiation, worksite hazards, environmental pollution, genetics
3	Chronic lower respiratory diseases	Tobacco use, diseases
4	Cerebrovascular diseases (stroke)	Tobacco use, high blood pressure, elevated serum cholesterol, diabetes, obesity, genetics
5	Unintentional injuries (accidents)	Alcohol misuse, tobacco use (fires), product design, home hazards, handgun availability, lack of safety restraints, excessive speed, automobile design, roadway design
6	Alzheimer's disease	Age, family history, genetics, head injury, heart health, general healthy aging[a]
7	Diabetes mellitus	Obesity (for type II diabetes), diet, lack of exercise, genetics
8	Nephritis, nephrotic syndrome, and nephrosis	Infectious agents, drug hypersensitivity, genetics, trauma
9	Influenza and pneumonia	Tobacco use, infectious agents, biological factors
10	Suicide	Family history, previous suicide attempts, history of mental disorders, history of alcohol and substance abuse, cultural and religious beliefs, barriers to accessing mental health treatment[b]

Sources: [a]Alzheimer's Association. (2013). *Risk Factors*. Retrieved July 11, 2013, from http://www.alz.org/alzheimers_disease_causes_risk_factors.asp#riskfactors.

[b] Centers for Disease Control and Prevention. (2012). *Suicide: Risk and protective factors*. Retrieved July 11, 2013, from http://www.cdc.gov/violenceprevention/suicide/riskprotectivefactors.html.

Data from U.S. Department of Health and Human Services, National Center for Health Statistics (NCHS). (2013). *Health, United States, 2011 with Special Feature on Emergency Care*. Hyattsville, MD: Author.

causes" (McGinnis & Foege, 1993, p. 2207). McGinnis and Foege (1993) conducted a study to see if they could identify the root causes of death. What they found was that the leading *actual causes of death* were modifiable behaviors—behaviors that people could change. The behavior that was the leading actual cause of death was tobacco use, accounting for some 400,000, or 19 percent, of the mortality in 1990. A similar study to that of McGinnis and Foege was conducted by Mokdad, Marks, Stroup, and Gerberding in 2004 using 2000 mortality data. They also found tobacco to be the leading actual cause of death, but that poor diet and physical inactivity killed almost as many (see Figure 1.5). It is now estimated that tobacco is the primary cause of more than 480,000 deaths per year, about one in five deaths annually (CDC, 2015c). Figure 1.5 provides evidence that nearly half of all causes of death in the United States could be attributed to a number of largely preventable behaviors and that by improving healthy behaviors, we can significantly reduce the consequences of chronic diseases. "These findings, along with escalating health care costs and aging population, argue persuasively that

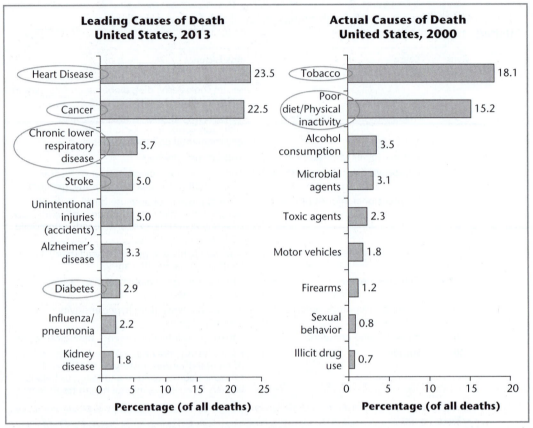

▲ **Figure 1.5** Leading versus actual causes of death in the United States

Source: The 2013 data from M. Heron, "Deaths: Leading causes for 2013." *National Vital Statistics Report 65*, 2 (February 16, 2016). The 2000 data from A. H. Mokdad, J. S. Marks, D. F. Stroup, and J. L. Gerberding, "Correction: Actual Causes of Death in the United States, 2000." *Journal of the American Medical Association 292*, 3 (2005): 293–294.

the need to establish a more preventive orientation in the U.S. health care and public health systems has become more urgent" (Mokdad et al., 2004, p. 1238).

THE CHAIN OF INFECTION

The **chain of infection** (see **Figure 1.6**) is a model used to explain the spread of a communicable disease from one host to another. The basic premise represented in the chain of infection is that individuals can break the chain (reduce the risk) at any point; thus, the spread of disease can be stopped. For example, the spread of some waterborne diseases is stopped when the first link of the chain is broken with the chlorination of the water supply, thus killing the pathogens that cause a disease. The risk is reduced because the pathogen is destroyed before it is consumed. The chain can also be broken by placing a barrier between the means of transmission and the portal of entry, as when healthcare providers protect themselves with surgical masks and rubber gloves. In this case, the risk is reduced because individuals are not exposing themselves to the pathogen. With such information, health education specialists can help create programs that are aimed at breaking the chain and reducing the risks.

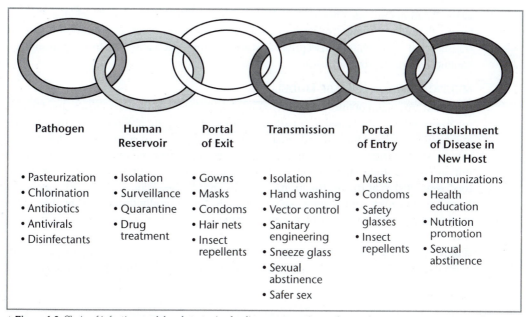

Pathogen	Human Reservoir	Portal of Exit	Transmission	Portal of Entry	Establishment of Disease in New Host
• Pasteurization • Chlorination • Antibiotics • Antivirals • Disinfectants	• Isolation • Surveillance • Quarantine • Drug treatment	• Gowns • Masks • Condoms • Hair nets • Insect repellents	• Isolation • Hand washing • Vector control • Sanitary engineering • Sneeze glass • Sexual abstinence • Safer sex	• Masks • Condoms • Safety glasses • Insect repellents	• Immunizations • Health education • Nutrition promotion • Sexual abstinence

▲ **Figure 1.6** Chain of infection model and strategies for disease prevention and control

Source: From J. F. McKenzie & R. R. Pinger, *An Introduction to Community & Public Health.* 8th ed. © 2015 Jones and Bartlett Publishers, Sudbury, MA. www.jbpub.com. Reprinted with permission.

COMMUNICABLE DISEASE MODEL

A second model used to describe the spread of a communicable disease is the **communicable disease model. Figure 1.7** presents the elements of this model—agent, host, and environment. These three elements summarize the minimal requirements for the presence and spread of a communicable disease in a population. The agent is the element (or, using the chain of infection labels, the pathogen) that must be present for a disease to spread—for example, a bacteria or virus. The host is any susceptible organism that can be invaded by the

▶ **Figure 1.7** Communicable disease model

Source: From J. F. McKenzie & R. R. Pinger. *An Introduction to Community & Public Health*, 8th ed. © 2015 Jones and Bartlett Publishers, Sudbury, MA. www.jbpub.com. Reprinted with permission.

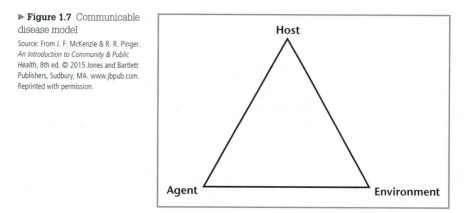

agent. Examples include plants, animals, and humans. The environment includes all other factors that either prohibit or promote disease transmission. Thus, communicable disease transmission occurs when a susceptible host and a pathogenic agent exist in an environment conducive to disease transmission.

MULTICAUSATION DISEASE MODEL

Obviously, the chain of infection and communicable disease models are most helpful in trying to prevent disease caused by a pathogen. However, they are not applicable to noncommunicable diseases, which include many of the chronic diseases such as heart disease and cancer. Most of these diseases manifest themselves in people over a period of time and are not caused by a single factor but by combined factors. The concept of "caused by many factors" is referred to as the **multicausation disease model** (see **Figure 1.8**). For example, it is known that heart disease is more likely to manifest itself in individuals who are older, who smoke, who do not exercise, who are overweight, who have high blood pressure, who have high cholesterol, and who have immediate family members who have had heart disease. Note that within this list of factors there are both modifiable and nonmodifiable risk factors. As when using the chain of infection model, the work of health education specialists is to create

▶ **Figure 1.8**
Multicausation
disease model

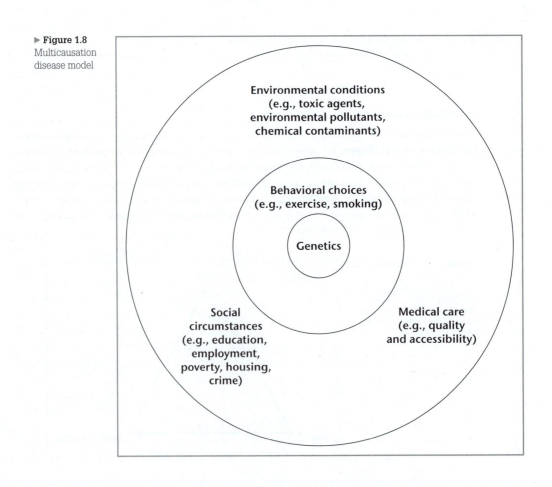

programs to help people reduce the risk of disease and injury by helping those in the priority population identify and control as many of the multicausative factors as possible. This model should look familiar to you because it is made up of the five determinants of health discussed previously in this chapter.

Other Selected Principles

Several other principles of health education/promotion have been noted by Cleary and Neiger (1998). They have identified, via the work of others, that health education specialists must address the principles of participation, empowerment, and cultural competency if health education/promotion is to be successful. We would like to add two other principles to this list, socio-ecological approach and advocacy. **Participation** refers to the active involvement of those in the priority population in helping identify, plan, and implement programs to address the health problems they face. Without such participation, ethical issues associated with program development come into play, and the priority population probably will not support and feel **ownership** of (responsibility for) the program. For example, if the health education specialists for a large corporation are creating a health promotion program for all employees, they should not begin to plan without the participation of (or at least representation by) each of the segments (clerical, labor, and management) of the employee population.

Health education/promotion activities have recently placed more emphasis on socio-ecological approaches to improving health. The underlying concept of the **socio-ecological approach** (sometimes referred to as the *ecological perspective*) is that behavior has multiple levels of influences. This approach "emphasizes the interaction between, and the interdependence of factors within and across all levels of a health problem" (Rimer & Glanz, 2005, p. 10). That is to say, seldom does behavior change based on influence from a single level. People live in environments (i.e., physical, social, political, cultural, and economic) that shape behaviors and access to the resources they need to maintain good health (Pellmar, Brandt, & Baird, 2002). Scholars who study and write about the levels of influence have used various labels to describe them. However, commonly used labels include individual and individual's characteristics (e.g., knowledge, attitudes, values, and skills), social relationships, organizational influences, community characteristics, and public policy (McLeroy, Bibeau, Steckler, & Glanz, 1988). Physical environment and culture have recently been added to levels of influence (Simons-Morton, McLeroy, & Wendel, 2012). In practice, behavior change often involves influences on multiple levels. For example, to get a person to begin an exercise program it may take a conversation with his or her physician (i.e., social influence), a company policy (i.e., organizational-level influence), and also the county commissioners voting to put walking paths in the community (i.e., community-level influence). Thus, a central conclusion of the socio-ecological approach "is that it usually takes the combination of both individual-level and environmental/policy-level interventions to achieve substantial changes in health behavior" (Sallis, Owen, & Fisher, 2008, p. 467). Therefore, health education specialists must do more than just educate to help to change behavior. They must now work in new ways and develop new skills. As a group these new skills are often called **population-based approaches**. They include policy development, policy advocacy, organizational change, community development, empowerment of individuals, and economic supports.

Consider this example to better understand how a population-based approach works. A state-level voluntary health organization was spending most of its time and resources helping individuals quit smoking or preventing others from starting to smoke. Recently the organization has developed a statewide advocacy network to respond to tobacco-related legislation. They are using a population-based approach to influence legislation and policy that will ultimately impact individual smoking behaviors. They still maintain the more individual approaches to dealing with the tobacco issue but have added the population-based approach.

Advocacy is another principle in which health education specialists have become more involved. **Advocacy** is defined "as the actions or endeavors individuals or groups engage in order to alter public opinion in favor or in opposition to a certain policy" (Pinzon-Perez & Perez, 1999, p. 29). Whereas **health advocacy** has been defined as "the processes by which the actions of individuals or groups attempt to bring about social, environmental and/or organizational change on behalf of a particular health goal, program, interest, or population" (Joint Committee, 2012, p. 17). Professional associations encourage health education specialists to get more involved in advocacy for the profession and for health-related issues (Auld & Dixon-Terry, 2010). As an example, the Coalition of National Health Education Organizations (CNHEO) (see Chapter 8 for more on this organization) sponsors the Health Education Advocate Web site (see the Weblink at the end of this chapter for the URL for this site). This site provides health education specialists with an easy link to contact their legislators whenever health education/promotion–related bills or concerns are considered by Congress.

If health education/promotion is going to create lasting change, then those in the priority population must be empowered as a result of the health education/promotion programming. **Empowerment** is a "social action process for people to gain mastery over their lives and the lives of their communities" (Minkler, Wallerstein, & Wilson, 2008, p. 294). Empowerment can take place at the individual, the organization or group, and the community level. Often, empowerment at one level can influence empowerment at the other levels. An example of empowerment occurred in Indiana—a community with a significantly high rate of obesity and cancer, which have been linked to a lack of physical activity. The Indiana Complete Streets Coalition formed to ensure that communities throughout Indiana have neighborhoods, public spaces, and transportation systems that can support physical activity and healthy living. As a result, individuals and families have been empowered to improve their health because they now live in neighborhoods where it is possible to walk and bike safely (CDC, 2016c). Social media is one growing strategy being used by health education specialists to advocate and empower individuals and communities. **Social media** is any type of "media that uses the Internet and other technologies to allow for social interaction (McKenzie et al., 2012, p. 448). Social media tools can include such things as online video sharing (e.g., YouTube), social networks (e.g., Facebook and Twitter), text messaging, podcasts, virtual worlds, blogs, and podcasts. The use of social media tools is a "powerful channel to reach target audiences with strategic, effective, and user-centric health interventions" (CDC, 2015d, ¶1). Because the Internet allows for a free flow of information, the CDC has developed guidelines, best practices, and toolkits for health education specialists using and developing social media materials (CDC, 2011b; CDC, 2015d). Becoming familiar with these various social media tools during your preparation as a health education specialist will prove valuable as doctors' offices, hospitals, state and local health departments, and voluntary agencies are using these tools to communicate with patients, volunteers, employees, and the general public.

There are many factors that impact the effectiveness of health education/promotion programming. Because of the health disparities that exist between and among the various subpopulations in the United States (Selig, Tropiano, & Greene-Moton, 2006) and because of the increasing diversification of the U.S. population (Pérez & Luquis, 2008), much more attention has been placed on understanding the impact of culture (i.e., values, beliefs, attitudes, traditions, and customs) on health and providing culturally appropriate programs (Davis & Rankin, 2006). Cultural factors arise from guidelines (both explicit and implicit) that individuals "inherit" from being a part of a particular society, racial or ethnic group, religious community, or other group. For health education specialists to be effective in a variety of communities, they need to strive to be culturally competent (Davis & Rankin, 2006; Luquis, Pérez, & Young, 2006; Selig et al., 2006). **Cultural competence** is "a developmental process defined as a set of values, principles, behaviors, attitudes, and policies that enable health professionals to work effectively across racial, ethnic and linguistically diverse populations" (Joint Committee, 2012, p. 16). Both health education specialists and the community health agencies providing health education/promotion programs need "to be able to communicate with different communities and understand how culture influences health behaviors" (McKenzie & Pinger, 2013, p. 198).

Summary

This introductory chapter presented many of the basic principles of the profession of health education/promotion including definitions of many of the key words and terms used in the profession, including *health, health education, health promotion, disease prevention, community health, global health, population health,* and *wellness*; a look at the current status of health education/promotion; an explanation of how health or health status has been measured, including mortality rates, life expectancy, YPLL, DALYs, HRQOL, and health surveys; an outline of the goal and purpose of the profession; the practice of health education/promotion, including planning, implementing, and evaluating programs; some of the basic underlying concepts and principles of the profession, including the health field concept, determinants of health, social determinants of health, levels of prevention, risk factors, and health risk reduction via understanding disease; and the principles of participation, ecological approach, advocacy, empowerment, social media, and cultural competence.

Review Questions

1. Define *health, health education, health promotion, disease prevention, public health, community health, global health, population health,* and *wellness.*

2. What is the status of health education/promotion?

3. Explain each of the following means of measuring health or health status:
   - Mortality rates. What is the difference among crude, adjusted, and specific rates?
   - Life expectancy
   - Years of potential life lost (YPLL)
   - Disability-adjusted life years (DALYs)
   - Health-related quality of life (HRQOL)
   - Health surveys

4. Of all the different measures of health presented in this chapter, which one do you think is the best indicator of health? Why?

5. Why are health-related data and epidemiology such an important discipline for health education/promotion?

6. In a given community with a midyear population estimate of 50,000, there were 21 deaths as a result of strokes in the year. What is the rate of stroke deaths per 100,000 population?

7. What is the goal of health education/promotion? What is its purpose?

8. What constitutes the basic practice of health education/promotion?

9. What is the difference between the leading causes of death and the actual causes of death?

10. Briefly explain the following concepts and principles of health education/promotion:
    - Health field concept; determinants of health
    - Levels of prevention
    - Risk factors
    - Health risk reduction
    - Chain of infection
    - Communicable disease model
    - Multicausation disease model
    - Selected principles of health education/promotion—participation, socio-ecological approach, advocacy, empowerment, social media, and cultural competence

Case Study

As a health education specialist with the Delaware County Health Department, Jordan has been asked by a local religious leader to give a presentation on preventing HIV and STDs to the Christian youth group (9th to 12th graders) of the community. The request has taken Jordan by surprise because for the past couple of years he has attempted to make similar presentations in the local schools but has been turned away because the superintendent said "the community was too conservative for such matters." Knowing that at least some of the people in the community think HIV and STD prevention education is too controversial, but also knowing the information is important for youth to have, Jordan wants to make sure he prepares and delivers a program that is well received. This is finally the chance he has been waiting for to make his entry into the youth population of the community. Jordan has decided to create a presentation on HIV and STD prevention that incorporates information on both risk factors and the chain of infection. To make sure that his presentation is on target, he has asked several other employees of the health department to sit down with him and brainstorm some ideas for his presentation. He begins his session with his colleagues by asking them all to write down information they think he should include in his presentation. Assume that you are one of these other employees of the health department in this meeting. What would you include on your list for Jordan? What would you advise Jordan not to include? Why? He then asks his colleagues for ideas on how to present the information (e.g., lecture, video, or role playing). What do you think would be the best method to use? Why did you select this method? How long do you think Jordan's presentation should be? Why?

Critical Thinking Questions

1. In this chapter, the term *public health* was defined. To what extent do you think that the government, at any level, has the right to legislate good health? For example, do you think a governmental body has the responsibility (or right) to require all motorcycle drivers to wear helmets because statistics show that wearing helmets can save lives? Defend your answer.

2. If you were asked by the CDC to come up with a new measure to describe the health status of an individual, what would you include in such a measure and why?

3. If you had the opportunity to develop three new health education/promotion programs, one at each level of the three levels of prevention (primary, secondary, and tertiary) for the community in which you live, what would they be? Who would be the priority population? Why did you pick the three that you did?

Activities

1. If you have not already done so, access the government document *Healthy People: The Surgeon General's Report on Health Promotion and Disease Prevention*. It provides a good background on the health promotion era in the United States.

2. Write your own definitions for *health, health education*, and *health promotion* using the concepts presented in the chapter.

3. Write one paragraph for each of the following:
   - Why do you think the health field concept was so important in getting people to think about health promotion?
   - At what level of prevention do you think it would be most difficult to change health behavior? Why?

4. In a PowerPoint presentation, use the chain of infection to outline three different means for preventing the spread of HIV.

5. In a photo story, use the multicausation disease model to explain how a person develops heart disease.

Weblinks

1. http://www.cdc.gov/nchs/

   National Center for Health Statistics (NCHS)

   This site is a rich source of data about health in the United States and the instruments used to collect the data.

2. http://www.cdc.gov/brfss/

   Behavioral Risk Factor Surveillance System (BRFSS)

   The BRFSS, the world's largest telephone survey, tracks health risks in the United States. Information from the survey is used to improve the health of U.S. citizens. At this site, you will find general information about the BRFSS, data generated by the BRFSS, copies of the data collection instruments, and more.

3. http://www.cdc.gov/healthyyouth

   Youth Risk Behavioral Surveillance System (YRBSS)

   At this site, you will find general information about the YRBSS, data generated by the YRBSS, copies of the data collection instruments, and more.

4. http://www.healtheducationadvocate.org

   Health Education Advocate

   The Health Education Advocate site is sponsored by the Coalition of National Health Education Organizations (CNHEO). The site was designed to provide a timely source of advocacy information related to the field of health education/promotion. Included on the site are a number of items to assist health planners with advocacy activities as well as information about how to identify and contact senators and congressional representatives, the status of specific bills, health resolutions and policy statements of sponsoring agencies, and advocacy resources.

5. https://www.thinkculturalhealth.hhs.gov/

   Think Cultural Health

   This is a page at the U.S. Department of Health and Human Services, Office of Minority Health Web site that presents information on cultural competence for health professionals. The site has a tag line of "advancing health equity at every point of contact." Included at the site are educational programs, resources, and other materials.

6. http://www.bls.gov/ooh/

   Occupational Outlook Handbook

   This is a page at the U.S. Department of Labor, Bureau of Labor Statistics Web site that provides the occupational outlook for a wide range of professions. Search for "health educators" to see short explanations of the nature of the work; training, other qualifications, and advancement; employment; job outlook and projections; earnings; wages; and sources of additional information about health education specialists.

7. http://www.countyhealthrankings.org/

   County Health Rankings

   This Web site presents the *County Health Rankings*. This site is a collaboration between the Robert Wood Johnson Foundation and the University of Wisconsin Population Health Institute.

8. http://www.teachepidemiology.org

   Teach Epidemiology

   This is a Web site sponsored by the Robert Wood Johnson Foundation that provides middle and high school teachers with ideas about how to incorporate the teaching of epidemiology into their curriculum.

References

American College Health Association (ACHA). (2016). *About ACHA-NCHA*. Retrieved March 9, 2016, from http://www.acha-ncha.org/overview.html.

Auld, M. E., & Dixon-Terry, E. (2010). The role of health education associations in advocacy. In J. M. Black, S. Furney, H. M. Graf, & A. E. Nolte (Eds.), *Philosophical foundations of health education* (pp. 311–318). San Francisco: Jossey-Bass.

Breslow, L. (1999). From disease prevention to health promotion. *Journal of the American Medical Association, 281* (11), 1030–1033.

Centers for Disease Control and Prevention (CDC). (1994). *Chronic disease in minority populations*. Atlanta, GA: Author.

Centers for Disease Control and Prevention (CDC). (2011a). *Health-related quality of life*. Retrieved March 7, 2106, from http://www.cdc.gov/hrqol/concept.htm.

Centers for Disease Control and Prevention (CDC). (2011b). *The health communicator's social media toolkit*. Retrieved March 10, 2016, from http://www.cdc.gov/socialmedia/tools/guidelines/pdf/socialmediatoolkit_bm.pdf.

Centers for Disease Control and Prevention (CDC). (2012a). *About Health Care Surveys*. Retrieved March 9, 2016, from http://www.cdc.gov/nchs/dhcs/about_dhcs.htm.

Centers for Disease Control and Prevention (CDC). (2014). *About BRFSS*. Retrieved March 9, 2016, from http://www.cdc.gov/brfss/about/index.htm.

Centers for Disease Control and Prevention (CDC). (2015a). *Youth Risk Behavior Surveillance System*. Retrieved March 9, 2016, from http://www.cdc.gov/healthyyouth/data/yrbs/index.htm.

Centers for Disease Control and Prevention (CDC). (2015b). *Social determinants: Frequently asked questions*. Retrieved March 9, 2016, from http://www.cdc.gov/socialdeterminants/faqs/index.htm.

Centers for Disease Control and Prevention (CDC). (2015c). *Tobacco-related mortality*. Retrieved March 9, 2016, from http://www.cdc.gov/tobacco/data_statistics/fact_sheets/health_effects/tobacco_related_mortality/.

Centers for Disease Control and Prevention (CDC). (2015d). *Social Media at CDC*. Retrieved March 10, 2016, from http://www.cdc.gov/socialmedia/tools/guidelines/index.html.

Centers for Disease Control and Prevention (CDC). (2016a). *Chronic disease overview*. Retrieved March 7, 2016, from http://www.cdc.gov/chronicdisease/overview.

Centers for Disease Control and Prevention (CDC). (2016b). *National health and nutrition examination survey*. Retrieved March 9, 2016, from http://www.cdc.gov/nchs/nhanes.htm.

Centers for Disease Control and Prevention (CDC). (2016c). *National comprehensive cancer control program: Success stories*. Retrieved March 22, 2016, from http://www.cdc.gov/cancer/ncccp/state.htm.

Cleary, M. J., & Neiger, B. L. (1998). *The certified health education specialist: A self-study guide for professional competency* (3rd ed.). Allentown, PA: The National Commission for Health Education Credentialing.

Coalition for National Health Education Organizations (CNHEO). (2007). *Employer's guide*. Retrieved March 9, 2016, from http://www.cnheo.org/publications.html.

Cottrell, R. R., & McKenzie, J. F. (2011). *Health promotion & education research methods: Using the five chapter thesis/ dissertation model* (2nd ed.). Sudbury, MA: Jones and Bartlett Publishers.

Davis, P. C., & Rankin, L. L. (2006). Guidelines for making existing health education programs more culturally appropriate. *American Journal of Health Education, 37* (4), 250–252.

Glanz, K., & Rimer, B. K. (2008). Perspectives on using theory: Past, present, and future. In K. Glanz, B. K. Rimer, & K. Viswanath (Eds.), *Health behavior and health education: Theory, research, and practice* (pp. 509–517). San Francisco: Jossey-Bass.

Green, L. W., & Ottoson, J. M. (1999). *Community and population health* (8th ed.). Boston: WCB/McGraw-Hill.

Hancock, T., & Minkler, M. (2005). Community health assessment or healthy community assessment: Whose community? Whose health? Whose assessment? In M. Minkler (Ed.), *Community organizing and community building for health* (2nd ed., pp. 138–157). New Brunswick, NJ: Rutgers University Press.

Hanlon, J. J. (1974). *Public Health*. St. Louis: Mosby.

Heron M. (2016). Deaths: Leading causes for 2013. *National vital statistics reports, 65* (2). Hyattsville, MD: National Center for Health Statistics.

Hezel Associates. (2007). *Marketing the health education profession: Knowledge, attitudes, and hiring practices of employers*. Retrieved March 7, 2016, from http://www.cnheo.org/.

Institute of Medicine (IOM). (2001). *Health and behavior: The interplay of biological, behavioral, and societal influences*. Washington, DC: Academy Press.

Institute of Medicine (IOM); Committee on Assuring the Health of the Public in the 21st Century; Board on Health and Disease Prevention; (2002). *The future of the public's health in the 21st century*. Washington, DC: The National Academies Press.

Johns, E. B. (1973). Joint Committee on Health Education Terminology: Report of the Joint Committee on Health Education Terminology. *Health Education, 4* (6), 25.

Joint Committee on Health Education and Health Promotion Terminology. (2001). Report of the 2000 Joint Committee on Health Education and Health Promotion Terminology. *American Journal of Health Education, 32* (2), 89–103.

Joint Committee on Health Education and Health Promotion Terminology. (2012). *Report of the 2011 Joint Committee on Health Education and Promotion Terminology.* Reston, VA: AAHE.

Joint Committee on Health Education Terminology. (1991a). Report of the 1990 Joint Committee on Health Education Terminology. *Journal of Health Education, 22* (2), 105–106.

Joint Committee on Health Education Terminology. (1991b). Report of the 1990 Joint Committee on Health Education Terminology. *Journal of School Health, 61* (6), 251–254.

King, N. (2009). Health inequalities and health inequities. In E. E. Morrison (Ed.), *Health care ethics: Critical issues for the 21st century* (pp. 339–354). Sudbury, MA: Jones & Bartlett.

Laframboise, H. L. (1973). Health policy: Breaking it down into more manageable segments. *Journal of the Canadian Medical Association, 108* (Feb. 3), 388–393.

Lalonde, M. (1974). *A new perspective on the health of Canadians: A working document.* Ottawa, Canada: Ministry of National Health and Welfare.

Luquis, R., Pérez, M., & Young, K. (2006). Cultural competence development in health education professional preparation programs. *American Journal of Health Education, 37* (4), 233–241.

Mason, J. O., & McGinnis, J. M. (1990). Healthy People 2000: An overview of the national health promotion disease prevention objectives. *Public Health Reports, 105* (5), 441–446.

McGinnis, J. M. (1985). The limits of prevention. *Public Health Reports, 100* (3), 255–260.

McGinnis, J. M. (2001). United States. In C. E. Koop (Ed.), *Critical issues in global health* (pp. 80–90). San Francisco: Jossey-Bass.

McGinnis, J. M., & Foege, W. H. (1993). Actual causes of death in the United States. *Journal of the American Medical Association, 270* (18), 2207–2212.

McGinnis, J. M., Williams-Russo, P., & Knickman, J. R. (2002). The case for more active policy attention to health promotion. *Health Affairs, 21* (2), 78–93.

McGovern, L., Miller, G., & Hughes-Cromwick, P. (2014). Health policy brief: The relative contribution of multiple determinants of health outcomes. *Health Affairs,* August 21, 2014, 1–9.

McKenzie, J. F., Neiger, B. L., & Thackeray, R. (2013). *Planning, implementing, and evaluating health promotion programs: A primer* (6th ed.). San Francisco: Pearson.

McKenzie, J. F., & Pinger, R. R. (2013). *An introduction to community health: Brief edition.* Boston: Jones and Bartlett Publishers.

McKenzie, J. F., & Pinger, R. R. (2015). *An introduction to community & public health* (8th ed.). Boston: Jones and Bartlett Publishers.

McKenzie, J. F., Pinger, R. R., & Kotecki, J. E. (2012). *An introduction to community health* (7th ed.). Boston: Jones and Bartlett Publishers.

McLeroy, K. R., Bibeau, D., Steckler, A., &. Glanz, K. (1988). An ecological perspective for health promotion programs. *Health Education Quarterly, 15* (4), 351–378.

Minkler, M., Wallerstein, N., & Wilson, N. (2008). Improving health through community organizing and community building. In K. Glanz, B. K. Rimer, & K. Viswanath (Eds.), *Health behavior and health education practice: Theory, research, and practice* (4th ed., pp. 287–312). San Francisco: Jossey-Bass.

Mokdad, A. H., Marks, J. S., Stroup, D. F., & Gerberding, J. L. (2004). Actual causes of death, in the United States, 2000. *Journal of the American Medical Association, 291* (10), 1238–1245.

Montagu, A. (1968). *Man observed.* New York: G. P. Putnam.

Moss, B. (1950). Joint Committee on Health Education Terminology. *Journal of Physical Education, 21,* 41.

Murray, C. J. L., & Lopez, A. D. (Eds.). (1996). *Summary of the global burden of disease: A comprehensive assessment of mortality and disability from diseases, injuries, and risk factors in 1990 and projected to 2020.* Geneva, Switzerland: World Health Organization.

Nash, D. B., Fabius, R. J., Skoufalos, A., Clarke, J. L., & Horowitz, M. R. (2016). *Population health: Creating a culture of wellness* (2nd ed.). Burlington, MA: Jones & Bartlett Learning.

National Center for Health Statistics (NCHS). (2015). *Health, United States, 2014: With special feature on adults aged 55-64.* Hyattsville, MD: Author.

National Commission for Health Education Credentialing, Inc. (NCHEC). (1996). *A competency-based framework for professional development of certified health education specialists.* Allentown, PA: Author.

Pellmar, T. C., Brandt, E. N. Jr., & Baird, M. (2002). Health and behavior: The interplay of biological, behavioral, and social influences: Summary of an Institute of Medicine Report. *American Journal of Health Promotion, 16* (4), 206–219.

Pérez, M. A., & Luquis, R. R. (2008). Changing U.S. demographics: Challenges and opportunities for health educators. In M. A. Perez & R. R. Luquis (Eds.). *Cultural competence in health education and health promotion* (pp. 1–21). San Francisco: Jossey-Bass.

Pinzon-Perez, H., & Perez, M. A. (1999). Advocacy groups for Hispanic/Latino health issues. *The Health Educator Monograph Series, 17* (2), 29–31.

Raphael, D., Brown, I., Renwick, R., & Rootman, I. (1997). Quality of life: What are the implications for health promotion? *American Journal of Health Behavior, 21* (2), 118–128.

Rimer, B. K., & Glanz, K. (2005). *Theory at a glance: A guide for health promotion practice* (2nd ed). NIH Pub. No. 05-3896. Washington, DC: National Cancer Institute.

Rugen, M. (1972). *A fifty year history of the public health section of American Public Health Association; 1922–1972.* Washington, DC: American Public Health Association, Inc.

Sallis, J. F., Owen, N., & Fisher, E. B. (2008). Ecological models of health behavior. In K. Glanz, B. K. Rimer, & K. Viswanath (Eds.), *Health behavior and health education practice: Theory, research, and practice* (4th ed., pp. 465–485). San Francisco: Jossey-Bass.

Selig, S., Tropiano, E., & Greene-Moton, E. (2006). Teaching cultural competence to reduce health disparities. *Health Promotion Practice, 7* (3), 247S–255S.

Simons-Morton, B. G., McLeroy, K. R., & Wendel, M. L. (2012). *Behavior theory in health promotion practice and research.* Burlington, MA: Jones & Bartlett Learning.

Sultz, H. A., & Young, K. M. (2011). *Health care USA: Understanding its organization and delivery* (7th ed.). Sudbury, MA: Jones & Bartlett.

Turnock, B. J. (2012). *Public health: What it is and how it works* (5th ed.). Burlington, MA: Jones & Bartlett Learning.

U.S. Department of Health, Education, and Welfare (USDHEW). (1980). *Promoting health/preventing disease: Objectives for the nation.* Washington, DC: U.S. Government Printing Office.

U.S. Department of Health and Human Services (USDHHS). (1991). *Health status of minorities and low-income groups* (3rd ed.). Washington, DC: U.S. Government Printing Office.

U.S. Department of Health and Human Services (USDHHS). (2014a). *Healthy People 2020: Determinants of health.* Retrieved March 9, 2016, from https://www.healthypeople.gov/2020/about/foundation-health-measures/Determinants-of-Health.

U.S. Department of Health and Human Services (USDHHS). (2014b). *Healthy People 2020: Social Determinants of Health.* Retrieved March 9, 2016, from https://www.healthypeople.gov/2020/topics-objectives/topic/social-determinants-of-health.

Williams, J. F. (1934). Report of the Health Education Section of the American Physical Education Association: Definitions of terms in health education. *Journal of Physical Education, 5* (16–17), 50–51.

World Health Organization (WHO). (1947). *Constitution of the World Health Organization.* Retrieved March 7, 2016, from http://apps.who.int/gb/bd/PDF/bd47/EN/constitution-en.pdf.

World Health Organization (WHO). (1986). *Health promotion sante: Ottawa charter.* Retrieved March 7, 2016, from http://www.euro.who.int/en/who-we-are/policy-documents/ottawa-charter-for-health-promotion,-1986.

World Health Organization (WHO). (2008). *The global burden of disease: 2004 update.* Retrieved March 7, 2016, from http://www.who.int/healthinfo/global_burden_disease/GBD_report_2004update_full.pdf.

World Health Organization (WHO). (2016a). *Public health.* Retrieved March 7, 2016, from http://www.who.int/trade/glossary/story076/en/.

World Health Organization (WHO). (2016b). *Epidemiology.* Retrieved March 7, 2016, from http://www.who.int/topics/epidemiology/en/.

World Health Organization (WHO). (2016c). *Risk factors.* Retrieved March 9, 2016, from http://www.who.int/topics/risk_factors/en/.

Yoho, R. (1962). Joint Committee on Health Education Terminology: Health education terminology. *Journal of Physical Education and Recreation, 33* (Nov.), 27–28.

The History of Health and Health Education/Promotion

Chapter Objectives

After reading this chapter and answering the questions at the end, you should be able to:

- Discuss how health beliefs and practices have changed from the earliest humans to the present day.
- Identify the dual roots of modern health education/promotion.
- Explain why a need for professional health education specialists emerged.
- Trace the history of public health in the United States.
- Relate the history of school health from the mid-1800s to the present.
- Identify important governmental publications from 1975 to the present and describe how these publications have impacted health promotion and education.

Although the history of health education/promotion as a profession is slightly more than 100 years old, the concept of educating about health has been around since the dawn of humans. This chapter discusses the history of health, health care, and health education/promotion from the earliest human records to the present. The main focus is on Northern Africa and Europe. These areas had the greatest influence on the development of health knowledge and health care in the United States. Although other parts of the world—for example, the Far East, Africa, Central America, and South America—contributed to the history of health and health care, their accounts are not as directly relevant to the history of health in the United States.

It is important that students recognize the difference between "educating about health," which can be done by anyone who believes he or she has knowledge about health to share with someone else, and "health education/promotion," which is done by a professionally trained health education specialist. The need for professional health education specialists emerged as human knowledge of health and health care increased. This chapter emphasizes the health education/promotion profession during the past 150 years as it evolved from the dual roots of school health and public health. You cannot fully appreciate the health education/promotion profession without understanding its origin. History reveals how progress was made over time. It also depicts the obstacles faced by those who promoted health improvements throughout the years. "At the same time, historical study shows us that despite the difficulties, change is possible, given dedication, organization and persistence. . . . Historical case studies may be able to teach us useful lessons about successful strategies used by public health reformers in the past" (Fee & Brown, 1997, p. 1763).

▷ Early Humans

We assume that the earliest humans learned by trial and error to distinguish between things that were healthful and those that were harmful. They were able to observe how animals bathed to cool their bodies and remove external parasites, apply mud to calm insect bites, consume certain herbs to provide medicinal benefits and avoid other herbs that were poisonous (Goerke & Stebbins, 1968, p. 5).

It does not stretch the imagination too far to see how education about health first took place. Someone may have eaten a particular plant or herb and become ill. That person would then warn (educate) others against eating the same substance. Conversely, someone may have ingested a plant or an herb that produced a desired effect. That person would then encourage (educate) others to use this substance. Through observation, trial, and error, other types of health-related knowledge were discovered. Eventually, this knowledge was transformed into rules or taboos for a given society. Rules about preserving food and how to bury the dead may have been implemented. Perhaps taboos against defecation within the tribe's communal area or near sources of drinking water were established (McKenzie & Pinger, 2015). The trial and error method, which undoubtedly produced serious illness and even death among some early humans, gradually became less needed. Knowledge was passed verbally from one generation to the next, preventing at least some of the potential ill effects of everyday life. As society progressed even further, this knowledge was written down and saved (see **Figure 2.1**).

▶ **Figure 2.1** Preparation of medicine from honey (the leaf from an Arabic translation of the *Materia Medica of Dioscorides*, dated 1224 Iraq, Baghdad School)

There was still much more unknown than known about protecting health. Disease and death were probably much more common than health and longevity. To early humans, it was puzzling when disease and death occurred for no apparent reason. In an attempt to make these events seem more rational, early man often attributed disease and accidents to magical spirits, which were believed to live in trees, animals, the earth, and the air. When these spirits were angered they would punish individuals or communities with disease and death (Goerke & Stebbins, 1968). To prevent disease, sacrifices were made to please the gods, taboos were obeyed, amulets were worn, and "haunted" places were avoided. Charms, spells, and chants were also used to protect from disease (Duncan, 1988). Again, it is likely that some form of rudimentary education about health was taking place to inform people how to keep from provoking the spirits and, thus, prevent disease.

▷ Early Efforts at Public Health

Evidence of broad-scale public health activity has been found in the earliest of civilizations. In India, sites excavated at Mohenjo-Daro and Harappa dating back 4,000 years indicate that bathrooms and drains were common. The streets were broad, paved, and drained by covered sewers (Rosen, 1958). Archeological evidence also shows that the Minoans (3000–1430 B.C.E.)

BOX 2.1

The Rights and Duties of the Surgeon of 2080 B.C.E.: From the *Code of Hammurabi*

"If a physician operate on a man for a -severe wound (or make a severe wound upon a man), with a bronze lancet, and save the man's life; or if he open an -abscess (in the eye) of a man, with a bronze lancet, and save the man's eye, he shall receive ten shekels of silver (as his fee)."

"If he be a freeman,* he shall receive five shekels."

"If it be a man's slave, the owner of the slave shall give two shekels of silver to the physician."

"If a physician operate on a man for a severe wound, with a bronze lancet, and cause the man's death; or open an abscess (in the eye) of a man with a bronze lancet, and destroy the man's eye, they shall cut off his hands."

"If a physician operate on a slave of a freeman for a severe wound, with a bronze lancet, and cause his death, he shall restore a slave of equal value."

"If he open an abscess (in his eye), with a bronze lancet, and destroy his eye, he

shall pay silver to the extent of one half of his price."

"If a physician set a broken bone for a man or cure his diseased bowels, the patient shall give five shekels of silver to the physician."

"If he be a freeman, he shall give three shekels."

"If it be a man's slave, the owner of the slave shall give two shekels of silver to the physician."

"If a veterinary physician operates on an ox or ass for a severe wound and save its life, the owner of the ox or ass shall give the physician, as his fee, one sixth of a shekel of silver."

"If he operate on an ox or an ass for a severe wound, and cause its death, he shall give to the owner of the ox or ass one fourth its value."

Freeman indicates a rank intermediate between that of "man" (or gentleman) and that of "slave."

Source: From R. F. Harper, *The Code of Hammurabi*, 1904, Chicago.

and Myceneans (1430–1150 B.C.E.) built drainage systems, toilets, and water flushing systems (Pickett & Hanlon, 1990). The oldest written documents related to health care are the **Smith Papyri**, dating from 1600 B.C.E., which describe various surgical techniques. The earliest written record concerning public health is the *Code of Hammurabi* (see **Box 2.1**), named after the king of Babylon. It contained laws pertaining to health practices and physicians, including the first known fee schedule (Rubinson & Alles, 1984).

▷ Early Cultures

The medical lore of the distant past was handed down from generation to generation. In virtually every culture for which there are documented historical accounts, people turned to some type of a physician or medicine man for health information (education about health), treatments, and cures (Green & Simons-Morton, 1990). In Egypt, as in many other cultures, this role was held by the priests. Eventually, the various incantations, spells, exorcisms, prescriptions, and clinical observations were compiled into written format, some of which survive in our museums and libraries (Libby, 1922).

The Egyptians made substantial progress in the area of public health. They possessed a strong sense of personal cleanliness and were considered to be the healthiest people of their time (see **Figure 2.2**). They used numerous pharmaceutical preparations and constructed earth privies for sewage, as well as public drainage pipes (Pickett & Hanlon, 1990). Nevertheless, they relied primarily on priests for their health information and used remedies such as "dung of the gazelle and the crocodile, the fat of a serpent, mammalian entrails and other excreta, tissues and organs" (Libby, 1922, p. 6).

In approximately 1500 B.C.E., the Hebrews extended Egyptian hygienic thought and formulated (in the biblical book of Leviticus) what is probably the world's first written hygienic code. It dealt with a variety of personal and community responsibilities, including cleanliness of the body, protection against the spread of contagious diseases, isolation of lepers, disinfection of dwellings after illness, sanitation of campsites, disposal of excreta and refuse,

▶ **Figure 2.2** The Egyptians were known for their cleanliness and were considered the healthiest people of the time.

protection of water and food supplies, and specific hygiene rules for menstruating women and women who had recently delivered a child.

The history of health and health care in the Greek culture (1000–400 B.C.E.) is intriguing as well as relevant to modern healthcare philosophy. The Greeks were perhaps the first people to put as much emphasis on disease prevention as they did on the treatment of disease conditions. Balance among the physical, mental, and spiritual aspects of the person was emphasized. Among the early Greeks, religion played an important role in health care. However, the role of physician began to take on a more defined shape, and a more scientific view of medicine emerged.

In the early stages of Greek culture, as represented in the *Iliad* and the *Odyssey*, the priesthood played a role in the healing arts. In the *Iliad*, **Asclepius** was a Thessalian chief who had received instruction in the use of drugs. By the beginning of the eighth century B.C.E., tradition had enshrined him as the god of medicine. He had two daughters who also had health-related powers. **Hygeia** was given the power to prevent disease, whereas **Panacea** was given the ability to treat disease. Hygeia was the more prominent figure and was often pictured with her father in sculptures and illustrations of the time (Schouten, 1967) (see **Figure 2.3**). The words *hygiene* and *panacea* can be traced back to these daughters of Asclepius (Libby, 1922).

Eventually, hundreds of elaborate temples were built throughout Greece to worship Asclepius. These temples were typically on beautiful sites overlooking the sea or beside healing fountains. The temple priests practiced their healing arts, which often involved fraud. The temple priests should not be confused with the **Asclepiads**. The Asclepiads were a brotherhood of men present at the temples who initially claimed descent from Asclepius. Although some of the Asclepiads probably helped the priests with their trickery, others broke away from

▶ **Figure 2.3** Asclepius and Hygeia

▶ **Figure 2.4** Illustration of a caduceus, a symbol that shows two snakes braided around a staff. It is representative of the medical profession and has its earliest association with Asclepius, the Greek healer.

the priests and began to practice medicine based on more rational principles. These ancient temples of Asclepius left their symbol as a permanent reminder of the past—the staff and serpent of the physician, known as the **caduceus** (Rubinson & Alles, 1984) (see **Figure 2.4**).

The famous Greek physician **Hippocrates** came from the Asclepian tradition. He lived from about 460 B.C.E. until 375 B.C.E. (See **Figure 2.5**.) Hippocrates developed a theory of disease causation consistent with the philosophy of nature held by leading philosophers of his

▶ **Figure 2.5** Hippocrates, 460–375 B.C.E., "Father of Western Medicine"

day. Hippocrates taught that health was the result of balance, and disease was the result of an imbalance. To the Greeks, the ideal person was perfectly balanced in mind, body, and spirit. Thus, study and practice related to philosophy, athletics, and theology were all important to maintain balance. To do this, however, took a tremendous commitment of time and energy. Each day required physical activity, study, and philosophical discussion while maintaining proper nutrition and rest. Few people could afford to lead such a life. Those who did were the aristocratic upper class leading a life of leisure supported by a slave economy (Rosen, 1958). The ideal Greek human being that is so often mentioned was, in fact, a small percentage of the Greek population.

Hippocrates holds an important place in the history of medicine. His theory of health and disease was still being taught in medical schools as a valid theory of disease causation as recently as the first quarter of the 20th century. Hippocrates, however, did more than just theorize about disease. He carefully observed and recorded associations between certain diseases and such factors as geography, climate, diet, and living conditions. Duncan (1988) noted, "One of his [Hippocrates's] most noteworthy contributions is the distinction between 'endemic' diseases, which vary in prevalence from place to place, and 'epidemic' diseases, which vary in prevalence over time" (p. 12). The traditional Hippocratic Oath is still used today and is the basis for medical ethics. Hippocrates and the Asclepiads moved health care away from religion and priests and attempted to establish a more rational basis to explain health and disease. Hippocrates's concept of balance in life is still promoted today as the best means for maintaining health and well-being.

Hippocrates has been credited as being the first epidemiologist and the father of modern medicine (Duncan, 1988). It is not hard to imagine that he was also a health educator. One can easily see Hippocrates educating his friends and patients about diet, exercise, rest, and the importance of balance in preventing disease and promoting health.

The Romans conquered the Mediterranean world, including the Greeks. In doing so, however, the Romans did not destroy the cultures they conquered but learned from them. The Romans accepted many Greek ideas, including those related to health and medicine. "As clinicians, the Romans were hardly more than imitators of the Greeks, but as engineers and administrators, as builders of sewerage systems and baths, and as providers of water supplies and other health facilities, they set the world a great example and left their mark in history" (Rosen, 1958, p. 38). (See **Figure 2.6**.)

The Roman Empire (500 B.C.E.–C.E. 500) built an extensive and efficient aqueduct system. Evidence of some 200 Roman aqueducts remains today, from Spain to Syria and from Northern Europe to North Africa (McKenzie & Pinger, 2015). The total capacity of the 13 aqueducts delivering water to the city of Rome has been estimated at 222 million gallons every 24 hours. At the height of the Empire this would have been enough to provide each citizen of Rome with at least 40 gallons of fresh water per day. Additionally, attention was paid to water purity. At specific points along the aqueduct, generally near the middle and end, settling basins were located, in which sediment might be deposited (Rosen, 1958).

The Romans also developed an extensive system of underground sewers. These served to carry off both surface water and sewage. The main sewer in Rome that emptied into the Tiber River was 10 feet wide and 12 feet high; it was still part of the Roman sewer system during the 20th century.

The Romans made other health advancements. They observed the effect of occupational hazards on health, and they were the first to build hospitals. By the second century C.E., a

▲ **Figure 2.6** Roman aqueducts

public medical service was set up whereby physicians were appointed to various towns and institutions. A system of private medical practice also developed during the Roman era (Rosen, 1958).

The Romans furthered the work of the Greeks in the study of human anatomy and the practice of surgery. Some Roman anatomists even dissected living human beings to further their knowledge of anatomy (Libby, 1922). In quoting the Latin writer Cornelius, Libby noted that these anatomists "procured criminals out of prison, by royal permission, and dissecting them alive, contemplated, while they were still breathing, the parts which nature had before concealed, considering their position, color, figure, size, order, hardness, softness, smoothness, and asperity" (Libby, 1922, p. 54). Although some opposed this hideous practice, others supported it, holding "it is by no means cruel as most people represent it, by the tortures of a few guilty, to search after remedies for the whole innocent race of mankind in all ages" (Libby, 1922, p. 54).

▷ Middle Ages

The era from the collapse of the Roman Empire to about C.E. 1500 is known as the Middle Ages or Dark Ages. This was a time of political and social unrest, when many health advancements of previous cultures were lost. Rosen (1958) notes that, "the problem that confronted the medieval world was to weld together the culture of the barbarian invaders with the classical heritage of the defunct [Roman] Empire and with the beliefs and teachings of the Christian religion" (p. 52). This proved to be no easy task.

With the Roman Empire no longer able to protect settlements, each city had to defend itself against its enemies. For safety, people lived within city walls along with their domesticated animals. As the population grew, expansion was difficult and overcrowding common (Rosen, 1958). Lack of fresh water and sewage removal were major problems for many medieval cities; Roman public health advancements were lost.

To make matters worse, there was little emphasis on cleanliness or hygiene. The new religion, Christianity,

> found its disciples among the lower classes, where personal hygiene was not practiced, and as a consequence, an entirely different attitude toward the human body developed. Excessive care of the body, that is, man's earthly and mutable part, was unimportant in the Christian dualistic concept, which separated body from soul. For some Eastern churchmen and holy men, living in filth was regarded as evidence of sanctity: cleanliness was thought to betoken pride, and filthiness humility. (Goerke & Stebbins, 1968, p. 9)

Fortunately, as Christianity matured so did its concept of the human body. Eventually, Christians came to believe that the body is the soul's earthly dwelling; thus, permitting better care of it.

Early Christians also reinforced the notion that disease was caused by sin or disobeying God. This propelled priests and religious leaders back into the position of preventing and treating disease. The health-related advancements of the Greco-Roman era were abandoned and shunned. Entire libraries were burned, and knowledge about the human body was seen as sinful.

The Middle Ages were characterized by great epidemics. Perhaps the cruelest of these was leprosy, a disease characterized by severe facial and extremity disfigurement. A highly contagious and virulent disease, all Western countries issued edicts against anyone suspected of having leprosy and regulated every aspect of the sufferer's life. In some communities, lepers were given the last rites of the church, forced to leave the city, made to wear identifying clothing, and required to carry a rod identifying them as lepers. Other lepers were forced to wear a bell around their necks and to ring it as a warning when other people came near. Such isolation usually brought about a relatively quick death resulting from hunger and exposure (Goerke & Stebbins, 1968). Eventually, leprosy hospitals were founded to treat the afflicted. It has been estimated that by C.E. 1200, there were 1,900 leper houses and leprosaria in Europe (Rosen, 1958).

The bubonic plague, known as the Black Death, may have been the most severe epidemic the world has ever known. The death toll was higher and the disruption of society greater than from any war, famine, or natural disaster in history. "At Constantinople, the plague raged with such violence that 5,000, and even 10,000 persons are said to have died in a single day" (Donan, 1898, p. 94). Estimates of casualties vary from 20 to 35 million, with Europe losing one quarter to one third of its entire population. In Avignon, France, 60,000 people died. As a result, the pope was forced to consecrate the Rhone River so that bodies might be thrown into it, because the churchyards were filled (Goerke & Stebbins, 1968).

Imagine what it must have been like to live through the plague. Literally one out of every three or four people you knew contracted the disease and died. The cause of the disease was unknown, creating widespread fear and superstition. Often, religious leaders and doctors were some of the first victims. They were exposed to the disease early in the epidemic through their contact with infected sufferers. This left many communities with no religious or medical leadership.

People reacted to the plague in different ways. Some became extremely pious, turned away from earthly pleasures, and practiced extreme self-denial in hopes of pleasing God. Others took the opposite approach, lost faith in God, and disregarded legal, moral, and sexual restraints (Goerke & Stebbins, 1968). The Brotherhood of the Flagellants was a group of religious zealots who believed the plague could be avoided by admitting to their sins and then ritual-istically beating themselves in atonement. Today, such a group would most likely be labeled a religious cult. Members of this group marched in long, two-column lines from city to city. In each city, they would chant a litany and conduct their ritualistic ceremony. At a signal from the group's master, the Flagellants would strip to the waist and march in a circle until they received another signal from the master. Upon receiving the second signal, they would throw themselves to the ground with their body position indicating the specific sin they had committed. The master would move among the bodies, thrashing those who had commit-ted certain sins or had offended the discipline of the Flagellants in some way. This would be followed by a collective flagellation in which the group members would rhythmically beat their own backs and breasts with a heavy scourge made of three or four leather thongs tipped with metal studs. According to eyewitness accounts, the Flagellants lashed themselves until their bodies became swollen and blue, and blood dripped to the ground. Further complicat-ing the health consequences of such punishment was a rule prohibiting bathing, washing, or changing clothes. When joining the Brotherhood, group members had to pledge to scourge themselves three times daily for 33 days and eight hours, which represented one day for each year of Christ's earthly life (Ziegler, 1969). In other words, to complete the Flagellant pledge, one would have to undergo the ritualistic beating 100 times.

Debate existed during the Middle Ages concerning the cause of the plague. In 1348, Jehan Jacme wrote that the disease was caused by five factors: (1) the wrath of God, (2) the corrup-tion of dead bodies, (3) waters and vapors formed in the interior of the earth, (4) unnatural hot and humid winds, and (5) the conjunction of stars and planets (Winslow, 1944).

Another story concerning the origins of the disease had Italian merchants trapped in a city on the Black Sea that was under siege by a local Mongol prince. The prince was forced to call off the siege because large numbers of his army were dying of a strange disease. Before leav-ing, the prince ordered his army to catapult the dead, diseased bodies into the city. Within days, the people inside the city began to die. Afraid, the Italian merchants set sail for Italy, but not before infected rats had boarded the ship. Soon many of the sailors became sick. The ship tried to dock in several cities but was denied permission because of the illness. Finally permission was granted to dock in Sicily where the rats came on shore and the plague began (De'ath, 1995).

Despite the disagreement that existed on the cause of the disease, contemporaries believed that the disease was contagious. In other words, it was passed from person to person in some unknown way. Although this concept of contagion had been around for many years and was discussed in the Bible, it was not until the Middle Ages and the epidemics of leprosy and bubonic plague that it started to become more universally accepted. The contagion concept opened the door to new interest in science and severely weakened the argument of those pro-moting the sin-disease theory.

The Middle Ages also saw epidemics of other communicable diseases, including smallpox, diphtheria, measles, influenza, tuberculosis, anthrax, and trachoma. The last major epidemic disease of this period was syphilis, which appeared in 1492. As with other epidemics, syphilis killed thousands of people (McKenzie & Pinger, 2015).

Although there were no professional health education specialists during the Middle Ages, education about health continued to exist. Priests, medical doctors, and community lead-ers attempted to "educate" anyone who would listen to their ideas about health and disease prevention. Given the rudimentary level of health knowledge and the lack of consensus on prevention and causation of disease, a professional health education specialist would probably have contributed little to the general population's health in the Middle Ages.

▷ Renaissance

The Renaissance, which means "rebirth," lasted roughly from C.E. 1500 to 1700. This time period was characterized by a gradual change in thinking. People began to view the world and humankind in a more naturalistic and holistic fashion. Although progress was slow, science again emerged as a legitimate field of inquiry, and numerous scientific advancements were made. The world did not change overnight from the superstitious and backward beliefs of the Dark Ages to a completely enlightened society in the Renaissance. Disease and plague still ravaged Europe and overall medical care was still rudimentary. Bloodletting was a major form of treatment for everything from the common cold to tuberculosis. Popular remedies included crabs' eyes, foxes' lungs, oil of anise, oil of spiders, and oil of earthworms. A major means of diagnosing a patient's condition consisted of examining the urine for changes in color. The inspection of a patient's urine by a true physician was known as "water casting." For many years, this was the principal diagnostic test of the medical profession.

Much surgery and dentistry was performed by barbers because they had the best chairs and sharpest instruments available. Some barbers dispensed health information, as can be seen in the following example from a Danish barber-surgeon: "It is very good for persons to drink themselves intoxicated once a month for the excellent reasons that it frees their strength, furthers sound sleep, eases the passing of water, increases perspiration, and stimulates general well-being" (Durant, 1961, pp. 495–496). Unfortunately, few were probably moderate enough to restrict their binges to once a month.

Rosen (1958) notes that, although the Renaissance "is characterized by the rapid growth and spread of science in various fields, public health as a practiced activity received very little, if any, direct benefit from these advances" (p. 84). Evidence of the poor public health conditions can be seen in this note describing the average English household floor of the 16th century:

> As to floors, they are usually made with clay, covered with rushes that grow in the fens and which are so seldom removed that the lower part remains sometimes for twenty years and has in it a collection of spittle, vomit, urine of dogs and humans, beer, scraps of fish and other filthiness not to be named. (Pickett & Hanlon, 1990, p. 25)

Although living conditions among the English royalty were certainly better than for those of the laboring class, health-related problems were still prevalent. Disposal of human waste was a major problem. Those who lived in old castles located their latrines in large projections on the face of walls. The excrement was discharged from these projections into deep-walled pits, moats, or streams near the walls of the castle. Those less fortunate used chamber pots and simply tossed their contents out the nearest window. Even among royalty, basic hygiene left much to be desired. Few monarchs bathed more frequently than once a week. Much of the material used in royal apparel, such as silk, velvet, and ermine, could not be washed; thus, it simply accumulated dirt and perspiration. Cloaking scents were used to try to renew the clothing, but they were not effective (Hansen, 1980).

On the positive side, the Renaissance was a period of exploration and expanded trade. The search for knowledge, characteristic of the Greek and Roman eras, was revitalized. Superstitions of the Middle Ages were slowly replaced with a more systematic inquiry into cause and effect. In the middle of the 15th century, learning gained momentum as a result of Johannes Gutenberg's invention of the printing press with moveable type. This allowed the great classical works of Hippocrates and Galen to be reproduced and distributed to larger audiences (Gordon, 1959).

There were also scientific advancements during the Renaissance. The human body was again considered appropriate for study, and realistic anatomical drawings were produced. John Hunter, the father of modern surgery, undertook a more orderly exploration of the workings of the human body. Antonie van Leeuwenhoek discovered the microscope and proved there were life forms too small for the human eye to see. These life forms, however, were not yet associated with disease. John Graunt forwarded the fields of statistics and epidemiology. Through studying the *Bills of Mortality*, published weekly in London, Graunt found more males than females were born, higher death rates during the first years of life than later in life, and higher death rates among urban dwellers than rural dwellers (Goerke & Stebbins, 1968).

In Italy, many cities had instituted health boards to fight the plague. It did not take long, however, for their responsibilities to be expanded. By the middle of the 16th century, numerous matters had fallen under the control and jurisdiction of these health boards. These included "the marketing of meat, fish, shellfish, game, fruit, grain, sausages, oil, wine and water; the sewage system; the activity of the hospitals; beggars and prostitutes; burials, cemeteries, and pesthouses; the professional activity of physicians, surgeons and apothecaries; the preparation and sale of drugs; the activity of hostelries and the Jewish community" (Cipolla, 1976, p. 32).

▷ Age of Enlightenment

The 1700s were a period of revolution, industrialization, and growth of cities. Both the French and American Revolutions took place during this century. Plague and other epidemics continued to be a problem. Science had not yet discovered that these diseases were produced by microscopic organisms. The general belief was that disease was formed in filth and that epidemics were caused by some type of poison that developed in the putrefaction process. The vapors, or "miasmas," rising from this rotting refuse could travel through the air for great distances and were believed to result in disease when inhaled. This concept, known as the **miasmas theory**, remained popular throughout much of the 19th century. As preventive measures, herbs and incense were often used to perfume the air, supposedly filling the nose and crowding out any miasmas (Duncan, 1988). It was still not known that contaminated water could cause disease infection.

Scientific advancements continued throughout the period. Dr. James Lind, a Royal Navy surgeon, discovered that scurvy could be controlled on long sea voyages by having sailors consume lime juice. To this day, British sailors are known as "limeys." Edward Jenner discovered a vaccine procedure against smallpox. Bernardino Ramazzini wrote on trade and industrial diseases. Theorists of the time conceived of the mind and body not as separate entities, but as dependent on each other. Philosophers of the 18th century, such as Diderot, Locke, Rousseau, and Voltaire, all "promoted the worth of each human life and the importance of individual health for the well being of society" (Rubinson & Alles, 1984, p. 5).

Although progress was made during this time, health education/promotion in itself still did not emerge as a profession. With the rudimentary state of medical knowledge in the 16th, 17th, and 18th centuries, there would have been little for a health education specialist to do other than promote the misconceptions and half-truths that predominated during the time period. However, health boards, the forerunner of today's health departments, did develop as scientific and medical knowledge increased. The roots of modern health education/promotion were planted, and the first sprouts would soon emerge.

▷ The 1800s

In the first half of the 1800s, little happened to improve the public's health. In England, the streets of London were filthy with animal and human waste. Overcrowding and industrialization added to the problem. These conditions, under which so many people lived and worked, had dire results. Smallpox, cholera, typhoid, tuberculosis, and many other diseases reached high endemic levels (Pickett & Hanlon, 1990).

In 1842, a momentous event occurred in the history of public health when Edwin Chadwick published his *Report on an Inquiry into the Sanitary Conditions of the Labouring Population of Great Britain*. In the report, he documented the deplorable living conditions of Britain's laboring class, made a strong case that these conditions were the cause of much disease and suffering, and called for government intervention. This report eventually led to the formation of a General Board of Health for England in 1848 (Goerke & Stebbins, 1968).

Extraordinary advancements in biology and bacteriology took place by the middle of the 19th century in England and throughout Europe. In 1849, Dr. John Snow, who laboriously studied epidemiological data related to a cholera epidemic in London, hypothesized that the disease was caused by microorganisms in the drinking water from one particular water pump located on Broad Street (see **Figure 2.7**). He removed the pump's handle to keep people from using the water source, and the epidemic abated. Snow's action was remarkable because it predated the discovery that microorganisms cause disease and was in opposition to the prevailing miasmas theory of the time (Johnson, 2006).

▶ **Figure 2.7** By removing the handle of this pump, which is still in place on Broad Street in London, John Snow interrupted a cholera epidemic.

In 1862, Louis Pasteur of France proposed his germ theory of disease. After this, advancements in bacteriology greatly accelerated. Over the next 20 years, Pasteur discovered how microorganisms reproduce, introduced the first scientific approach to immunization, and developed a technique to pasteurize milk. Robert Koch, a German scientist, developed the criteria and procedures necessary to establish that a particular microbe, and no other, caused a particular disease. Joseph Lister, an English surgeon, developed the antiseptic method of treating wounds by using carbolic acid, and he introduced the principle of asepsis to surgery. These are just a few of the tremendous advancements in bacteriology made during the second half of the 19th century. As a result, the years from 1875 to 1900 became known as the **bacteriological period of public health** (McKenzie & Pinger, 2015).

▷ Public Health in the United States

1700s

During the 1700s, health conditions in the United States were similar to those in Europe—deplorable. Diseases such as smallpox, cholera, and diphtheria were prevalent. Because of the slave trade, diseases such as yaws, yellow fever, and malaria were common in southern states (Marr, 1982). Large numbers of immigrants were entering the ports, cities were growing, overcrowding was common, and the Industrial Revolution was about to begin.

The primary means of controlling disease were quarantine and regulations on environmental cleanliness. For example, as early as 1647, the Massachusetts Bay Colony enacted regulations to prevent pollution of Boston Harbor. In 1701, Massachusetts passed laws allowing for the isolation of smallpox patients and for ship quarantine, as needed. However, there was no overseeing body or agency to enforce compliance.

In an attempt to address health problems, some cities formed local health boards (Pickett & Hanlon, 1990). Prominent citizens who advised elected officials on health-related matters made up these boards. They had no paid staff, no budget, and no authority to enforce regulations. According to tradition, the first health board was formed in Boston in 1799, with Paul Revere as chairman. This is contested, however, by other cities claiming earlier health boards, including Petersburg, Virginia (1780), Baltimore (1793), Philadelphia (1794), and New York (1796).

Life expectancy is one measure of health status for a given population. It is defined as "the average number of years a person from a specific cohort is projected to live from a given point in time" (McKenzie & Pinger, 2015, p. 608). The first life expectancy tables were developed for the United States in 1789 by Dr. Edward Wigglesworth (Ravenel, 1970). **Table 2.1** shows Wigglesworth's table. It provides strong evidence of the prevailing health conditions. In 1789, life expectancy at birth was only 28.15 years. By 2020, the projected life expectancy at birth in the United States will be 79.5 years (U.S. National Center for Health Statistics, 2009).

1800s

From 1800 to 1850, health status improved little. Conditions of overcrowding, poverty, and filth worsened as the Industrial Revolution encouraged more and more people to move to the cities. Epidemics of smallpox, yellow fever, cholera, typhoid, and typhus were common. Tuberculosis and malaria reached exceptionally high levels. For example, in 1850, the Massachusetts tuberculosis death rate was 300 per 100,000 population, and the infant

TABLE 2.1 **Expectation of life according to Wigglesworth life table—1789**

Expectation	Years	Expectation	Years
At birth	28.15	At age 50	21.16
At age 5	40.87	At age 55	18.35
At age 10	39.23	At age 60	15.43
At age 15	36.16	At age 65	12.43
At age 20	34.21	At age 70	10.06
At age 25	32.32	At age 75	7.83
At age 30	30.24	At age 80	5.85
At age 35	28.22	At age 85	4.57
At age 40	26.04	At age 90	3.73
At age 45	23.92	At age 95	1.62

Source: Ravenel, M. P. (Ed.). (1970). *A Half Century of Public Health.* New York: Arno Press and *The New York Times*. Originally published in 1921 by American Public Health Association.

mortality was about 200 per 1,000 live births. Conditions were so bad that life expectancy actually decreased in some cities during this period of time. In Boston, the average age at death dropped from 27.85 years in 1820–1825 to 21.43 in 1840–1845. In New York during the same period, the average age of death decreased from 26.15 to 19.69 (Shattuck, 1850).

Public health reform in the United States was slow to begin. Interestingly, a major report helped jump-start the public health reform movement in the United States, just as Chadwick's landmark 1842 report stimulated public health reform in Britain. Lemuel Shattuck's 1850 *Report of the Sanitary Commission of Massachusetts* contained remarkable insights about the public health issues of Massachusetts, including how to approach and solve these problems. Shattuck was a bookseller and publisher from Boston. He retired early at age 46 and dedicated the remainder of his life to his interest in community affairs (American Public Health Association [APHA], 1959). His report is remarkable because no national or state public health programs existed at the time, and local health agencies that did exist were functioning at a minimal level. Shattuck visualized how to improve the public's health through the initiation of state and local level health departments. "Of the 50 recommendations which Shattuck listed, 36 have become accepted principles of public health practice" (Goerke & Stebbins, 1968, p. 28). Among his many recommendations were the keeping of vital statistics, environmental sanitation, control of food and drugs, teaching prevention and sanitary science in medical schools, smoke control in cities, control of alcoholism, the supervision of mental disease, exposure of nostrums, preaching health from pulpits, routine physical exams, and the establishment of nurse training schools (APHA, 1959; Pickett & Hanlon, 1990).

The publication of Shattuck's report did not mean an end to the public health problems in the United States. In fact, the report went largely unnoticed for 19 years until 1869, when the Commonwealth of Massachusetts established a state board of health made up of physicians and laymen exactly as Shattuck had envisioned. One year later, Virginia and California formed their own state boards of health (Ravenel, 1970). By 1900, 38 states had established state boards of health. Today, every U.S. state has a state board or department of health.

Despite the formation of state boards of health, these state-level agencies could not meet health needs on a more local level. With limited resources, there was simply too much to accomplish. As a result, the first full-time county health departments were formed in Guilford County, North Carolina, and Yakima County, Washington, in 1911. Some sources have cited Jefferson County, Kentucky, as the first county health department, set up in 1908 (Pickett & Hanlon, 1990).

As states initiated boards of health, board members had to interact, communicate, and develop their skills. These needs led to the founding of the American Public Health Association (APHA). (See Chapter 8 for more APHA information.) Following a series of national conventions on quarantine held from 1857 through 1860, "Stephen Smith invited a group of 'refined gentlemen' to discuss informally the possibility of a national sanitary association" (Bernstein, 1972, p. 2). Smith's suggestion of an association for health officials and interested citizens was well received. A decision was made to establish a committee to work on a permanent organization. One year later, in 1873, the first annual meeting was held in Cincinnati, Ohio, and 70 new members were elected. Smith remained active in the association throughout his life. At the age of 99, he walked to the podium unassisted to speak at the 50th anniversary celebration of the APHA.

The federal government started a public health service that dates back to 1798, when Congress passed the Marine Hospital Service Act. Previously, sailors in the merchant marine had nowhere to turn for health care. Because they paid no local or state taxes, ill or injured sailors generally were not welcomed in port cities. The Marine Hospital Service Act required the owners of every ship to pay the tax collector 20 cents per month for every seaman they employed. This money was used to build hospitals and provide medical services in all major seaport cities (see **Figure 2.8**). This act "represented the first prepaid medical and hospital

▲ **Figure 2.8** Old Marine Hospital in Charleston, South Carolina, 1934

insurance plan in the world, under the administrative supervision of what eventually became a public health agency" (Pickett & Hanlon, 1990, p. 34).

Successive legislation throughout the 19th century gradually expanded the scope of the Marine Hospital Service. In 1902, Congress retitled it the Public Health and Marine Hospital Service and gave it a definite organizational structure under the direction of the surgeon general. In 1912, "Marine Hospital" was dropped from the name, and the service became known as it is today, the U.S. Public Health Service. "The mission of the U.S. Public Health Service Commissioned Corps is to protect, promote, and advance the health and safety of our Nation" (U.S. Public Health Service, 2016). The Commissioned Corps comprises over 6,500 health professionals that proudly wear the uniform of the U.S. Public Health Service (see **Figure 2.9**).

In 1879, Congress created the National Board of Health. The board was composed of seven members appointed by the president, including representatives of the Army, Navy, Marine Hospital Service, and Justice Department. Its functions were to obtain information on all matters related to public health, and provide grants-in-aid to state boards of health. The National Board also provided money to university scientists for health-related research. Unfortunately, the board was short-lived. In administering quarantine functions, the board incurred opposition from state agencies and private shipping concerns. Others in positions of power were not in favor of the research grant program and felt such expenditures were extravagant. Thus, in 1882, the board's appropriations were transferred to the Marine Hospital Service, which carried on with the quarantine functions but discontinued the grant program (U.S. Department of Health, Education, and Welfare [USDHEW], 1976).

1900 to Present

The period from 1900 to 1920 is known as the **reform phase of public health** (McKenzie & Pinger, 2015). During this time, urban areas expanded, and many people lived and worked in deplorable conditions. To address these concerns, federal regulations were passed concerning

▶ **Figure 2.9** Uniform of the U.S. Public Health Service.

the food industry, states passed workers' compensation laws, the U.S. Bureau of Mines and the U.S. Department of Labor were created, and the first clinic for occupational diseases was established. By the end of the 1920s, the movement for healthier workplace conditions was well established, and the average life expectancy had risen to 59.7 years.

Also during this period, the first national voluntary health agencies were formed. They were run primarily by volunteers along with a few paid staff. Each of these agencies was designed to address a specific health problem. For example, the National Association for the Study and Prevention of Tuberculosis was established in 1902, and the American Cancer Society was founded in 1913. Today, volunteer agencies continue to be important players in the prevention of disease and the promotion of health (McKenzie & Pinger, 2015). They often hire health education specialists.

The 1920s were a relatively quiet period in public health. Progress continued, but at a slower pace. However, the Public Health Education Section of the APHA was founded in 1922 (Bernstein, 1972). This is the APHA section to which most health education specialists belong. Its mission is, "To be a strong advocate for health education, disease prevention and health promotion directed to individuals, groups and communities in all activities of the Association." (APHA, 2016).

The need for health education/promotion existed in the early 20th century as many questionable and fraudulent health practices were being promoted. Moore's (1923) book about public health in the United States included two chapters on questionable and unreliable health activities. One of the most interesting examples involved a cure-all product known as Tanlac. The May 11, 1917, edition of the *Holyoke Daily Transcript* contained Fred Wicks' testimonial in a Tanlac advertisement, as well as his obituary (Moore, 1923, pp. 173–174).

Other examples of questionable health practices abound. William Harvey Kellogg and his younger brother W. K., founders of the Kellogg cereal company, were best known in the early 1900s for the sanitarium they established and operated in Battle Creek, Michigan. The rich and famous came from all over the world to be treated at the sanitarium. Many of the treatment modalities, however, would be considered questionable and even quackery by today's standards. For example, they used some 200 different types of hydrotherapy along with therapeutic enemas, electric horses, vibrators, and cold air (Butler, Thornton, & Stoltz, 1994). However, the sanitarium did promote exercise and good nutrition as ways to prevent and treat disease. (See **Figure 2.10**.) The concept of prevention was again gaining prominence.

Tension between preventive medicine and curative medicine began to appear in the United States during the early 20th century. Moore (1923) related a story about a town in which public health work had banished malaria. A physician was asked how his profession had been affected by this public health advancement. He replied off-handedly, "If it hadn't been for the influenza, I'd have gone broke. That saved us" (p. 373).

In a more rational manner, Newsholme (1936) noted three reasons that treatment formed a larger part of public health efforts than prevention and why it would continue to do so in the future. First, the knowledge to prevent disease and death was only partial. Medical workers simply did not have the knowledge and skills to prevent many disease states. Second, even when knowledge to prevent disease did exist, many people did not know about it, and those that did found it difficult to make those changes necessary to prevent disease. Third, there were such a large number of sick people needing prompt medical treatment that it was difficult to focus attention on prevention. Many of the same arguments are used today to account for the emphasis on traditional medical interventions instead of prevention.

▶ **Figure 2.10** Kellogg Sanitarium in Battle Creek, Michigan.

From 1930 through World War II, the role of federal government in social programs expanded. Prior to the Great Depression, medical services were self funded or funded by relatives and friends, as well as by religious organizations and some voluntary agencies. During the Depression, however, private resources could not meet the demands of those requiring assistance. In 1933, President Franklin D. Roosevelt created numerous agencies and programs as part of his New Deal, which improved the plight of the disadvantaged. Much of the money was used for public health efforts, including the control of malaria, the building of hospitals, and the construction of municipal water and sewage systems.

The Social Security Act of 1935 was a real milestone and the beginning of the federal government's involvement in social issues, including health. The act provided support for state health departments and their programs. Funding was made available to develop sanitary facilities and to improve maternal and child health.

Two major public health agencies were formed at this time. On May 26, 1930, the Ransdell Act converted the Hygienic Laboratory to the National Institute of Health, with a broad mandate to learn the cause, prevention, and cure of disease (USDHEW, 1976). The National Institutes of Health, as it is called today, is now one of the premiere—if not *the* premiere—medical research facilities in the world. In 1946, the Communicable Disease Center was established in Atlanta, Georgia. Now called the Centers for Disease Control and Prevention (CDC), it is one of the world's leading epidemiological centers. (See **Figure 2.11**.) The CDC is also a major training facility for health communications and educational methods (Pickett & Hanlon, 1990). The CDC's vision for the 21st century is "Health Protection . . . Health Equity" (CDC, 2016f). Its mission is "Collaborating to create the expertise, information, and tools that people and communities need to protect their health—through health promotion, prevention of disease, injury and disability, and preparedness for new health threats" (CDC, 2016f).

Following World War II, concern rose over the number of healthcare facilities and the adequacy of the care they provided. In 1946, Congress passed the National Hospital Survey and Construction Act, also known as the Hill-Burton Act, to improve the distribution and enhance the quality of hospitals. From the passage of the Hill-Burton Act through the 1960s,

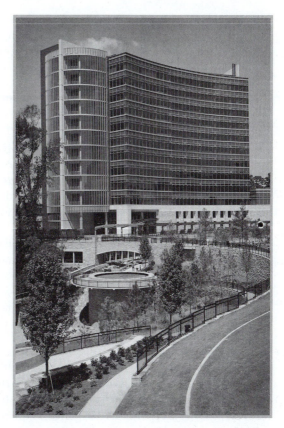

▶ **Figure 2.11** CDC's "Arlen Specter Headquarters and Emergency Operations Center" located on CDC's Roybal campus in Atlanta, Georgia

new hospital construction occurred rapidly. Little thought, however, was given to planning. As a result, hospitals were built too close together and provided overlapping and unnecessary services (McKenzie & Pinger, 2015).

In 1954, Dr. Mayhew Derryberry, the first chief of health education in the federal government, noted, "The health problems of greatest significance today are the chronic diseases . . . . The extent of chronic diseases, various disabling conditions, and the economic burden that they impose have been thoroughly documented" (*Voices From the Past,* 2004, p. 368). Before the 1950s, the major emphasis of public health had been on communicable or contagious diseases. However, through improved public health services, medical care, and immunization programs, many contagious diseases no longer threatened as they once had, and the focus shifted ever so slowly to the prevention of chronic diseases. Derryberry predicted how this change of focus would impact health education: "Health education and health educators will be expected to contribute to the reduction of the negative impact of such major health problems as heart disease, cancer, dental disease, mental illness and other neurological disturbances, obesity, accidents and the adjustments necessary to a productive old age" (*Voices From the Past,* 2004, p. 368). Although the seed may have been planted for health education specialists to play a greater role in the prevention of chronic diseases, it was not until the 1970s that the seed finally sprouted.

In 1965, the federal government again passed major legislation designed to improve the health of the U.S. population. Although major improvements were made in health facilities and the quality of health care, there were still many underserved people. Most of these people were either poor or elderly. In response, Congress passed the Medicare and Medicaid bills as amendments to the Social Security Act of 1935. **Medicare** was created to assist in the payment of medical bills for the elderly, whereas **Medicaid** did the same for the poor. These bills provided medical care for millions of people who could not otherwise have obtained such services.

It was evident by the 1970s that disease prevention held the greatest potential improving Americans' health and reducing healthcare costs. The first national effort to promote the health of citizens through a more preventive approach took place in Canada. In 1974, the Canadian Ministry of Health and Welfare released a publication titled *A New Perspective on the Health of Canadians* (Lalonde, 1974). This document, often called the *Lalonde Report*, presented epidemiological evidence that supported the importance of lifestyle and environmental factors. It called for numerous national health promotion strategies encouraged Canadians to be more responsible for their own health. (See Chapter 1 for information on the Health Field Concept associated with this publication.) The Lalonde Report influenced many U.S. health professionals to rethink current assumptions that focus on high-technology, treatment-based medicine. So important was this report that Bates and Winder (1984) likened it to a re-emergence of Hygeia and the beginning of the second public health revolution (p. 24).

HEALTHY PEOPLE INITIATIVES AND PUBLIC HEALTH STANDARDS

In the United States, the government publication *Healthy People* was the first major recognition of the importance of lifestyle in promoting health and well-being (U.S. Public Health Service, 1979). This publication supported a shift from the traditional medical model toward lifestyle and environmental strategies that emphasized prevention.

In 1980, *Promoting Health/Preventing Disease: Objectives for the Nation* was released. This federal document contained 226 U.S. health objectives for the United States divided into three areas: preventive services, health protection, and health promotion. These objectives provided the framework for public health efforts during the 1980s. They allowed public health professionals to focus on key areas while providing baseline data for measuring progress (U.S. Department of Health and Human Services [USDHHS], 1980). Although not all of these objectives were met, the planning and evaluation process used to develop them became a valuable way to measure progress in U.S. health and healthcare services. This led to the practice of developing U.S. health objectives each decade. In 1990, *Healthy People 2000: National Health Promotion and Disease Prevention Objectives* was released, and in 2000, *Healthy People 2010: Understanding and Improving Health* was released.

The Healthy People initiative has evolved into an important strategic planning tool for public health professionals at the federal, state, and local levels. Formal reviews measure the progress of these objectives at mid-course (halfway through the 10-year period) and again at the end of 10 years.

Healthy People 2020 was released in December 2010 and will guide U.S. public health practice and health education specialists for the next 10 years. The Healthypeople.gov Web site is user friendly and permits the entire report to be searched and accessed. The vision statement, mission statement, and four overarching goals of *Healthy People 2020* can be seen in

TABLE 2.2 *Healthy People 2020* **Vision, Mission, and Goals**

Vision

A society in which all people live long, healthy lives.

Mission

Healthy People 2020 strives to:

- Identify nationwide health improvement priorities;
- Increase public awareness and understanding of the determinants of health, disease, and disability, and the opportunities for progress;
- Provide measurable objectives and goals that are applicable at the national, state, and local levels;
- Engage multiple sectors to take actions to strengthen policies and improve practices that are driven by the best available evidence and knowledge;
- Identify critical research, evaluation and data collection needs.

Overarching Goals

- Attain high quality, longer lives free of preventable disease, disability, injury, and premature death.
- Achieve health equity, eliminate disparities, and improve the health of all groups.
- Create social and physical environments that promote good health for all.
- Promote quality of life, healthy development and healthy behaviors across all life stages.

Source: U.S. Department of Health and Human Services. (2010). *Developing Healthy People 2020*.

Table 2.2 (CDC, 2016a). The meat of the report includes numerous objectives spread over 42 different topic areas (see **Table 2.3** on next page) (CDC, 2016e).

For *Healthy People 2020* to be effective, programs must be developed and initiated to meet the established goals. This means that partner states, counties, communities, organizations, and individuals must get involved. The CDC uses a simple but powerful model to guide partners in establishing effective programs known as MAP-IT. (See **Figure 2.12**.) The MAP-IT model guides partners through five steps: mobilize, assess, plan, implement, and track (CDC, 2016c). It is important to note that the five MAP-IT steps are similar to four of the seven responsibilities of a health education specialist that you will learn more about later in this text (Chapter 6). The health education specialist responsibilities are to assess, plan, implement, and evaluate.

Another important initiative designed, in part, to improve the effectiveness of public health departments working on Healthy People objectives is the National Public Health Performance Standards Program (NPHPSP) (CDC, 2016d). This is a partnership initiative to develop performance standards; collect, monitor, and analyze data; and ultimately improve public health performance. It is the first time that a common, systematic strategy for measuring public health performance has been available. The goals of the program are to:

- provide performance standards for public health systems and encouraging their widespread use;

▲ **Figure 2.12** MAP-IT

Source: http://healthypeople.gov/2020/implement/mapit.aspx

TABLE 2.3 *Healthy People 2020* Topic Areas

1. Access to Health Services
2. Adolescent Health
3. Arthritis, Osteoporosis, and Chronic Back Conditions
4. Blood Disorders and Blood Safety
5. Cancer
6. Chronic Kidney Diseases
7. Dementias, Including Alzheimer's Disease
8. Diabetes
9. Disability and Health
10. Early and Middle Childhood
11. Educational and Community-Based Programs
12. Environmental Health
13. Family Planning
14. Food Safety
15. Genomics
16. Global Health
17. Healthcare Associated Infections
18. Health Communication and Health Information Technology
19. Health-Related Quality of Life and Well-Being
20. Hearing and Other Sensory or Communication Disorders
21. Heart Disease and Stroke
22. HIV
23. Immunization and Infectious Diseases
24. Injury and Violence Prevention
25. Lesbian, Gay, Bisexual, and Transgender Health
26. Maternal, Infant, and Child Health
27. Medical Product Safety
28. Mental Health and Mental Disorders
29. Nutrition and Weight Status
30. Occupational Health
31. Older Adults
32. Oral Health
33. Physical Activity
34. Preparedness
35. Public Health Infrastructure
36. Respiratory Diseases
37. Sexually Transmitted Diseases
38. Sleep Health
39. Social Determinants of Health
40. Substance Abuse
41. Tobacco Use
42. Vision

Source: U.S. Department of Health and Human Services. (2013). *Healthy People 2020 Topic Areas.* Retrieved May 29, 2013, from www.cdc.gov/nchs/healthy_
people/hp2020_topic_areas.htm.

- encourage and leverage national, state, and local partnerships to build a stronger foundation for public health preparedness;
- promote continuous quality improvement of public health systems;
- strengthen the science base for public health practice improvement (CDC, 2016d).

Local and state health departments are encouraged to use these performance standard assessments to conduct their own self-assessments. Through this process, weaknesses can be identified and improvements made to enhance the overall performance of public health departments (CDC, 2016d).

HEALTH EDUCATION/PROMOTION: A RECOGNIZED PROFESSION

One more important historical event for health education/promotion occurred on October 27, 1997, when the Standard Occupational Classification (SOC) Policy Review Committee approved the creation of a new, distinct classification for the occupation of health educator (Auld, 1997/1998). Health educators had pursued this goal for more than 25 years. Health educators were previously included in the category "Instructional Coordinator," a broad, primarily education-related category that failed to consider the many varied and unique responsibilities of health educators. Approval of health education as a separate occupational classification means that the Department of Labor's Bureau of Labor Statistics, the Department of Commerce's Bureau of the Census, and all other federal agencies that collect occupational data now collect data on health education specialists. Many state and local governments also maintain data on health education/promotion. For the first time, it is possible to determine the number of health education specialists employed and the outlook for future health education/promotion positions. This approval is one more sign that health education/promotion is gaining the respect and recognition it deserves.

In summary, tremendous advancements in public health and health education/promotion took place during the 20th century. It could reasonably be argued that the total number of advancements in public health during the 20th century were equal to or greater than the total number of public health advancements in all prior time. In reflecting on these great successes of public health, the Department of Health and Human Services identified 10 public health achievements they believed had the greatest impact on major causes of morbidity and mortality of the 20th century. **Box 2.2** lists these 10 achievements. Imagine what life would be like today if none of these achievements had been realized. Think of the role health education/promotion has played in these advancements.

BOX 2.2

10 Great Public Health Achievements in the United States, 1900–1999

- Vaccination
- Motor vehicle safety
- Safer workplaces
- Control of infectious diseases
- Decline in deaths from coronary (heart) disease and stroke
- Safer and healthier foods
- Healthier mothers and babies
- Family planning
- Fluoridation of drinking water
- Recognition of tobacco use as a health hazard

Source: U.S. Department of Health & Human Services (1999). "Changes in the Public Health System," *Morbidity and Mortality Weekly Report*, 48, 50, 1141.

▷ School Health in the United States

Life in early America was hard, and there was little time for education. The labor of building homes, clearing forests, tilling fields, hunting, and preparing food filled the days. Most people lived under primitive conditions. Settlements were few and far apart. Travel and transportation were costly, slow, and limited to foot, horseback, boat, or wagon.

In the mid-1600s, as communities became more established, the call for education was soon heard. Religion had always been an important part of life in America, and it was the religious leaders who led the drive for education. They believed that Satan benefited when people were illiterate, because they could not read the scriptures. In 1647, Massachusetts passed the "Old Deluder" law to prevent Satan from deluding the people by keeping them from reading the Bible. The law specified that a town with 50 families should establish an elementary school, and a town with 100 households should set up a Latin grammar secondary school (Means, 1962).

The curriculum in these early schools was largely derived from the educational practices in England. Essentially, reading, as the avenue to religious understanding, was the primary subject. Writing, spelling, grammar, and arithmetic supplemented reading. Later, geography and history were added, but the teaching of health was not part of the early education system in the United States.

Because only boys attended these early schools, and working for the family was still a major concern, daily sessions were by necessity of short duration. The length of the school term was usually only a few months. Teachers were lacking in preparation, with their basic qualifications being only to (1) read, (2) know more of the Bible than the students, (3) work cheap, and (4) keep the students under control. Teachers were totally dependent on the rod for classroom management (Means, 1962). Girls were not sent to school as it was generally felt they could learn everything they needed to know about cleaning, sewing, cooking and tending to a home and family from their mothers.

School buildings typically were inadequate (see **Figure 2.13**). They were poorly built, inaccessible, and sometimes temporary structures. Their interiors were inadequately lighted, were

▶ **Figure 2.13** An old one-room schoolhouse

furnished with uncomfortable seating, had no sanitary facilities, and were heated with wood-burning stoves. These schools were not even close to meeting modern standards for school construction (Means, 1962).

The schools and their curricula remained much the same until the 1800s. By the mid-1800s, most schools had become tax supported, and attendance was compulsory. Those concerned about public health pointed out the numerous health and safety problems in the schools. These concerns helped bring attention to the conditions of the schools and ultimately paved the way for health instruction in the curriculum (Means, 1962).

Horace Mann, whose writings and speeches promoted the importance of education in general, was perhaps the first spokesperson for teaching health in schools. He was elected secretary of the Massachusetts State Board of Education in 1837. Beginning in 1837 with the publication of his *First Annual Report* and continuing through the publication of the *Sixth Annual Report* in 1843, Mann called for mandatory hygiene programs that would help students understand their bodies and the relationship between their behaviors and health (Rubinson & Alles, 1984).

Another momentous event in the development of school health occurred in 1850, when Lemuel Shattuck from Massachusetts wrote his *Report on the Sanitary Commission of Massachusetts* (1850). (This is the same report discussed previously in reference to public health.) Although the report has become a classic in the field of public health, it also provided strong support for school health (Means, 1975). In the report, Shattuck (1850) eloquently supports the teaching of physiology, as the term *health education* had yet to be coined:

> It has recently been recommended that the science of physiology be taught in the public schools; and the recommendation should be universally approved and carried into effect as soon as persons can be found capable of teaching it. . . . Every child should be taught early in life, that to preserve his own life and his own health and the lives and health of others, is one of the most important and constantly abiding duties. By obeying certain laws or performing certain acts, his life and health may be preserved; by disobedience, or performing certain other acts, they will both be destroyed. By knowing and avoiding the causes of disease, disease itself will be avoided, and he may enjoy health and live; by ignorance of these causes and exposure to them, he may contract disease, ruin his health, and die. Every thing connected with wealth, happiness and long life depend upon health; and even the great duties of morals and religion are performed more acceptably in a healthy than a sickly condition. (pp. 178–179)

Aside from local and state attempts to promote the teaching of health-related curricula in the schools, no concerted national effort existed until that of the Women's Christian Temperance Union. Originally founded in 1874, the union expounded on the evils of alcohol, narcotics, and tobacco through every conceivable means and was one of the most effective lobbying organizations ever (Means, 1962). Between 1880 and 1890, every state in the union passed a law requiring instruction concerning the effects of alcohol and narcotics due to stimulus from the Temperance Movement (Turner, Sellery, & Smith, 1957).

Other national movements soon followed. In 1915, the National Tuberculosis Association introduced the "Modern Health Crusade" as a device for promoting the health of school children. It was based on promotion to "knighthood" for those that followed certain health habits. The Child Health Organization of America encouraged the nation to adopt more functional health education/promotion programs. One of its active leaders, Sally Lucas Jean, was ultimately responsible for changing the name from hygiene education to health education (Means, 1962). With this name change, the focus of health education shifted from that of physiology and hygiene, which was factual and unrelated to everyday living, to an emphasis on healthy living and health behavior.

Despite these advancements, health education from 1900 to 1920 was generally characterized by inconsistency and awkward progress. World War I provided the impetus for widespread acceptance of school health education as a discipline in its own right (Turner et al., 1957). Out of 2,510,706 men examined as potential military draftees during World War I, 730,756 (29 percent) were rejected on physical grounds. A large portion of these physical deficiencies could have been prevented if the schools had been doing their part to train children concerning health and fitness (Andress & Bragg, 1922). In the immediate postwar years, 16 states required hygiene instruction in their public schools; 12 of these states made provisions for the preparation of health teachers in the teacher training schools supported by the state (Rogers, 1936).

Significant research and demonstration projects related to school health education were conducted in the 1920s and 1930s. Examples include the Malden, Massachusetts project, done in cooperation with the Massachusetts Institute of Technology; the Mansfield, Ohio, project supported by the American Red Cross; the Fargo, North Dakota, project sponsored by the Commonwealth Fund; and the Cattaraugus County, New York, project financed by the Milband Memorial Fund. According to Turner and colleagues (1957), "these programs showed that habits could be changed and health improved through health education" (p. 27).

In the 1930s, the drive for health education from the public slowed. Health education continued to address the major health issues of the time but without the enthusiasm brought on by World War I. Notable research studies supplemented authoritative opinion in helping to point out difficulties and offer solutions related to the teaching of health education. Several important conferences were held on health education and youth health at the national level (Means, 1962). The profession was moving forward.

Professional organizations emerged during the 1900s that still exist today. School health education, long associated with physical education, received official recognition in 1937, when the American Physical Education Association became the American Association for Health and Physical Education which eventually evolved into the American Association for Health, Physical Education, Recreation and Dance (AAHPERD). In the 1990s, AAHPERD changed from an association to an alliance of national and district associations. The national association that represented health education specialists was the American Association for Health Education (AAHE). For many years AAHE was a major force in the health education field. At their 2013 National Convention, AAHPERD dropped the association structure and went back to one organization. The name AAHPERD was changed to "SHAPE America" with a mission to, " advance professional practice and promote research related to health and physical education, physical activity, dance and sport." (SHAPE America, 2016). This means that AAHE is no longer in existence. Although SHAPE America still intends to service those school health educators that also teach physical education, most health education specialists, including those focused on school health, have joined another professional association such as the Society for Public Health Education, which represents all health education specialists in all practice settings, or the American School Health Association.

The American School Health Association evolved from the American Association of School Physicians, which was founded in 1927. Over the next 10 years this association of school physicians expanded its functions, interests, and scope of activity. As a result, it broadened its membership to include school health personnel other than physicians. In 1938, its name was changed to the American School Health Association to reflect these changes. Today, the mission of the American School Health Association is to "transform all schools into places where every student learns and thrives" (American School Health Association, 2016).

The American Public Health Association had long been an organization interested in and supportive of school health. In fact, many of the earliest supporters of health education in the schools had been leaders in public health. Appropriately, the organization established a separate section within its administrative structure to focus on school health interests. In 1942, the School Health Section of the American Public Health Association was formed. (Chapter 8 discusses all these professional associations in greater detail.)

With the bombing of Pearl Harbor on December 7, 1941, the United States found itself at war. Once again, national focus turned to physical fitness and health. With no major threats of war in the previous 20 years, the physical status of young U.S. men had again degenerated. Of the approximately 2 million men examined for induction into the nation's armed forces, almost 50 percent were disqualified. Of those disqualified, 90 percent were found to be physically or mentally unfit (American Youth Commission, 1942). This unfortunate situation helped greatly to stimulate interest in the health of high school students and provided strong motivation for health education/promotion classes.

After World War II, school health education continued to grow as a profession. As Means (1975) observed, "This period from 1940 into the 1970s was one of appraisal, re-evaluation, and consolidation with respect to research accomplished in school health education. During this time leaders in the field attempted to look back, review, and take stock of what was known as a determinant of future action" (p. 107).

The **School Health Education Study** was a major study of significance to school health education. Directed by Dr. Elena M. Sliepcevich (1964), the study included 135 randomly selected school systems involving 1,460 schools and 840,832 students in 38 states. Health behavior inventories were administered to students in grades 6, 9, and 12. The results were appalling. Health misconceptions among students at all levels prevailed. Questionnaires were distributed to school administrators throughout the country to obtain data on organizational procedures and instructional practices related to school health education. Again the results indicated major problems in the organization and administration of health programs. Cortese (1993) noted, " . . . some health topics were omitted while others were repeated grade after grade at the same level of sophistication. No logical rationale placed learning exercises at various grade levels, and a need existed for a challenging and meaningful curriculum" (p. 21).

The second phase of the School Health Education Study established a curriculum writing team to develop a school health education curriculum based on needs identified from the first phase of the study. The team consisted of prominent names in school health education at the time, including Gus T. Dalis, Edward B. Johns, Richard K. Means, Ann E. Nolte, Marion B. Pollock, and Robert D. Russell (Means, 1975). Over the next eight years, the writing team developed a comprehensive curriculum package that still influences school health curricula today.

The **School Health Education Evaluation Study** of the Los Angeles Area was one more important study. Its purpose was to evaluate the effectiveness of school health work in selected schools and colleges of the area. More specifically, the project aimed at the appraisal of the entire school health program, including administrative organization, school health services, health instruction, and healthful school environment. Further, it examined the students' health knowledge, attitudes, and behavior. The study resulted in 11 conclusions and 17 important recommendations for the field (Means, 1975).

School health programs have continued to evolve from the mid-1970s to the present. Several important events and trends have impacted school health education and overall school health programs. In 1978, the Office of Comprehensive School Health was established within the U.S. Department of Education. The primary purpose of the office was policy development for health issues that affected children and youth. Although the office held great promise for school health education efforts, unfortunately, it was never fully funded. A director was named, Peter Cortese, but the office was finally deactivated with the budget cuts during President Ronald Reagan's administration (Rubinson & Alles, 1984).

The 1980s saw the emergence of two important concepts: coordinated school health programs and comprehensive school health instruction. Based on the initial ideas of Turner and colleagues (1957), and later refined by Allensworth and Kolbe (1987), a **coordinated school health program** consisting of eight interactive components that work together to enhance the health and well-being of the students, faculty, staff, and community was devised (see **Figure 2.14**). The eight components consist of health education, physical education, health services, nutrition services, counseling, psychology and social services, healthy school environment, staff health promotion and family and community involvement.

The original eight component coordinated school health program model has been expanded and revised to now include 10 components, and is known as the Whole School, Whole Community, Whole Child Model (WSCC) (CDC, 2016g). To arrive at the 10 WSCC components, the original Healthy School Environment component was split into the social and emotional climate component and the physical environment component. The original

▶ **Figure 2.14** CDC diagram of Whole School, Whole Community, Whole Child (WSCC)

Source: Centers for Disease Control and Prevention. 2016. *Whole School, Whole Community, Whole Child.* www.cdc.gov/healthyschools/wscc/index.htm

---

BOX 2.3

Characteristics of an Effective Health Education Curriculum

1. Focuses on clear health goals and related behavioral outcomes.
2. Is research based and theory-driven.
3. Addresses individual values, attitudes, and beliefs.
4. Addresses individual and group norms that support health-enhancing behaviors.
5. Focuses on reinforcing protective factors and increasing perceptions of personal risk and harmfulness of engaging in specific unhealthy practices and behaviors.
6. Addresses social pressures and influences.
7. Builds personal competence, social competence, and self-efficacy by addressing skills.
8. Provides functional health knowledge that is basic, accurate, and directly contributes to health-promoting decisions and behaviors.
9. Uses strategies designed to personalize information and engage students.
10. Provides age-appropriate and developmentally appropriate information, learning strategies, teaching methods, and materials.
11. Incorporates learning strategies, teaching methods and materials that are culturally inclusive.
12. Provides time for instruction and learning.
13. Provides opportunities to reinforce skills and positive health behaviors.
14. Provides opportunities to make positive connections with influential others.
15. Includes teacher information and plans for professional development and training that enhance effectiveness of instruction and student learning.

Source: Centers for Disease Control and Prevention (CDC). (2016). *Characteristics of an Effective Health Education Curriculum* Available at: http://www.cdc.gov/healthyyouth/SHER/characteristics/index.htm

---

family/community involvement component was split into the community involvement component and family engagement component (CDC, 2016b). The WSCC model recognizes the importance of establishing healthy behaviors in youth. To accomplish this the model promotes the cooperation and collaboration of government agencies, community organizations, schools, community members and families.

Comprehensive school health education is actually the health curriculum component of the coordinated school health program. **Box 2.3** identifies factors that need to be in place for the development and delivery of a planned, sequential, effective school health education program. Emphasis should be placed on six specific adolescent risk behaviors that are monitored by the Youth Risk Behavior Surveillance System (YRBSS) (CDC, 2016h). These six behaviors contribute to the leading causes of death and disability among youth and adults. These behaviors usually are established during childhood, persist into adulthood, are interrelated, and are preventable. These risk behaviors are as follows:

- Behaviors that contribute to unintentional injuries and violence
- Sexual behaviors that contribute to unintended pregnancy and sexually transmitted diseases, including HIV infection
- Alcohol and other drug use
- Tobacco use
- Unhealthy dietary behaviors
- Inadequate physical activity (CDC, 2016h)

BOX

2.4

National Health Education Standards

Health Education Standard 1—Students will comprehend concepts related to health promotion and disease prevention to enhance health.

Health Education Standard 2—Students will analyze the influence of family, peers, culture, media, technology, and other factors on health behaviors.

Health Education Standard 3—Students will demonstrate the ability to access valid information and products and services to enhance health.

Health Education Standard 4—-Students will demonstrate the ability to use interpersonal communication skills to enhance health and avoid or reduce health risks.

Health Education Standard 5—Students will demonstrate the ability to use decision-making skills to enhance health.

Health Education Standard 6—Students will demonstrate the ability to use goal-setting skills to enhance health.

Health Education Standard 7—Students will demonstrate the ability to practice health-enhancing behaviors and avoid or reduce health risks.

Health Education Standard 8—Students will demonstrate the ability to advocate for personal, family, and community health.

Source: Reprinted with permission from the American Cancer Society. *National Health Education Standards Achieving Excellence, Second Edition.* (Atlanta, GA: American Cancer Society; 2007), 8, http://www.cancer.org/bookstore

---

In 2006, with support from the American Cancer Society, the Joint Committee on National Health Education Standards was formed. Committee members included representation from the American Association for Health Education, The American Public Health Association, The American School Health Association and the Society of State Leaders of Health and Physical Education. The standards can be seen in **Box 2.4**. The goal of the National Health Education Standards is improved educational achievement for students and improved health in the United States. The standards promote **health literacy**, the capacity of individuals to access, interpret, and understand basic health information and services, and the skills to use the information and services to promote health. The standards provide a foundation for curriculum development, instruction, and assessment of student performance. A rationale and numerous performance indicators, broken down by grade-level groupings, accompany each of the eight standards. The National Health Education Standards also provide an important guide for colleges and universities to enhance pre-professional preparation as well as the continuing education of health education/promotion teachers.

The National Board for Professional Teaching Standards, founded in 1987, developed national standards for school health education teachers. These standards go beyond the requirements for state teacher licensure. Since fall 2008, individuals with three years of full-time health education/promotion teaching experience and a valid state teacher's license for those three years may voluntarily complete a rigorous evaluation process to become a National Board Certified Health Education Teacher. This National Board Certification places school health education on an equal level with other teaching fields and allows highly qualified and dedicated health education teachers to be recognized for their work. Some states or districts may provide salary bonuses for these highly qualified teachers who obtain National

Board Certification (National Board for Professional Teaching Standards, 2016). It is expected that many exceptional and highly dedicated health education/promotion teachers will seek National Board Certification.

Since 1987, the concept of a coordinated school health program has dominated the school health arena. At first glance, it would seem that schools would be excited to initiate comprehensive school health programs. How could they not embrace a concept that would bring together multiple components of the school in an integrated attempt to improve the health of faculty, staff, students, and the community? A healthy child taught by a healthy teacher in a health-conscious community should forward the school's overall mission to provide each child with the best education possible. Unfortunately, the full potential of co-ordinated school health programs has never been realized in most school districts. Factors may include the low priority placed on health by many school administrators; a lack of lead-ership to promote, coordinate, and oversee school health programs; and an overemphasis on competency testing. Another dynamic could be the adverse reactions from conservative groups that perceive coordinated school health as a means of incorporating sex education into the curriculum. New optimism has emerged with release of the Whole School, Whole Community, Whole Child movement (CDC, 2016g). Time will tell if this expanded and more comprehensive model will gain further traction than the coordinated school health program model of the past.

Another positive support for the future of school health is the bipartisan passage of the 2015 Every Child Achieves Act which recognizes both health education and physical edu-cation as "core subjects" in schools (SOPHE, 2015). Health education specialists had been calling for this recognition for many years (Gambescia, 2006). Previously both health educa-tion and physical education were not considered "core subjects" by federal mandates which allowed schools to minimize their importance while placing more focus on those subjects such as math, science and English that were considered core subjects. The passage of this act reflects a growing awareness of the importance of health education to the academic success and overall well-being of students. It will be interesting to watch how passage of this act will actually influence school health education in the future.

Despite the apparent lack of success with coordinated school health programs, schools still hold tremendous promise for health education/promotion efforts. With nearly all young people under 19 years of age attending schools, health education specialists must remain dili-gent in their effort to bring effective health promotion and education programs to this popu-lation. Every health education specialist should be advocating for the Whole School, Whole Community, Whole Child movement with national and state education agencies, federal and state government representatives, and local school boards.

▷ Patient Protection and Affordable Care Act

On March 23, 2010, amid both fanfare and criticism, President Barack Obama signed into law the Patient Protection and Affordable Care Act (referred to as the Affordable Care Act or ACA). Through a combination of cost controls, subsidies, and mandates, it expands health-care coverage to 31 million uninsured Americans (Open Congress, 2010). Another impor-tant feature is the act's focus on prevention and prevention services (Koh & Sebelius, 2010;

Society for Public Health Education [SOPHE], 2013). The bill provides better access to clinical prevention services by removing cost barriers. Further, the bill encourages and promotes worksite wellness programs, encourages evidence-based community prevention and wellness programs, and provides strong support for school-based health centers. (See **Table 2.4**

TABLE 2.4 **Wellness and Prevention Provisions in the Patient Protection and Affordable Care Act (H.R. 3590)**

Immediate Effects 2010

- Establish the National Prevention, Health Promotion and Public Health Council
- Create a Prevention and Public Health Fund—500 million in FY 2010
- Create task forces on prevention services and community preventive services
- Establish a grant program to support the delivery of evidence-based and community-based prevention and wellness services
- Conduct a national worksite health policies and programs survey
- Award grants to support the operation of school-based health centers—50 million in FY 2010
- Eliminate cost sharing for tobacco cessation counseling and prescriptions for pregnant women in Medicaid and Medicare

2011

- National strategy to improve nation's health due March 2011
- Prevention & Public Health Fund receives up to $750 million
- School-based health centers receive another $50 million
- Improve access by eliminating cost sharing for prevention services in Medicare and Medicaid
- Provide grants to small employers to establish wellness programs
- Require chain restaurants and food from vending machines to disclose nutritional content

2012

- Worksite survey results due
- Prevention & Public Health Fund receives up to $1 billion
- School-based health centers receive up to $50 million

2013

- Prevention & Public Health Fund receives up to $1.25 billion
- School-based health centers receive up to $50 million

2014

- Permit employers to offer employee rewards in the form of premium discounts, waivers of cost sharing, or other benefits for participating in a wellness program and meeting certain health-related standards
- Establish 10-state pilot program allowing states to apply similar rewards as noted above for employers
- Prevention & Public Health Fund receives up to $1.5 billion
- School-based health centers receive up to $50 million

2015 and Beyond

- Prevention & Public Health Fund receives up to $1.25 billion
- School-based health centers receive up to $50 million

Source: From Society for Public Health Education (SOPHE). 2010. What does health care reform do for prevention and wellness? http://www.sophe.org/advocacy_matters.cfm. Reprinted by permission.

for a summary of the act's prevention provisions.) This bill should create new and expanded opportunities for health education specialists to promote health. More importantly, it is good for the health of Americans. As Koh and Sebelius (2010) state: "In short, to prevent disease and promote health and wellness, the Act breaks new ground. . . . Moving prevention toward the mainstream of health may well be one of the most lasting legacies of this landmark legislation" (p. 5).

As of 2015, the ACA has been met with much criticism and has faced several legal challenges. To date, it remains mostly intact and has had some positive effects. As of 2015, 16.4 million Americans have gained health insurance coverage through the ACA (Wilensky & Teitelbaum, 2017). It is estimated that by 2023, the number of uninsured in the United States will be half the size as in 2012. As the 2016 Presidential elections approach, the ACA will once again be a topic of interest with some Presidential candidates promising repeal of the ACA if elected.

Summary

The history of health and health education/promotion is important to the professional development of health education specialists. By understanding the past, you can appreciate the present and become a leader in this emerging profession.

Today's concept of health education/promotion is relatively new, dating back only to the middle to late 1800s. Since ancient times, however, humans have been searching for ways to keep themselves healthy and free of disease. Without knowledge of disease causation or medical treatment, it was only natural to rely on superstition and spiritualism for answers. The concept of prevention was intriguing, but the knowledge and skills to prevent disease were unknown.

Progress in preventing and treating disease is evident in the early civilizations of Egypt, Greece, and Rome. These cultures recognized a need for humans to maintain sound minds and bodies. Systems of rudimentary pharmacology, better waste disposal, and safer drinking water were among some of the most noteworthy improvements.

During the Middle Ages, much of what had been previously learned was lost. Society took a giant step backward. Science and knowledge were shunned, while religion gained new favor as the preferred means of preventing and treating disease. Great epidemics struck the European continent, and millions of people lost their lives.

The Renaissance witnessed a rebirth of interest in knowledge. Science again flourished, and healthcare advancements were made. Understanding of disease, however, was still rudimentary, and the effects of treatments were often worse than the diseases. Sanitary conditions were deplorable and would remain so through the 1800s. The emergence of health education/promotion as a profession was still more than a century away.

The Age of Enlightenment saw tremendous growth in cities as the Industrial Revolution got under way in both England and the United States. Unfortunately, this population growth compounded sanitation problems related to overcrowding. Epidemics were still prevalent. In addition, employment conditions of the working class were frequently unsafe and unhealthy.

By the mid-1850s, conditions were ripe for the birth of public health in Great Britain and the United States. The contagion theory of disease emerged, and early reformers called for the government to take control of environmental conditions that led to disease. Health departments at city, state, and county levels were established and began to monitor and regulate food safety, water quality, and waste disposal. Professional organizations for health personnel were created, and voluntary agencies were formed. Major pieces of legislation were passed as the government sought to improve working conditions and took greater responsibility for the poor and infirm. During the mid-1900s, emphasis was placed on building new medical facilities and enhancing the technology required to treat disease.

By the 1970s, the cost of medical treatment had escalated, and concern for prevention was enhanced. This set the stage for the development of national health objectives for the decades of the 1980s, 1990s, and 2000s. *Healthy People 2020* is now in place and identifies the objectives for the current decade. Health education/promotion has made and continues to make great strides as a profession.

In the mid-1800s, as public health was starting to make important strides, school health education was also budding. In addition to reading, writing, and arithmetic, early pioneers saw the need to educate students about health-related matters. In the early 1900s, groups such as the National Tuberculosis Association, the American Cancer Society, and the Women's Christian Temperance Union strongly supported educating school children about health. Both World War I and World War II provided important impetus for health-related instruction and physical training in the schools.

During the 1960s and 1970s, several important studies supported the need for school health education and documented its effectiveness. Coordinated school health programs, created in the 1980s and 1990s, have evolved into the expanded whole school, whole community, whole child concept. School Health Program Guidelines, national health education standards, and identifying the six leading causes of death and disability helped promote health education/promotion.

Although health and school health education have made great strides since the first humans contemplated how to treat and prevent disease, there is still a long way to go. Both in the United States and worldwide there are many people who do not have access to medical care or the important information and skills of professionally trained health education specialists. Heart disease, cancers, diabetes, obesity, and HIV are prevalent in both developed and developing countries, and traditional infectious diseases, parasitic infections, poor sanitation, unsafe water and malnutrition continue to affect people in developing low and middle income countries.

As in the past, health education professionals of today must envision what *can* be and strive to make that vision a reality. Turner et al. (1957) noted,

> As society looks ahead, it can conceive the hope that someday almost every human being will be well, intelligent, physically vigorous, mentally alert, emotionally stable, socially reasonable and ethically sound. At least, society must concern itself with progress toward that goal. (p. 18)

Health education specialists must be important players in this process. The recent Affordable Health Care Act should expand opportunities for health education specialists to impact Americans' health through community, worksite, and school-based programs.

Review Questions

1. Describe the earliest efforts at health care and informal health education/promotion.

2. Compare and contrast the great societies of ancient Egypt, Greece, and Rome. How are these cultures similar in relation to health? How are they different?

3. What were the major epidemics of the Middle Ages? Why were they so feared? What factors contributed to their spread? What were some strategies people used to prevent these diseases?

4. Discuss the Renaissance and why it is important to the history of health and health care.

5. Who wrote the *Report of the Sanitary Commission of Massachusetts* (1850)? Explain how this report was important to the history of both school health and public health.

6. Identify at least five major groups or events that forwarded school health programs.

7. What Canadian publication and its U.S. counterpart helped focus attention on the importance of disease prevention and health promotion?

8. What are *national health objectives?* Where can they be found? Why are they so important?

9. Describe the initiatives that have shaped school health education programs over the past 10 years.

10. Explain how the Affordable Health Care Act may serve to improve the public's health and advance the health education/promotion profession in the United States.

Case Study

Angelita is a health education professor employed by a state university. The local newspaper wants to interview her about the Affordable Health Care Act's prevention components, including how the act may enhance the health of their readers. The newspaper reporter also wants her to talk about previous governmental initiatives designed to prevent disease and improve the public's health. In preparation for the interview, Angelita wants to develop an outline of important points she would like to make. Your task, as Angelita's graduate assistant, is to develop the first draft of these important points.

Critical Thinking Questions

1. If a health educator is simply considered as someone who informs others about health, who would be considered humanity's first health educators? Defend your answer.

2. If a health education specialist trained in the year 2013 could time-travel back to the Middle Ages, what impact could that person have on the health problems of that era? What positive factors would work in the health education specialist's favor? What negative factors would work against the health education specialist?

3. When the first schools were being started in Massachusetts, do you believe health education/promotion would have been accepted as an academic subject? Why or why not? Do you believe health education/promotion is accepted as an academic subject at the present time? Why or why not?

4. Go online and find a copy of the new *Healthy People 2020* objectives. Read the introduction and overview. Find the objectives for one of the topic areas and review them. Next, select one objective in that topic area that you feel strongly about, and explain why you feel it will or will not be met by the year 2020. What role might a health education specialist have in meeting the objective you selected?

▷ Activities

1. Develop a timeline using 100-year increments from the early Egyptians to the current year. Mark all of the important health-related events as they occurred along the timeline. Next, continue your timeline 100 years into the future. Predict and mark important health-related events. Explain why you believe these predictions will come true.

2. Imagine what it would have been like to live through an outbreak of the Black Death in the Middle Ages. Write a 5-day personal diary, with daily entries depicting what you might have seen or heard and how you might have felt.

3. Interview several individuals who are at least 80 years old concerning the health care they received as young children. Ask them to describe any health education/promotion they can remember. When was it? Where did it take place? Who provided the education? Was it effective?

4. Contact your high school health teacher. Ask if he or she is aware of the National Standards for Health Education and to what extent the curriculum in the school district has been based on these standards. Ask the health teacher if he or she is aware of the whole school, whole community, whole child movement. If so, what has been done to implement this model at the local level? Who coordinates the effort? What programs or initiatives are a result of the effort? If nothing has been done, ask why? Try to determine the barriers to initiating the whole school, whole community, whole child program in the district.

▷ Weblinks

1. http://www.cdc.gov/museum/timeline/index.html

   Centers for Disease Control and Prevention

   This CDC Web site provides a timeline to learn about important events in the history of the CDC from its founding in 1946 to the present. Take note of the many important contributions to public health by this illustrious organization.

2. https://history.nih.gov/exhibits/history/index.html

   National Institutes of Health, Office of History

   This National Institutes of Health (NIH) Web site provides a brief history of this organization, highlighting some of its more important accomplishments.

3. **https://www.youtube.com/watch?v=zZG94c7xQmE**

   See a short video with leaders in public health talking about the importance of *Healthy People 2020* goals and what needs to happen for these goals to be met.

4. **http://www.healthypeople.gov/**

   Healthy People 2020

   This is the home page for the *Healthy People 2020* goals and objectives. From this page you should be able to access the actual *Healthy People 2020* documents, as well as information on how the objectives are developed.

5. **http://www.cdc.gov/healthyschools/wscc/index.htm**

   This site provides additional details on the Whole School, Whole Community, Whole Child initiative including a description of various components and how they can be integrated into the school program. Additional information on health and academics, data and statistics, tools, and resources are available at this site. This information is important for health education specialists who want to work in schools and make a difference in the lives of their students.

6. **https://www.youtube.com/watch?v=0ZEKSHBJtdc**

   A full length movie about Father Damien and the Kalaupapa, Molokai, Leper Colony, the last leper colony still functioning in the United States.

7. **https://vimeo.com/32226544**

   Watch this video on the history of public health in the United States.

References

Allensworth, D., & Kolbe, L. (1987). The comprehensive school health program: Exploring an expanded concept. *Journal of School Health, 57,* 409–412.

American Public Health Association. (May, 1959). Lemuel Shattuck (1793–1859): Prophet of American Public Health. *American Journal of Public Health Nations Health. 49* (5), 676–677.

American Public Health Association. (2016). *Public Health Education and Health Promotion.* Retrieved January 26, 2016, from https://www.apha.org/apha-communities/member-sections/public-health-education-and-health-promotion.

American School Health Association. (2016). *About the American School Health Association.* Retrieved January 30, 2016, from: http://www.ashaweb.org/about/.

American Youth Commission. (1942). *"Health and fitness," youth and the future.* Washington, DC: American Council on Education.

Andress, M. J., & Bragg, M. C. (1922). *Suggestions for a program for health teaching in the elementary schools.* U.S. Department of the Interior, Bureau of Education, Health Education No. 10, Washington, DC: U.S. Government Printing Office.

Auld, E. (Winter 1997/1998). Executive edge. *SOPHE News&Views, 24* (4), 4.

Bates, I. J., & Winder, A. E. (1984). *Introduction to health education.* San Francisco: Mayfield.

Bernstein, N. R. (1972). *APHA: The first one hundred years.* Washington, DC: American Public Health Association.

Butler, M., Thornton, F., & Stoltz, D. (1994). *The Battle Creek idea.* Battle Creek, MI: Heritage Publications.

Centers for Disease Control and Prevention (CDC). (2016a). *About Healthy People.* Retrieved January 29, 2016, from http://www.healthypeople.gov/2020/About-Healthy-People.

Centers for Disease Control and Prevention (CDC). (2016b). *Expanding the coordinated school health approach.* Retrieved January 30, 2016, from http://www.cdc.gov/healthyschools/wscc/approach.htm.

Centers for Disease Control and Prevention (CDC). (2016c). *MAP-IT: A guide to using Healthy People 2020 in your community.* Retrieved January 30, 2016, from http://www.healthypeople.gov/2020/tools-and-resources/Program-Planning.

Centers for Disease Control and Prevention (CDC). (2016d). *The National Public Health Performance Standards Program.* Retrieved January 30, 2016, from http://www.cdc.gov/nphpsp/index.html.

Centers for Disease Control and Prevention (CDC). (2016e). *Topic areas at a glance.* Retrieved January 29, 2016, from http://www.cdc.gov/nchs/healthy_people/hp2020/hp2020_topic_areas.htm.

Centers for Disease Control and Prevention (CDC). (2016f). *Vision, mission, core values, and pledge.* Retrieved January 29, 2016, from http://www.cdc.gov/media/subtopic/factsheet.htm.

Centers for Disease Control and Prevention (CDC). (2016g). *Whole School, Whole Community, Whole Child.* Retrieved January 30, 2016, from http://www.cdc.gov/healthyschools/wscc/index.htm.

Centers for Disease Control and Prevention (CDC). (2016h). *Youth Risk Behavior Surveillance System.* Retrieved January 30, 2016, from http://www.cdc.gov/healthyyouth/data/yrbs/index.htm.

Cipolla, C. M. (1976). *Public health and the medical profession in the Renaissance.* Cambridge, England: Cambridge University Press.

Cortese, P. A. (1993). Accomplishments in comprehensive school health education. *Journal of School Health, 63* (1), 21–23.

De'ath, E. (1995). *The Black Death—1347 AD.* [Film]. Available from Ambrose Video Publishing Inc., 1290 Avenue of the Americas, Suite 2245, New York, NY 10104.

Donan, C. (1898). *The Dark Ages 476–918.* London: Rivingtons.

Duncan, D. (1988). *Epidemiology: Basis for disease prevention and health promotion.* New York: Macmillan.

Durant, W. (1961). *The Age of Reason begins.* Vol. 7. *The story of civilization.* New York: Simon and Schuster.

Fee, E., & Brown, T. M. (1997). Editorial: Why history? *American Journal of Public Health, 87* (11), 1763–1764.

Gambescia, S.F. (2006). Health education and physical education are core academic subjects. Health Promotion Practice. 7(4), 369–371.

Goerke, L. S., & Stebbins, E. L. (1968). *Mustard's introduction to public health* (5th ed.). New York: Macmillan.

Gordon, B. (1959). *Medieval and Renaissance medicine.* New York: Philosophical Library.

Green, W. H., & Simons-Morton, B. G. (1990). *Introduction to health education.* Prospect Heights, IL: Waveland Press.

Hansen, M. (1980). *The royal facts of life.* Metuchen, NJ: The Scarecrow Press.

Johnson, S. (2006). *The ghost map: The story of London's most terrifying epidemic—and how it changed science, cities, and the modern world.* New York: Penguin Books.

Koh, H. K., & Sebelius, K. G. (2010). Promoting prevention through the Affordable Care Act. *The New England Journal of Medicine.* Retrieved September 3, 2010, from http://www.nejm.org/doi/full/10.1056/NEJMp1008560.

Lalonde, M. (1974). *A new perspective on the health of Canadians.* Ottawa: Government of Canada.

Libby, W. (1922). *The history of medicine in its salient features.* Boston: Houghton Mifflin.

Marr, J. (1982). Merchants of death: The role of the slave trade in the transmission of disease from Africa to the Americas. *Pharos, 45*(1), 31–35.

McKenzie, J. F., & Pinger, R. R. (2015). *An introduction to community & public health* (8th ed.). Burlington, MA: Jones and Bartlett Learning.

Means, R. K. (1962). *A history of health education in the United States.* Philadelphia: Lea & Febiger.

Means, R. K. (1975). *Historical perspectives on school health.* Thorofare, NJ: Charles B. Slack.

Moore, H. H. (1923). *Public health in the United States.* New York: Harper & Brothers.

National Board for Professional Teaching Standards. (2016). *Eligibility and Policies.* Retrieved January 30, 2016, from http://boardcertifiedteachers.org/about-certification.

Newsholme, A. (1936). *The last thirty years in public health.* London: Arno Press & *New York Times.*

Open Congress. (2010). *H.R.3590—Patient Protection and Affordable Care Act: Open Congress summary.* Retrieved September 3, 2010, from http://www.opencongress.org/bill/111-h3590/show#.

Pickett, G., & Hanlon, J. J. (1990). *Public health administration and practice* (9th ed.). St. Louis: Times Mirror/Mosby.

Ravenel, M. P. (Ed.). (1970). *A half century of public health.* New York: Arno Press & *New York Times.*

Rogers, J. F. (1936). *Training of elementary teachers for school health work.* U.S. Department of the Interior, Office of Education, Pamphlet No. 67. Washington, DC: U.S. Government Printing Office.

Rosen, G. (1958). *A history of public health.* New York: MD Publications.

Rubinson, L., & Alles, W. F. (1984). *Health education foundations for the future.* St. Louis: Times Mirror/Mosby.

Schouten, J. (1967). *The rod and serpent of Asclepius.* Amsterdam: Elsevier.

SHAPE America. (2016). *About SHAPE America: Our Mission.* Retrieved January 30, 2016, from http://www.shapeamerica.org/about/.

Shattuck, L. (1850). *Report of the Sanitary Commission of Massachusetts.* Boston: Dutton and Wentworth.

Sliepcevich, E. M. (1964). *School health education study: A summary report.* Washington, DC: SHES.

Society for Public Health Education (SOPHE). (2013). *What does health care reform do for prevention and wellness?* Retrieved January 30, 2016, from http://www.sophe.org/advocacy_matters.cfm.

Society for Public Health Education (SOPHE). (2015). *SOPHE applauds passage of Every Child Achieves Act.* Press Release July 17, 2015. Retrieved April 9, 2016 from: http://www.sophe.org/ECAAPassagePR.cfm

Turner, C. E., Sellery, C. M., & Smith, S. A. (1957). *School health and health education* (3rd ed.). St. Louis: Mosby.

U.S. Department of Health, Education, and Welfare (USDHEW). (1976). *Health in America: 1776–1976.* (DHEW Publication No. (HRA) 76–616). Washington, DC: U.S. Government Printing Office.

U.S. Department of Health and Human Services (USDHHS). (1980). *Promoting health/preventing disease: Objectives for the nation.* Washington, DC: U.S. Government Printing Office.

U.S. National Center for Health Statistics, National Vital Statistics Reports (NVSR). (2009). *Deaths: Final data for 2006,* Vol. 57, No. 14, April 17, 2009.

U.S. Public Health Service. (1979). *Healthy people: The surgeon general's report on health promotion and disease prevention.* Washington, DC: U.S. Government Printing Office.

U.S. Public Health Service. (2016). *The Mission of the Commissioned Corps.* Retrieved January 26, 2016, from http://www.usphs.gov/aboutus/mission.aspx.

Voices From the Past. (2004). Today's health problems and health education. *American Journal of Public Health, 94* (3), 368–369.

Wilensky, S. E., & Teitelbaum, J. B. (2017). *Annual health reform update. Burlington, MA: Jones & Bartlett Learning.*

Winslow, C. A. (1944). *The conquest of epidemic disease.* Princeton, NJ: Princeton University Press.

Ziegler, P. (1969). *The Black Death.* New York: Harper & Row.

Chapter

3

Philosophical Foundations

Chapter Objectives

After reading this chapter and answering the questions at the end, you should be able to:

- Define the terms *philosophy, wellness, holistic,* and *symmetry,* and identify common elements between them.

- Discuss the importance of developing a personal philosophy about life.

- Compare and contrast the advantages and disadvantages of having similar life and occupational philosophies.

- Formulate a statement that describes your personal philosophy of life and identify the influences that account for your philosophy.

- Identify and explain the differences between the following health education/promotion philosophies:

  a. behavior change philosophy
  b. cognitive-based philosophy
  c. decision-making philosophy
  d. freeing or functioning philosophy
  e. social change philosophy
  f. eclectic philosophy

- Explain how a health education specialist might use each of the six health education/promotion philosophies listed above to address a situation in a scenario.

- Create and defend your own philosophy of health education/promotion.

Kristy has been exploring health-related careers and is interested in pursuing a major in health education/promotion. Her interest has been partially piqued by the fact that her parents' lives improved when they began to lower their cholesterol and increase their exercise by incorporating information and strategies presented to them by a health education specialist employed by their physician. The health education specialist worked with Kristy's parents on a regular basis for nearly six months, and they gave rave reviews on that specialist's methodologies. As a result, her parents were able to reduce or eliminate several of the medications they had been taking. Kristy also had to admit that the entire family's health had benefited from her parents' "new" lifestyle.

In thinking about a career as a health education specialist, Kristy formulated several questions. Her inquiry included the philosophies, styles, and methods of practice held or used by health education specialists. Others were related to the profession as a whole and how someone decides whether becoming a health education specialist is a good match for her or his philosophy of life.

This chapter addresses some of the same questions that Kristy contemplated in relation to the practice of health education/promotion and possibly becoming a health education specialist. To that end, we will explore questions such as

- What is a philosophy?
- Why does a person need a philosophy?
- What are some of the philosophies or philosophical principles associated with the notion of *health*?
- What philosophical viewpoints related to health education/promotion are held by some of the past and current leading health education specialists?
- How is a philosophy developed?
- What are the predominant philosophies used in the practice of health education/ promotion today?
- How will adopting any of the health education/promotion philosophies impact the way health education specialists practice in their chosen setting?

The purpose of discussing the development of a health education/promotion philosophy is not to provide a treatise on "the nature of the world," so to speak, but to emphasize the importance of a guiding philosophy to the practice of any profession. Smith (2010) notes, "When a health educator identifies and organizes concepts deemed as valuable in relation to health outcomes, he or she can begin to form a philosophical framework for functioning comfortably and effectively" (p. 51). Gambesia (2013) adds, "Our philosophy of public health education, therefore, will strongly influence our approach as to what we do as health education specialists" (p. 11).

The term *philosophy* may seem to some to describe an almost ethereal, esoteric academic exercise. In actuality, however, a well-considered philosophy provides the underpinnings that serve to bridge theory and practice. Although various general types of philosophies of health education/promotion are covered later in the chapter, the following example might help you begin to see the importance of how a health education specialist's philosophy helps in determining his or her practice approach in working with individuals and communities.

Consider the case of Julieta, a 30-year-old mother of two, who smokes, does not exercise regularly, eats many of her meals at fast-food restaurants, and has a family history of heart disease. Julieta is enrolled in a required personal health course at a local university. She is going back to school to become a bilingual elementary school teacher. Because a health risk appraisal is a required part of the class, she has made an appointment to visit Javier, one of the health education specialists in the health promotion center on campus.

Javier has adopted the philosophy of behavior change. As a proponent of this approach, he believes that all people are capable of changing their health behavior if they can be shown the steps to success. Initially, he would use a behavior change contract method to get Julieta to try to eliminate one or two of her negative health behaviors. As a part of this process, some preliminary analysis would be done in an attempt to identify the triggers that cause her to engage in negative health behaviors. He would help her identify short-term and long-term goals. Together they would establish specific and measurable objectives to reach those goals, and strategies to reach the objectives. He would also try to ensure that she receives some appropriate reward for every objective and goal she accomplishes. During the visit, Javier also shares with Julieta that there are other health education specialists at the center who employ different philosophies from his and that she might benefit from also visiting one of them. The results of Julieta's visits to the other health education specialists are covered later in this chapter.

▷ What Is a Philosophy?

The word *philosophy* comes from Greek and literally means "the love of wisdom" or "the love of learning." The term **philosophy** in this chapter means a statement summarizing the attitudes, principles, beliefs, values, and concepts held by an individual or a group. In an academic setting, a philosopher studies the topics of ethics, logic, politics, metaphysics, theology, or aesthetics. It is certainly not imperative that a person be an academic philosopher to have a philosophy. All of us have convictions, ideas, values, experiences, and attitudes about one or more of the philosophy topics listed above as they apply to life. These are the building blocks (sometimes known as principles) that make up any philosophy.

A person who has generated his or her personal philosophy of how life operates for him or her often is inquisitive about what facts or factors help explain an issue so that the true meaning can help inform both opinion and approach to addressing the issue. Alternative explanations behind issues are explored. Without a philosophy, a person may well fall into the trap of thinking that opinion is the same as fact. When opinion is equated with fact (reality), it becomes much more difficult for a person, regardless of occupation, to be open to new ideas or concepts or other ways of looking at the world (see **Figure 3.1**). Gambescia (2013) states, "Health education specialists should promote diverse ideas and encourage critical thinking. We should seek a high level of tolerance . . ." (p. 13).

You most likely have already developed certain philosophical viewpoints or notions about what is real and true in the world as you know it. The manner in which you consistently act toward other people often reflects your philosophy concerning the importance of people in general. That you are studying to become a health education specialist says something about your philosophical leanings in terms of a career. For example, the profession of health education/promotion is considered a helping profession. Gambescia (2007) states that health education "is an enabling good that helps individuals and communities flourish" (p. 722). Those who work in the profession should value helping others.

In today's society there are many examples of the use of a philosophical position. Corporations, for example, create slogans espousing their purported philosophy. Of course, more than a few of them are also trying to sell a product or service at the same time. Many of us recognize certain companies by phrases such as "Just Do It" (Nike), or "Think Different" (Apple). The use of caring slogans and catchy phrases is meant to convey to the public that the company is in business solely because it is interested in the welfare of people everywhere and is

▲ **Figure 3.1** Young Man Contemplating the Tree of Life: What Will It Hold for Me?

responsive to their needs. If the company's actions match the slogan, the public is more likely to perceive the slogan as a true representation of the corporate philosophy.

Additionally, many not-for-profit and for-profit agencies and companies often have mission statements. A mission statement is meant to convey a philosophy and direction that form a framework for all actions taken by that organization. For example, the mission statement for the Central District Health Department in Boise, Idaho, is "Healthy People in Healthy Communities."

After reading this statement there is little doubt that the overriding philosophy in this department is one of promoting prevention for both individuals and communities. For individuals who have a philosophy that emphasizes prevention and early intervention, this is likely to be a place where they might find employment that is personally rewarding and professionally fulfilling.

Just as often, insight into a person's philosophy can be gained by hearing, reading, or analyzing that person's quotes or sayings. For example, the following quote from actor Michael J. Fox (2010) embodies his philosophy of life in the face of an incurable disease: "Parkinson's demanded of me that I be a better man, a better husband, father, and citizen. I often refer to it as a gift. With a nod to those who find this hard to believe, especially my fellow patients who are facing great difficulties, I add this qualifier—it's the gift that keeps on taking . . . but it's a gift" (p. 89). As you will see later and as can be noted from Fox's statement, a philosophy is rarely stagnant, but rather continuous because it is formulated by considering values, beliefs, experiences, and consequences of actions. Composing a philosophy statement allows a person to reflect on what is important to him or her when viewing the world in its many manifestations.

The thoughts stated previously are well summarized by Loren Bensley (1993), one of the most influential health education specialists of the latter half of the 20th century:

> Philosophy can be defined as a state of mind based on your values and beliefs. This in turn is based on a variety of factors which include culture, religion, education, morals, environment, experiences, and family. It is also determined by people who have influenced you, how you feel about yourself and others, your spirit, your optimism or pessimism, your independence and your family. It is a synthesis of all learning that makes you who you are and what you believe. In other words, a philosophy reflects your values and beliefs which determine your mission and purpose for being, or basic theory, or viewpoint based on logical reasoning. (p. 2)

Please note that a philosophy does not have to be abstract. Pondering the reason for being gives people a chance to integrate their past, present, and future into a coherent whole that guides them through life.

▷ Why Does One Need a Philosophy?

The answer to the question "Why does one need a philosophy?" is both simple and complex. Each of us already has a view of the world and what is true for us. This image helps shape the way we experience our surroundings and act toward others in our environment. In other words, a person's philosophy helps form the basis of reality for her or him.

Of course, some philosophical change is probably inevitable. New experiences, new insights, and new learnings create the possibility that some of the tenets composing the philosophy might need retooling. This is a normal part of growth. Most people's philosophical views are altered somewhat as they study, grow older, and experience the world in different ways. Gambescia (2013) concurs when he writes, "experienced health education specialists should seriously think about updating their philosophy statement as it is tangible evidence of one's growth in the field of public health" (p. 110).

Usually a person's philosophy (e.g., determining how to treat others, what actions are right or wrong, and what is important in life) needs to be synchronous in all aspects of life. This means that a person's philosophical viewpoint holds at home, at school, in the workplace, and at play. If incongruence develops between a person's philosophy and the philosophy of the leaders in the workplace, problems can occur.

As an example, consider the career of a public health education specialist working in HIV/AIDS prevention education who is employed by a state department of education. Assume that this individual has a philosophical view that all human life is sacred and education is the best source of prevention. Also assume that the person's work both on and off the job reflects consistency and a commitment to those ideals. In other words, the person's actions are synchronous with the aforementioned philosophy. As long as the administration in the state department of education and family and friends remain supportive of this health education specialist's role and philosophy, chances are that this person will do well. If, however, the state department leadership changes and the new superintendent is opposed to the idea that individuals infected with HIV are worth saving (because they chose their behaviors) or refuses to allow condoms to be mentioned as an age-appropriate secondary source of prevention, the specialist may have a difficult time remaining in that environment. The reason for this statement is that this educator is now not allowed to act according to his or her beliefs, ideals, and knowledge. There is a disharmony between the philosophical stance and the ability to act in concert with that stance.

Certainly, there are exceptions to this rule. Health education specialists might hold philosophies on how they personally live, yet they might have to educate those who have made choices that are opposed to their belief system. This situation begins to cross the bounds of a general philosophy and get into ethics (right behavior—see Chapter 5). Although a possible moral-philosophical conflict seems apparent in this situation, health education specialists need to remember that their primary concern is to protect and enhance the health of those they serve. The health of any one of us affects the health of all of us in some manner (legally, monetarily, physically, or emotionally). At the very least, the health education specialist should refer this situation to another trained individual who can fulfill the obligation to the public.

The late U.S. Surgeon General C. Everett Koop was confronted with the same dilemma when he was in office during the advent of the AIDS epidemic, 1981–1989. Although he was a strong conservative Christian leader and against the use of drugs and premarital sex, he championed the cause of HIV/AIDS education by stressing that the epidemic was a health problem that required a health-based prevention message. Through the power of his office, he insisted that HIV/AIDS prevention education include the merits of abstinence, the dissemination of needles to inner-city addicts, and the increased availability of condoms to individuals who choose to be sexually active or have multiple sexual partners (see **Figure 3.2**).

A further example that illustrates the impact of a philosophy on the practice of a profession comes from an article by Governali, Hodges, and Videto (2005) in which they state, "philosophical thought is central to the delivery of health education. For a profession to stay vital and relevant, it is important to assess its activities, regularly evaluate its goals, and assess its philosophical direction" (p. 211). The emphasis the authors place on the influence of activities and goals related to philosophy is a direct reflection of their personal and professional

▲ **Figure 3.2** The current U.S. Surgeon General, Vivek H. Murthy, is a strong supporter of the value of health education and promotion in creating a more prevention-focused approach to health.

philosophical foundation formed over the years. A well-reasoned philosophy often plays an important role in the choice of a career path.

A study identifying factors that influence career choices further validates that statement. Tamayose, Farzin, Schmieder-Ramirez, and Rice (2004) surveyed public health students enrolled at a west coast university to determine what major influences led them to pursue careers in public health. Researchers found that the top two items mentioned by the students were "enjoyment of the profession/commitment to health improvement" and "provide a health/community service to others." Both of these statements reflect a common philosophical thread that permeates the thinking of a majority of individuals currently practicing in the field of health education/promotion with whom we have come in contact.

In summary, the formation of a philosophy is one of the key determining factors behind the choice of an occupation, a spouse, a religious conviction, a political persuasion, and friends. A firm philosophical foundation serves as a beacon that lights the way and provides guidance for many of the major decisions in life.

▷ Principles and Philosophies Associated with Health

In Chapter 1, the meaning of the term *health* was discussed. Recall that, although the term *health* is elusive to define, nearly all definitions include the idea of a multidimensional construct that most people value, particularly when health deteriorates. Some see health as an end to itself; others see health as being important in large part because its presence enables the freedom to act as one desires without major physical or mental impediments. Over the past 30 to 50 years, educators have identified several philosophies or philosophical principles that tend to be associated with the establishment and maintenance of health. These philosophies provide a set of guiding principles that help create a framework to better understand the depth of the term *health*.

Rash (1985) mentions that, although health is often not an end in itself, good health does bring a richness and enjoyment to life that will make service to others more possible. He feels that those who seek to enhance the health of others through education should espouse a **philosophy of symmetry**; that is, health has physical, emotional, spiritual, and social components, and each is just as important as the others. Health education specialists should seek to motivate their students or clients toward symmetry (balance) among these components.

Oberteufer (1953) rejected the notions of a dualistic (human = mind + body) or a triune (human = mind + body + spirit) nature for humanity. Instead, he embraced the ideal of a **holistic philosophy** of health when he stated, "The mind and body disappear as recognizable realities and in their stead comes the acknowledgment of a whole being . . . man is essentially a unified integrated organism" (p. 105). Thomas (1984) is convinced that the holistic view of health produces health professionals who are more passionate about creating a society in which the promotion of good health is seen as a positive goal.

Greenberg (1992), Donatelle (2011), Edlin and Golanty (2004), and Hales (2004), among others, have elevated the construct of wellness to the level of a philosophy. **Wellness**, always a positive quality (as opposed to illness being always a negative), is visualized as the integration of the spiritual, intellectual, physical, emotional, environmental, and social dimensions of health to form a whole "healthy person." Those who subscribe to this philosophy believe that all people can achieve some measure of wellness, no matter what limitations they have,

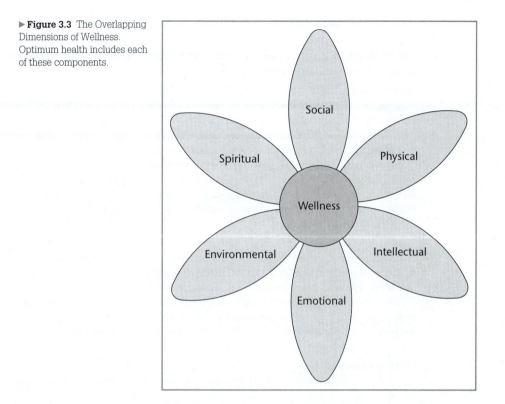

▶ **Figure 3.3** The Overlapping Dimensions of Wellness. Optimum health includes each of these components.

and that achieving optimal health is an appropriate journey for everyone. The optimum state of wellness occurs when people have developed all six of the dimensions of health to the maximum of their ability (see **Figure 3.3**).

To be sure, there are those who differ in their philosophical view of health being composed of all the dimensions of wellness. For example, Balog (2005) believes that health must by nature be seen solely as a physical state because "health must reside in the person" (p. 269), and it is not possible for a person to be truly healthy if the systems of the body are not functioning optimally in the way they were intended to operate. He argues that any other view of health is really not objective but introduces subjective views of what others value (the good life). In Balog's view, it is important for health education specialists to distinguish that which affects health from that which is health. In other words, he cautions against confusing "good life" with "good health."

The philosophies previously mentioned are not meant to be all inclusive. The purpose for discussing them is to help provide a framework to further assist the reader in developing a philosophy about health and, ultimately, health education/promotion.

▷ Leading Philosophical Viewpoints

Over the past 25 years, several publications and numerous articles have focused on recounting the philosophical positions of past and present leading health education specialists. To assist you in formulating your own health education/promotion philosophy, we present here a small sample of the philosophies expressed in these publications. As previously mentioned, one way a philosophical approach is developed is through the influence of role models, or mentors. The viewpoints that follow may help stimulate your thoughts and provide guidance as you begin developing your own health education philosophy and as you consider whether a career in health education/promotion is for you.

BECKY SMITH (2010)

Studying the definitions of health from the perspectives of scholars such as Dubos, Fromm, Maslow, Montagu, Tillich, and Tournier.

. . . helped me develop a personal understanding of how individuals express health and how the potential for health can manifest despite severe limitations in one or more dimension(s). . . . when internal and external elements that facilitate the development of human potential are available, individuals are more likely to experience optimal health. . . . I prefer to look for that expression of health as a starting point for professional interaction, education, and enhancement of health rather than focus on existing debilitation. (p. 52)

JOHN ALLEGRANTE (2006)

I have always believed that the goal of health education is to promote, maintain, and improve individual and community health through the educational process. I believe that there are fundamental conceptual hallmarks and a social agenda that differentiate the practice of health education and that of medicine in achieving this goal. These hallmarks include the use of consensus strategies to identify health needs and problems, voluntary participation as an ethical requirement, and an obligation to foster social and political change. I also believe that our perspective and methodologies require that we enter into a social contract with people that engages them as partners, not merely as patients. (p. 306)

MARIAN HAMBURG (1993)

Eta Sigma Gamma has given me the chance to expound on a few of my beliefs about health education.

1. You can't plan everything. Unexpected opportunities appear and it is important to be ready to take advantage of them. (p. 68)
2. I believe in mentorship. Its power incorporated into health education programming has enormous strength for influencing positive health behaviors. (p. 70)
3. I believe that effective health education programming requires appropriate inter-sectoral cooperation, and that health educators, regardless of the source of their professional preparation, must be its facilitators. School-community can be one world. (p. 71)
4. I believe that we need to put more of our resources into joint efforts and coalition building. Much of health education's future as a profession depends upon the support that health educators, regardless of their specialized training, provide for the maintenance and expansion of certification. (p. 73)
5. It is not surprising to me that the concept of networking has become an important basis for health education practice. We bring together people with common problems to seek solutions through the sharing of feelings and information. (p. 73)

JOHN SEFFRIN (1993)

I believe the most fundamental outcome of health education is the enabling of individuals to achieve a level of personal freedom not very likely to be obtained otherwise. Freedom means being able to avoid any unnecessary encumbrance on one's ability to make an enlightened choice (p. 110). . . . We need to be resourceful and open to change. In doing so, however, we need to change in ways that do not violate certain basic principles:

1. appreciation for each individual's uniqueness;
2. respect for ethnic and cultural diversity;

3. protection for individual and group autonomy;

4. promotion and preservation of free choice; and

5. intervention strategies based on good science. (p. 114)

Philosophies are as individual as the people themselves, yet some common themes (development of individual potential, learning experiences that help in decision making, free choice, and enhancement of individual uniqueness) seem to emerge and hold true regardless of the health education specialist. Let us now examine how these philosophies are actually applied in the practice of health education/promotion.

▷ Developing a Philosophy

Now that it is clear that a philosophy is not some abstraction used only by individuals such as the Dalai Lama or Gandhi, let us explore the ways in which a philosophy is formed. In previous sections, it was noted that most practicing professionals and many organizations have developed certain philosophical stances that serve as their road map and guide for living and working in the world. What provides the basis for forming a philosophy?

Suppose you are searching through the Web sites of various health education/promotion programs, trying to determine which one might be best for you. In your search, you come across the Web site for the community health education program at the University of Wisconsin at La Crosse (see the Weblinks section at the end of the chapter for URL references). One of the prominent features of the site is a statement of the mission of this program.

The mission of the BS-PH CHE (Bachelor of Science—Public Health, Community Health Education) program at the University of Wisconsin-La Crosse (UW-La Crosse) (2016) is:

"To prepare leaders in school and community health through the bridging of competency and standard-based education, scholarship, advocacy, and service-related endeavors, thereby contributing to healthier people and healthier communities."

The process of developing this mission statement most likely involved several meetings of faculty, staff, students, community leaders, and administrators. During the meetings, the core beliefs and principles regarding health education/promotion of those in attendance were probably assessed. After coupling the list of beliefs with the required list of core competencies, the mission statement was formulated.

In drafting your own philosophy statement, you should employ a similar process (without the committee, of course). Think about what a health education specialist does and what the result of his or her work should be. Construct lists of your thoughts under headings such as (1) personal values and beliefs (see the Weblinks section for examples of values), (2) what *health* means to you, (3) attributes of people you admire and trust, (4) results of health studies and readings that you find meaningful, and (5) outcomes you would like to see from the process of health education/promotion (e.g., better decision making, more community involvement, promotion of positive behaviors, and healthier communities). From your lists, some common themes will emerge and the identification of these themes is a key to drafting your own health education/promotion philosophy statement. Exploring why you value the topics represented within these themes should enable you to compose a philosophy statement that will reflect a way of thinking, acting, and viewing the world that works for you.

Please note, however, that using this approach to formulate a philosophy is not a guarantee that the philosophy will remain stable. As a matter of fact, there is a strong likelihood that some changes will occur because of new learnings, activities, and experiences (e.g., working in a different culture, experiencing the premature death of a child or spouse, losing a job as a result of downsizing, or encountering a new mentor). A philosophy reflects the sum of knowledge, experience, and principles from which it was formed.

As a further aid to formulating a philosophy statement about health and health education/promotion, we would like to reference a series of questions that Dr. Julie Dietz of Eastern Illinois University gives her students when they are assigned to write their personal philosophy of health education. These questions do a great job of capturing the interface between a personal philosophy of health and a professional philosophy of the profession of health education/promotion. They are

Statement of Personal Health Philosophy

- What does it mean to be *healthy*?
- What are your health-related responsibilities and obligations to yourself?
- What are your health-related responsibilities and obligations to your community or society?
- What do you expect your community and society to do to keep you healthy?

Statement of Professional Health Education and Promotion Philosophy

- What is Health Education/Health Promotion, and what does it mean to be a professional in this field?
- What are your goals for yourself and your profession?
- What are your professional responsibilities to yourself, your community, and to your profession?
- How does community health education fit within these goals? (personal communication, May 2011)

We conclude this section with a short vignette that illustrates several concepts or principles that need to be considered when formulating a philosophy statement about life, health, and health education/promotion practice.

The story, adapted from the book *The Boy Who Harnessed the Wind* by Kamkwamba and Mealer (2009), is about the amazing accomplishments of William Kamkwamba of the African nation of Malawi. William was curious about how things worked (particularly electricity) and had read a book titled *Using Energy*, which he accessed in a makeshift library in his town; so he was able to construct a functioning windmill from parts of engines and wrecked automobiles he found in a local junkyard. Most people around him said his dream of supplying his family and his community with reliable electricity for lighting homes and pumping water was "crazy." Like many youths in Africa, William's formal education was cut short by the inability of his family to pay the $80 annual tuition. Yet he maintained the initiative to keep on trying and learning despite his family's suffering through famine, disease, and government graft.

Although rudimentary, the windmill he constructed worked well enough to supply power to light four small light bulbs in his home. Eventually, educators and scientists throughout Africa and beyond learned of the accomplishments of this self-taught scholar. As a result, William has been a featured lecturer at several international conferences, he has completed high school at an international school in South Africa (as a result of a grant), he graduated from Dartmouth College in 2014, and he recently received an ideo.org Global Fellowship. His refusal to abandon his dreams, fueled by his desire to make things better for his village and family, provided a stark contrast to many in his country (and around the world) who take for granted the educational opportunities they have or just give up and settle for the status quo. Given his story, William's philosophy must include values or ideals such as perseverance, ethical conduct, a heart for helping others, and initiative.

All too often, in determining abilities, it is our experience that people set their sights and dreams too low. A personal philosophy needs to incorporate the realization that life sometimes dishes out bumps and bruises. Acknowledging this fact may well prevent any of us from excessively limiting our assessment of our place in the world. In addition, personal philosophy is often a reflection of an individual's perspective of the world and how and why it seems to work that way.

Remember, the formation of a philosophy, whether personal or occupational, requires several steps. First, individuals need to answer the following questions in reference to themselves: What is important to me? What do I most value? What beliefs do I hold? Second, they need to identify ways the answers to the first questions influence the way they believe and act. Third, after carefully considering and writing down the answers to these questions, a philosophy statement can be formulated. The statement reflects and identifies the factors, principles, ideals, values, beliefs, and influences that help shape reality for the person authoring the philosophy statement.

The steps mentioned above can be used to formulate any type of philosophy statement. However, for those who are studying health education/promotion, there is one additional and important question to consider: Is this philosophy statement consistent with being a health education specialist? If the answer is "yes," then for that person health education/promotion is a profession worthy of further consideration.

▷ Predominant Health Education/Promotion Philosophies

Butler (1997) accurately points out that even though there are several definitions of the phrase *health education/promotion*, recurring themes in many of the definitions allow for a general agreement as to its meaning. He notes, however, that the methods used to accomplish health education/promotion are less clear. The manner in which a person chooses to conduct health education/promotion can be demonstrated to be a direct reflection of that person's philosophy of health education/promotion. With that in mind, have any predominant philosophies of health education/promotion emerged? If so, what are they?

Welle, Russell, and Kittleson (1995) conducted a study to determine the philosophies favored by health education specialists. As part of the background for their study, they conducted a literature review and identified five dominant philosophies of health education/promotion that have emerged during the last 50 to 60 years. The philosophies identified were behavior change, cognitive-based, decision-making, freeing or functioning, and social change.

1. The **behavior change philosophy** involves a health education specialist using behavioral contracts, goal setting, and self-monitoring to try to foster a modification in an unhealthy habit in an individual with whom he or she is working. The nature of this approach allows for the establishment of easily measurable objectives, thus enhancing

the ability to evaluate outcomes. Javier from earlier in the chapter uses this approach. (Example: setting up a contract to increase the number of hours of study each week)

2. A health education specialist who uses a **cognitive-based philosophy** focuses on the acquisition of content and factual information. The goal is to increase the knowledge of the individuals or groups so that they are better prepared to make decisions about their health. (Example: posting statistics about the number of people killed or injured in automobile accidents who were not wearing seat belts)

3. In using the **decision-making philosophy**, a health education specialist presents simulated problems, case studies, or scenarios to students or clients. Each problem, case, or scenario requires decisions to be made in seeking a "best approach or answer." By creating and analyzing potential solutions, the students develop skills needed to address many health-related decisions they might face. An advantage of this approach is the emphasis on critical thinking and lifelong learning. (Example: using a variety of case study examples of different popular diet programs to see competing perspectives of effectiveness)

4. The **freeing or functioning philosophy** was proposed by Greenberg (1978) as a reaction to traditional approaches of health education/promotion that he felt ran the risk of blaming victims for practicing health behaviors that were often either out of their control or not seen as in their best interests. The health education specialist who uses this philosophical approach has the ultimate goal of freeing people to make the best health decisions possible based on their needs and interests—not necessarily the interests of society. Some health education specialists classify this as a subset of the decision-making philosophy discussed previously. (Example: lessons on the responsible use of alcohol)

5. The **social change philosophy** emphasizes the role of health education specialists in creating social, economic, and political change that benefits the health of individuals and groups. Health education specialists espousing this philosophy are often at the forefront of the adoption of policies or laws that will enhance the health of all. (Example: no smoking allowed in restaurants, or new housing developments with pedestrian-friendly areas such as sidewalks and parks)

The previously listed philosophies of health education/promotion are the products of more than 50 years of study, experimentation, and dialogue within the profession. The research conducted by Welle et al. (1995) found that the philosophy most preferred by both health education/promotion practitioners and academicians was decision-making. Both groups listed behavior change as a second choice, and both agreed that their least favorite was cognitive-based. Ratnapradipa and Abrams (2012) report that crafting a philosophy of health promotion statement may well move a health education specialist away from the use of only cognitive-based strategies (lecture) to incorporate more problem-based approaches to learning (decision-making) for their clients and communities. The fact that health education specialists who are employed in the academic setting and those who are employed as practitioners in the field agreed on these choices as predominant philosophies speaks well for the interface between preparation programs and practice.

Another interesting finding from the study occurred when, as a part of the survey, the health education specialists were given health education/promotion vignettes to address or solve. In many cases, the respondents changed the philosophical approach they used depending on the setting (school, community, work site, or medical). The responding health

Practitioner's Perspective

PHILOSOPHY OF HEALTH EDUCATION/PROMOTION Travis C. Leyva

CURRENT POSITION/TITLE: Disease Prevention Program Manager

EMPLOYER: New Mexico Department of Health

DEGREE/INSTITUTION/YEAR: Bachelor in Community Health, New Mexico State University, 2004

MAJOR: Community Health

MINOR: Environmental Health

Describe your past and current professional positions and how you came to hold the job you now hold (How did you obtain the position?): A week prior to graduating with my Bachelor's in Community Health, I had come across a job posting online for a Disease Prevention Specialist (DPS)—Health Educator position that caught my interest. It was a position that would conduct surveillance and field investigations for all reportable sexually transmitted diseases (STDs) in the region. I applied, interviewed, and three months later I started my journey as a health educator.

After a year as a DPS, I was promoted to Regional Emergency Preparedness Specialist where I coordinated responses to public health emergencies and bioterrorism threats. After one year in that position, I was promoted as the Border Infectious Disease Surveillance (BIDS) Officer Epidemiologist, where I coordinated with Mexican health officials on Border Health Infectious Disease issues. Following two years in that position, I was promoted to Program Manager of Disease Prevention, where I now supervise all the positions I was in and more! I must say that all of my promotions started with a supervisor who encouraged and motivated me to work hard and promote myself to where I am today.

Describe the duties of your current position: I oversee six different program areas in my current position. They include STD and TB Surveillance and Field Investigation, Hepatitis Surveillance and Field Investigation, HIV Prevention, HIV Medical Case Management, Harm Reduction Program, and Emergency Preparedness Program.

My job is to ensure that all deliverables are obtained by setting goals and objectives for our staff to follow. In separate intervals, I strategize, implement, and evaluate certain activities conducted by our staff to optimize the output of our services. An activity that I am most proud of is the creation of a small group, video-based intervention titled "iHEAL—Integrated Health Education for Addictive Lifestyles." This intervention educates and creates risk-reduction plans for those who may be infected and/or affected by HIV, hepatitis C, STDs, or injection drug use. iHEAL is currently being presented at detention centers, state prisons, drug rehabilitation centers, probation and parole workshops, teen drug court programs, and some high schools. The intervention has now been requested to be presented throughout the state, and a DVD of the presentation is currently being made to distribute to health educators in the Disease Prevention field.

Describe what you like most about this position: The best thing about my position is the staff and clients I work with on a daily basis. All the staff that I work with have a unique, nonjudgmental attitude that focuses on helping people who may be infected or affected by a disease. Usually clients who we serve are unaware of how they became infected with a disease or how they could transmit a disease to others, and after we as health educators work with them, it is quite rewarding that we have made a difference in one person's life, sometimes even saving it.

Describe what you like least about this position: There is always change in public health. Although it can be a good thing at times, sometimes change can be difficult and uncertain. Working with grant-funded programs, there are always new deliverables that need to be met and at times it means to stop the processes that are in place and create new ones, usually without any new resources. Also, there is always a change in administration, which means there may be new directives and new priorities.

BOX

3.1

continued

How do you use your philosophy of health education/promotion in your position? My philosophy among my staff is to educate and promote healthy lifestyle choices to every individual as you would like for it to be done to you. Being non-judgmental and courteous is key to being a successful health educator. A major component to my philosophy is that we as health educators cannot direct an individual to make healthier lifestyle choices, but rather we can provide them with options for them to choose how to make healthier lifestyle choices for themselves. Those who choose to make a change or difference usually succeed and maintain those choices.

What recommendations/ advice do you have for current health education students? My advice to current health education students is to first find a niche in public health. Whether it be STDs, Children Medical Services, Family Planning, or Harm Reduction, once you find a niche, my best recommendation is to integrate all public health programs into your health education deliveries. Some of the best health educators I have seen and worked with are those who can educate on a topic and also refer to other areas that can only benefit and support the topic area they are presenting on. People recognize when a health educator is an integrated subject matter expert.

education specialists had earlier identified a specific health education/promotion philosophy they favored (Welle et al., 1995). These results indicate that health education specialists are adaptable and resourceful, and they will use any health education/promotion approach that seems appropriate to the situation, that is, an **eclectic health education/promotion philosophy**.

In a thought-provoking essay, Buchanan (2006) introduced a different philosophical paradigm calling for health education specialists to "return to their roots" and reconsider the meaning of the word *education* in the practice of health education/promotion. He feels that the practice of health education/promotion buys into the medical model so often that health education specialists have lost their bearings and are now more often purveyors who almost demand that persons or the public adopt behaviors that "we know" will lead to a healthier life.

Instead, he suggests that health education specialists should be "disseminators of factual information and facilitators of rational choice" (p. 301). Using this philosophy,

> The quality of a health educator's work would be evaluated not by its effectiveness in changing people's behavior but by whether their audiences find the dialogue valuable in helping them think about how they want to live their lives, the impact of their behaviors on the pursuit of their life goals, and the kinds of environmental conditions that community members find most conducive to living healthy and fulfilling lives. (p. 301)

In actuality, Buchanan's views seem to incorporate the use of the cognitive-based, the decision-making, and the freeing or functioning health education/promotion philosophies outlined previously. This is not surprising because in any list of philosophies there is always the possibility of one philosophy overlapping with another, so in practice not all is as clean as it might seem. In making a similar argument as Buchanan, Governali et al. (2005) call for an integrated behavioral ecological philosophy so that health education specialists use the multidimensional nature of the interaction of the individual and the environment. This approach also resembles the eclectic philosophical model.

▷ Impacting the Delivery of Health Education/Promotion

This section uses scenarios to help focus on the methods health education specialists might use, depending on their philosophical stance. The decision to use any philosophy involves understanding and accepting the foundation that helped create the philosophy in the first place. To this end, Welle et al. (1995) state,

> Health educators must remember that every single educational choice carries with it a philosophical principle or belief. Educational choices carry important philosophical assumptions about the purpose of health education, the teacher, and also the learner. Thus, health educators should take the time necessary for individual philosophical inquiry, in order to be able to clearly articulate what principles guide them professionally. . . . Different settings may produce the need for different philosophies. Every health educator should be aware of which elements of their individual philosophies they are willing to compromise. (p. 331)

At the outset, it is important to remember that one of the overriding goals of any health education/promotion intervention is the betterment of health for the person or the group involved. All the philosophies have that goal. They differ, however, in how to approach that objective.

Remember the case of Julieta discussed early in this chapter. Her encounter with Javier, a university-based health education specialist who used a behavior change philosophical approach, was also described earlier. We now continue this scenario with Julieta visiting the other university health education specialists.

Javier has referred Julieta to Nokomis, a health education specialist who advocates for a decision-making philosophy. This means that Nokomis believes in equipping her clients with problem-solving and coping skills, so that they make the best possible health choices. Initially, she might sit down with Julieta and hypothesize some situations that would necessitate Julieta thinking through the rationale behind the negative health behaviors she practices. Nokomis also would most likely try to encourage Julieta to see that some of her behaviors affect more people than just herself. The main goal is to move Julieta to a point where she admits that some of her health behaviors need to be changed and to help her identify the reasons that changing them would make her life better.

In her third and final visit, Julieta visits health education specialist Li Ming, an advocate of a freeing or functioning philosophy of health education/promotion. Li Ming feels that, too often, health education specialists fail to find out the needs and desires of the client. They simply "barge in" and either overtly or covertly blame the client for any negative health behaviors. Li Ming would advocate change only if the behavior were infringing on the rights of others. In the beginning, Li Ming would confer with Julieta and find out "how her life was going." She would ask Julieta to identify any behaviors she wanted to change, making certain that Julieta had all the information necessary to make an informed decision. Although Li Ming might believe that Julieta should stop smoking and start exercising, she would help Julieta change only those behaviors Julieta wanted to change.

One caveat needs to be mentioned at this time. The fact that Julieta was required to take a personal health course in her teacher preparation program and that the instructor required a health risk assessment illustrates the social change philosophy at work at a microlevel. If health were not a state requirement (legislation) in the first place, she might not have considered changing any of her negative health behaviors.

Julieta's situation demonstrates a point made previously—in practice, there often is a natural mixing of some of the philosophies. For example, all the approaches mentioned used portions of the cognitive-based health education/promotion philosophy. To reiterate, this philosophy is based on the premise that persons need to be provided with the most current information that impacts their health behaviors, and the acquisition of that information should create a dissonance and cause change.

The fifth philosophy, social change, is probably not as well suited to addressing the health behaviors of individuals. Proponents stress changes in social, economic, and political arenas to impact the health of populations. Of course, populations are made up of individuals, so changing the environment of a disadvantaged neighborhood to be healthier (e.g., creating jobs, ensuring adequate and safe housing and high-quality schools, and providing healthcare coverage for all) ultimately impacts the health of people at the individual level as well.

▷ Summary

The term *philosophy* means a statement summarizing the attitudes, principles, beliefs, and concepts held by an individual or a group. Forming both a personal and an occupational philosophy requires reflection and the ability to identify the factors, principles, ideals, and influences that help shape your reality. The decision to use any philosophy involves understanding and accepting the foundation that helped create the philosophy in the first place. A sound philosophical foundation serves as a guidepost for many of the major decisions in life.

The five predominant philosophies of health education/promotion that were identified in the chapter are (1) behavior change, (2) cognitive-based, (3) decision-making, (4) freeing or functioning, and (5) social change. Health education specialists might disagree on which philosophy works best. They might even use an eclectic or multidimensional philosophical approach, depending on the setting or situation. However, it is important to remember that one of the overriding goals of any health education/promotion intervention is the betterment of health for the person or community involved. All the philosophies have that goal. They simply differ in how to attain it.

▷ Review Questions

1. Define each of the following and explain their relationship to one another.
   - Philosophy
   - Wellness
   - Holistic
   - Symmetry

2. Why is it important to have a personal life philosophy?

3. Compare and contrast the value of having a personal life philosophy and a personal work philosophy that are similar.

4. Define and explain the differences between:
   - A behavior change philosophy and a cognitive-based philosophy

- A decision-making philosophy and a social change philosophy
- A freeing or functioning philosophy and an eclectic health education/promotion philosophy

5. Explain how a person might use each of the five major health education/promotion philosophies and the eclectic philosophy to address a societal problem that can be addressed by health education/promotion (e.g., smoking, seat belt use, air pollution, exercise, diet, medication compliance, and cancer risk reduction).

Case Study

You are entering the final semester of your senior year of study with a major in public health education. The health education/promotion program at your university requires seniors in their last semester to intern a minimum of 25 hours per week at a state or nonprofit agency. For this capstone experience, you have been assigned to the mayor's office in a medium-size city near the campus.

During an orientation on the first day, you overhear that one of the tasks you will be assigned will involve meeting with the leaders of several community groups with the goal of creating smoke-free public parks in the city. The smoke-free park concept represents one of the mayor's main objectives in her second term in office. You also hear that the mayor is excited to have a health education student intern because she greatly respects the skills that a health education specialist possesses.

The second day you have the opportunity to meet with the mayor, and, in fact, she does introduce to you the idea of a smoke-free public park system. During this meeting you discover that she is quite knowledgeable about the negative health effects of second- and third-hand smoke in part because her son, a lifetime nonsmoker who worked in a pub in town (smoking was allowed in pubs), died last year from lung cancer at the age of 36. At the close of the meeting, the mayor asks you to submit to her your philosophy of health education/promotion so that she can see what approach you might take with the community groups.

Using the model outlined in this chapter, write out your health education/promotion philosophy. Based on your philosophy statement and given the project that you will be assigned, is the mayor's office a good place for you to intern to hone your skills? Why or why not?

Critical Thinking Questions

1. Of the five basic health education/promotion philosophies identified by Welle et al. (1995), why do you think that the least favorite among health education specialists was the cognitive philosophy? Why do you think decision making was viewed as most popular?

2. What is the purpose of health education/promotion? How might the formulation of a purpose statement be reflected in your philosophy of health education/promotion?

3. You have been hired by a local pharmacy to provide health education/promotion services to customers and employees. Shortly after you begin work, however, you discover that much of your job is marketing nutritional supplements and nonpharmaceutical health-related services provided by the pharmacy and not the health

education/promotion you had envisioned. How might this apparent conflict of interest have been avoided?

4. Suppose that you are a proponent of the social change philosophy. How might this philosophy be employed by a health education specialist to reduce or eliminate exposure to the Zika virus? Defend your answer to a group that advocates for use of the cognitive philosophy as the best approach to address this problem.

5. An article by Bruess (2003) in the *American Journal of Health Education* discusses the notion of "role modeling" for health education specialists. (The reference for the article can be found at the end of this chapter.) After reading the article, summarize Dr. Bruess's main points and use your answer to determine which philosophical viewpoint(s) a health education specialist must hold to feel as Dr. Bruess does on the issue of role modeling. Finally, assess how you feel about the issue. Do you agree or disagree with him? Provide a rationale for your answer.

▶ Activities

1. Take a survey of your classmates to assess what predominant health education/promotion philosophy each of them might employ. Compare the results with those from the study by Welle et al. (1995) described in this chapter. What were the reasons for any differences? Similarities?

2. After reexamining the philosophies of health, write a paragraph that could be used to explain your philosophy of health to a friend or colleague.

3. Interview a school or community health educator in your city. Ask what his or her philosophy of health education/promotion is. Then ask about the influences that helped the educator form his or her philosophy. Summarize the interview in a one-page paper.

4. Use any three of the five philosophical approaches to health education/promotion discussed in the chapter and address the following situation: In the past week in your community, two teenagers have been killed in separate incidents while riding bicycles. In neither case was the teenager wearing a helmet. A local citizens group has asked you and two of your health education specialist colleagues to attend a meeting concerning what to do about this issue.

▶ Weblinks

1. http://www.uwlax.edu/

   Mission statement of the Department of Health Education and Health Promotion program at the University of Wisconsin, La Crosse.

   From the university's homepage, navigate to the Community Health Program. The program description provides a fine example of a mission and philosophy statement for health education and health promotion based on the seven responsibilities of health education specialists.

2. http://www.mindtools.com

   The Decision Making section of the Toolkit offers examples of terms that denote values and beliefs, thus assisting students to identify possible values or beliefs they might hold.

Having these terms delineated helps in the initial stages of the development of both a personal and a professional philosophy.

3. Log in to your university library and find the online version of Dr. Stephen Gambescia's Presidential keynote address to the 2007 Society for Public Health Education (SOPHE) convention (see below in references list). It provides an excellent "tour" through the thought processes of the rationale for forming a philosophy of health education for the profession of health education.

References

Allegrante, J. P. (2006). Commentary: In search of the new ethics for health promotion. *Health Education and Behavior, 33* (3), 305–307.

Balog, J. E. (2005). The meaning of health. *American Journal of Health Education, 36* (5), 266–271.

Bensley, L. B. (1993). This I believe: A philosophy of health education. *The Eta Sigma Gamma Monograph Series, 11* (2), 1–7.

Bruess, C. E. (2003). This I believe: A philosophy of health education. *American Journal of Health Education, 34* (4), 237–239.

Buchanan, D. R. (2006). Perspective: A new ethic for health promotion: Reflections on a philosophy of health education for the 21st century. *Health Education and Behavior, 33* (3), 290–304.

Butler, J. T. (1997). *The principles and practices of health education and health promotion.* Englewood, CO: Morton.

Donatelle, R. J. (2011). *Health: The basics, green edition.* San Francisco: Pearson Education.

Edlin, G., & Golanty, E. (2004). *Health and wellness* (8th ed.). Sudbury, MA: Jones and Bartlett.

Fox, M. J. (2010). *A funny thing happened on the way to the future: Twists and turns and lessons learned.* New York: Harper-Collins.

Gambescia, S. F. (2007). 2007 SOPHE presidential address: Discovering a philosophy of health education. *Health Education and Behavior, 34* (5), 718–722.

Gambescia, S. F. (2013). A process for updating a philosophy of education statement. *Health Promotion Practice, 14* (1), 10–14.

Governali, J. F., Hodges, B. C., & Videto, D. M. (2005). *American Journal of Health Education, 36* (4), 210–214.

Greenberg, J. S. (1978). Health education as freeing. *Health Education, 9* (2), 20–21.

Greenberg, J. S. (1992). *Health education: Learner centered instructional strategies* (2nd ed.). Dubuque, IA: William C. Brown.

Hales, D. (2004). *An invitation to health* (3rd ed.). Belmont, CA: Thomson-Wadsworth.

Hamburg, M. V. (1993). Would I do it all over? *The Eta Sigma Gamma Monograph Series, 11* (2), 67–74.

Kamkwamba, W., & Mealer, B. (2009). *The boy who harnessed the wind.* New York: Harper-Collins.

Oberteufer, D. (1953). Philosophy and principles of school health education. *Journal of School Health, 23* (4), 103–109.

Rash, J. K. (1985). Philosophical bases for health education. *Health Education, 16* (3), 48–49.

Ratnapradipa, D., & Abrams, T. (2012). Framing the teaching philosophy statement for health educators: What it includes and how it can inform professional development. *The Health Educator, 44* (1), 37–42.

Seffrin, J. R. (1993). Health education and the pursuit of personal freedom. *The Eta Sigma Gamma Monograph Series, 11* (2), 109–118.

Smith, B. J. (2010). Connecting a personal philosophy of health to the practice of health education. In J. M. Black, S. Furney, H. M. Graf, & A. E. Nolte, eds., *Philosophical foundations of health education* (pp. 49–54). San Francisco: Jossey-Bass.

Tamayose, T. S., Farzin, M., Schmieder-Ramirez, J., & Rice, G. T. (2004). Important issues when choosing a career in public health. *Californian Journal of Health Promotion, 2* (1), 65–73.

Thomas, S. B. (1984). The holistic philosophy and perspective of selected health educators. *Health Education, 15* (1), 15–20.

University of Wisconsin LaCrosse (2016). Mission statement from the Community Health Education major. Retrieved on June 11, 2016 from https://www.uwlax.edu/Health-Education-and-Health-Promotion/Community-Health-Education/

Welle, H. M., Russell, R. D., & Kittleson, M. J. (1995). Philosophical trends in health education: Implications for the 21st century. *Journal of Health Education, 26* (6), 326–333.

Theories and Planning Models

Chapter Objectives

After reading this chapter and answering the questions at the end, you should be able to:

- Define and explain the difference among *theory, concept, construct, variable,* and *model*.
- Explain the importance of theory to health education/promotion.
- Explain what is meant by behavior change theories and planning models.
- Describe how the concept of socio-ecological approach applies to using theories.
- Explain the difference between continuum theories and stage theories.
- Identify and briefly explain the behavior change theories and their components used in health education/promotion:
  - Health Belief Model
  - Theory of Planned Behavior
  - Elaboration Likelihood Model of Persuasion
  - Information-Motivation-Behavioral Skills Model
  - Transtheoretical Model of Change
  - Precaution Adoption Process Model
  - Social Cognitive Theory
  - Social Network Theory
  - Social Capital Theory
  - Diffusion Theory
  - Community Readiness Model
- Identify and briefly explain the planning models and their components used in health education/promotion:
  - PRECEDE-PROCEED
  - Multilevel Approach to Community Health (MATCH)
  - Intervention Mapping
  - CDCynergy
  - Social Marketing Assessment and Response Tool (SMART)
  - Mobilizing for Action through Planning and Partnerships (MAPP)
  - Generalized Model (GM)

Ａs noted in Chapter 1, the profession of health education/promotion evolved from other biological, behavioral, psychological, sociological, and health science disciplines. As this profession has grown, so has the number of theories and models used by health education specialists in their work. This chapter introduces the terms *theory, concept, construct, variable,* and *model.* It explains why theory is used in health education/promotion. It also presents an overview of theories that focus on behavior change, as well as the models associated with program planning. However, space does not permit comprehensive coverage of all theories and models used by health education specialists. For example, theories and models associated with implementation and evaluation processes are not covered in this chapter.

Because theories and models are dynamic, they change and evolve (Crosby, Kegler, & DiClemente, 2009). To that end, we will not attempt to introduce every possible theory or planning model in this chapter. Health education specialists continually deal with both revised and new theories and models. Future courses and the books, articles, and associated materials in those courses will likely expose you to more complete coverage of health education/promotion's theoretical base (e.g., DiClemente, Crosby, & Kegler, 2009; DiClemente, Salazar, & Crosby, 2013; Edberg, 2015; Glanz, Rimer, & Viswanath, 2008a; Goodson, 2010; Green & Kreuter, 2005; Hayden, 2014; Institute of Medicine [IOM], 2001; Sharma & Romas, 2012; Simons-Morton, McLeroy, & Wendel, 2012).

▷ Definitions

To understand the theoretical foundations presented in this chapter, you must be familiar with some key related terms. Let us begin with **theory**. One of the most frequently quoted definitions of this term was provided by Glanz, Rimer, and Viswanath (2008b), who modified a previous definition by Kerlinger (1986). It states: "A *theory* is a set of interrelated concepts, definitions, and propositions that presents a *systematic* view of events or situations by specifying relations among variables in order to *explain* and *predict* the events of the situations" (p. 26). Stated a little differently, "a theory is a systematic arrangement of fundamental principles that provide a basis for explaining certain happenings of life" (McKenzie, Neiger, & Thackeray, 2013, p. 163). Thus, "the role of theory is to untangle and simplify for human comprehension the complexities of nature" (Green et al., 1994, p. 398).

As applied to the profession of health education/promotion, a theory is a general explanation of why people act, or do not act, to maintain and/or promote the health of themselves, their families, organizations, and communities. The primary elements of theories are known as **concepts** (Glanz et al., 2008b). When a concept has been developed, created, or adopted for use with a specific theory, it is referred to as a **construct** (Kerlinger, 1986). In other words, "the key concepts of a theory are its constructs" (Rimer & Glanz, 2005, p. 4). The operational form (practical use) of a construct is known as a **variable**. A variable is a quantitative measurement of a construct.

A **model** "is a composite, a mixture of ideas or concepts taken from any number of theories and used together" (Hayden, 2014, p. 2). Stated a bit differently, "Models draw on a number of theories to help people understand a specific problem in a particular setting or context. They are not always as specific as theory" (Rimer & Glanz, 2005, p. 4). Unlike theories, models do "not attempt to explain the processes underlying learning, but only to represent them" (Chaplin & Krawiec, 1979, p. 68).

Consider how these terms are used in practical application. A personal belief is a *concept* related to various health behaviors. For example, people are more likely to behave in a healthy way—such as, exercise regularly—if they feel confident in their ability to actually engage in a healthy form of exercise. Such a concept is captured in a *construct* of the Social Cognitive Theory (SCT) called *self-efficacy*. (See the discussion of the SCT later in this chapter.) If health education specialists want to develop an intervention to assist people in exercising, the ability to measure a person's self-efficacy toward exercise will help create the intervention. The measurement may consist of a few questions that ask people to rate their confidence in their ability to exercise. This measurement, or operational form, of the self-efficacy construct is a *variable*. However, because of the complexity of getting a nonexerciser to become an exerciser, the health education specialist may need to use constructs from several theories (a *model*) to plan the intervention. In our example, it is possible that no one theory may work perfectly to assist the nonexerciser to begin and sustain a habit of exercising.

In the health education/promotion profession, the adjective *theory-based* (as in theory-based planning, theory-based practice, or theory-based research) commonly refers to both theories and models. In fact, some of the best-known and often used theories use "model" in their title (e.g., Health Belief Model). Goodson (2010) explains why "model" and "theory" are used inconsistently. She indicates that when some models were created, they were properly titled as models. They were created using constructs from several theories to explain specific phenomena. They had little empirical testing to prove their worth. Over time, these models were tested and refined, gaining theory status. Goodson (2010) concludes, "because we tend to borrow the theories we employ from other disciplines and fields and because our concern usually centers in applying these theories (or models) to practice or research, it seems to matter little to us whether we deal with theories or with models; it seems to matter even less what labels we attach to them" (p. 228).

▷ The Importance of Using Theory in Health Education/Promotion

Using theory is important in all professions, not just in health education/promotion. Theory helps organize various forms of knowledge (e.g., data, facts, and information) so that they take on meaning that would not occur if the pieces of knowledge were presented in isolation. Such meaning helps to guide the work of a practitioner (Timmreck, Cole, James, & Butterworth, 2010).

Theory helps health education specialists plan, implement, and evaluate programs. More specifically, it (1) indicates reasons why people are not behaving in healthy ways, (2) identifies information needed before developing an intervention, (3) provides a conceptual framework for selecting constructs to develop the intervention, (4) gives insights into how best to deliver the intervention, and (5) identifies measurements needed to evaluate the intervention's impact (Crosby et al., 2009; Glanz et al., 2008b; Salazar, Crosby, & DiClemente, 2013). Theory also "provides a useful reference point to help keep research and implementation activities clearly focused" (Crosby et al., 2009, p. 11), and it infuses ethics and social justice into practice (Goodson, 2010). In addition, "using theory as a foundation for program planning

BOX	**Other Behavior Change Theories**	
4.1	Community Organization Theory (Minkler et al., 2001)	Public Health Model (PHM) (Street, Hopkins, & Olson, 2002)
	Extended Parallel Processing Model (Gore & Bracker, 2005)	Resilience Theory (Ungar, 2008)
	Protection Motivation Theory (PMT) (Rogers, 1983)	

and development is consistent with the current emphasis on using evidence-based interventions in public health, behavioral medicine, and medicine" (Rimer & Glanz, 2005, p. 5).

In the rest of this chapter, some of the theories and models used by health education specialists are presented in two main groups. The first group contains theories that focus on behavior change. Through their constructs, these theories help explain how change might take place. The second group contains planning models, which give structure and organization to the program planning process. These models provide health education specialists with step-by-step procedures, "integrating multiple theories to explain and address health problems," (Rimer & Glanz, 2005, p. 36), as they plan, implement, and evaluate health education/promotion programs.

There is not space in this chapter to adequately describe all the theories that have been developed to explain how behavior change occurs. Several of the theories that are not explained in detail in this chapter and are used less frequently in the health education/promotion setting but are nevertheless important are listed in **Box 4.1**.

▷ Behavior Change Theories

There are a number of behavior change theories that can be used by health education specialists to design interventions to encourage behavior change. Each theory provides a distinct process for helping to explain and change health behavior (Crosby, Salazar, & DiClemente, 2013a), and each works better in some situations than in others, depending on which level of influence is used to plan a health education/promotion program.

"Levels of influence" are at the heart of the **socio-ecological approach** (also called the *ecological perspective*). This multilevel, interactive approach examines how physical, social, political, economic, and cultural dimensions influence behaviors and conditions. The socio-ecological approach "emphasizes the interaction between, and the interdependence of, factors within and across all levels of a health problem" (Rimer & Glanz, 2005, p. 10). In other words, changes in health behavior do not take place in a vacuum. "Individuals influence and are influenced by their families, social networks, the organizations in which they participate (workplaces, schools, religious organizations), the communities of which they are a part, and the society in which they live" (IOM, 2001, p. 26).

The concept of the socio-ecological approach comes from Bronfenbrenner's (1974, 1979) ecological paradigm that was created to understand human development. Several authors applied his work to health promotion/education. Those most often cited in the literature are McLeroy, Bibeau, Steckler, and Glanz (1988) who identified five levels of influence: "(1) the

TABLE 4.1 **An ecological perspective: Levels of influence**

Ecological Level	Definition
Intrapersonal	Individual characteristics that influence behavior, such as knowledge, attitudes, beliefs, and personality traits
Interpersonal	Interpersonal processes and primary groups, including family, friends, and peers that provide social identity, support, and role definition
Organizational	Rules, regulations, policies, and informal structures, which may constrain or promote recommended behaviors
Community	Social networks and norms, or standards, which exist as formal or informal among individuals, groups, and organizations
Public Policy	Local, state, and federal policies and laws that regulate or support healthy actions and practices for disease prevention, early detection, control, and management
Physical Environment	Natural and built environment
Culture	Shared beliefs, values, behaviors, and practices of a population

Sources: Rimer, B. K., & Glanz, K. (2005). *Theory at a glance: A guide for health promotion practice,* 2nd ed. (NIH Pub. No. 05-3896). Washington, DC: National Cancer Institute; Simons-Morton, B. G., McLeroy, K. R., & Wendel, M. L. (2012). *Behavior theory in health promotion practice and research.* Burlington, MA: Jones & Bartlett Learning.

individual and individual's characteristics, such as knowledge, attitudes, values, and skills; (2) social relationships, including family and friendship ties and connections; (3) organizational influences and factors; (4) community characteristics; and (5) public policy"; and two additional levels "(6) the physical environment and (7) culture" were added (Simons-Morton et al., 2012, p. 45). **Table 4.1** lists and defines each of the seven levels. **Figure 4.1** provides a visual representation of the socio-ecological framework. By examining a health problem using this multilevel approach, health education specialists can get a better understanding of how to "attack" the problem.

Consider how the levels of influence can be applied to cigarette smoking in the United States. At the *intrapersonal* (or *individual*) *level*, a large majority of smokers know that smoking is bad for them, and a slightly smaller majority have indicated they would like to quit. Many have tried to quit—some have tried on many occasions. At the *interpersonal level (or within groups)*, many smokers are encouraged to quit by those in their social networks, such as their physician and/or family and friends. Some smokers may attempt to quit on their own, or they may join a formal smoking cessation group.

At the *institutional* (or *organizational*) *level*, institutions, such as churches and businesses, often have policies that regulate smoking. These institutions may offer smoking cessation classes or support groups to assist those who "belong" to the organization, to quit smoking. At the *community level*, some towns, cities, and counties have ordinances that prohibit smoking in public places. At the *public policy* or *population level*, many states have high cigarette taxes and/or laws that limit smoking. Also at this level, the federal government spends many dollars for public service announcements (PSAs) and other forms of media advertising the dangers of tobacco use.

The *physical environment* can also impact smoking behavior. Some of the laws that are written to prohibit indoor smoking are written in such a way that people are permitted to smoke in certain areas of a building if it has a separate ventilation system. And finally, culture can

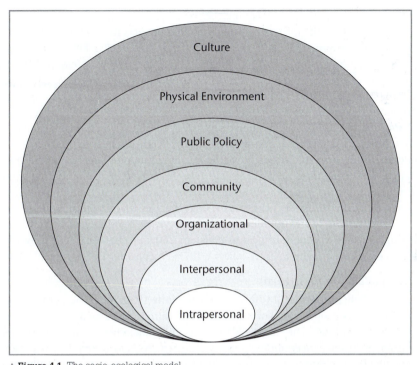

▲ **Figure 4.1** The socio-ecological model

Source: Simons-Morton, B. G., McLeroy, K. R., & Wendel, M. L. (2012). *Behavior theory in health promotion practice and research.* Burlington, MA: Jones & Bartlett Learning. p. 45.

play a part in smoking behavior. "Now that the Marlboro Man has passed away from lung cancer, and sex appeal of cigarettes has given way to photos of black lungs, the cigarette culture has lost its once powerful hold on American consumers" (Demerritt, 2013).

The following sections describe some of the theories and models that focus on behavior change. These theories/models are grouped according to the levels of influence where they may be most effective. To simplify the presentation of the socio-ecological model, Glanz and Rimer (1995) combined the levels of institutional, community, and public policy factors into a single "community" level. We have used it here as well.

Intrapersonal (Individual) Theories

Intrapersonal theories focus on factors within individuals such as knowledge, attitudes, beliefs, self-concept, developmental history, past experiences, motivation, skills, and behavior (Rimer & Glanz, 2005). Several of the theories used by health education specialists to develop interventions at the intrapersonal level are the Health Belief Model (HBM), the Protection Motivation Theory (PMT), the Theory of Planned Behavior (TPB), the Elaboration Likelihood Model of Persuasion (ELM), the Information-Motivation-Behavioral Skills Model (IMB), the Transtheoretical Model of Change (TMC), and the Precaution Adoption Process Model (PAPM).

Although all of the theories listed above fall into the intrapersonal theories category, they can be divided further into continuum theories, or stage theories. A **continuum theory** identifies variables that influence actions (i.e., beliefs, attitudes), quantifies the variables, and combines those variables into a single equation that predicts the likelihood of action (Weinstein, Rothman, & Sutton, 1998; Weinstein, Sandman, & Blalock, 2008). Thus, people can be "placed along a continuum of action likelihood" (Weinstein et al., 1998, p. 291). The HBM (Rosenstock, 1966), PMT (Rogers, 1975), TPB (Ajzen, 2006), ELM (Petty & Cacioppo, 1986), and IMB (Fisher & Fisher, 1992) are examples of continuum theories that are appropriate for use at the intrapersonal level.

A **stage theory** consists of an ordered set of categories into which people can be classified. It identifies factors that could induce movement from one category to the next (Weinstein & Sandman, 2002). More specifically, stage theories have four principal elements: (1) a category system to define the stages, (2) an ordering of stages, (3) barriers to change that are common to people in the same stage, and (4) different barriers to change, facing people in different stages (Weinstein et al., 1998). Advocates of stage theories "claim that there are *qualitative* differences among people and question whether changes in health behaviors can be described by a single prediction equation" (Weinstein et al., 2008, pp. 124–125). The most commonly reported stage theory is the TMC (Prochaska, 1979; Prochaska & DiClemente, 1983).

HEALTH BELIEF MODEL (HBM)

The **Health Belief Model (HBM)** was developed in the 1950s by a group of psychologists to help explain why people would or would not use health services such as tuberculosis screenings (Rosenstock, 1966). The HBM "addresses the individual's perceptions of the threat posed by a health problem (susceptibility, severity), the benefits of avoiding the threat, and factors influencing the decision to act (barriers, cues to action, and self-efficacy)" (Rimer & Glanz, 2005, p. 12). As you read the following example of why a person may or may not choose to enroll in a weight loss program, refer to the graphic representation of the HBM in **Figure 4.2**.

Suppose a person sees an advertisement about a weight loss program while reading Facebook. This is a **cue to action** that gets the person thinking about the possibility of losing weight. There may be some variables (demographic, socio-psychological, and structural) that cause the person to think about it a little more. The person remembers his or her college health course, which included information about weight gain and heart disease. This person knows she or he is at a higher than normal risk for heart disease because of family history, age, and less than desirable food and exercise choices. Therefore, he or she comes to the conclusion that she or he is susceptible to heart disease (**perceived susceptibility**). The person also believes that, if she or he develops a heart or vascular condition, it can be serious (**perceived seriousness/severity**).

Based on these factors, the person thinks that there is reason to be concerned about heart disease (**perceived threat**). This person knows that reducing his or her weight reduces the chances of a heart attack or stroke (**perceived benefits**). But continuing on a weight loss program takes time and effort, and this person does not always remember and is not always motivated to do it (**perceived barriers**). He or she must now analyze the difference between the benefits of and the barriers to enrolling in a weight loss program (**reduction of threat**). For this person, the **likelihood of taking action** (enrolling in the program) will be determined by considering the perceived threat against the reduction of threat.

When the HBM was first conceived, **self-efficacy** (confidence in one's own ability to perform a certain task or function) was not part of the model. However, because evidence showed self-efficacy was a meaningful concept in the perceived barriers construct, it was

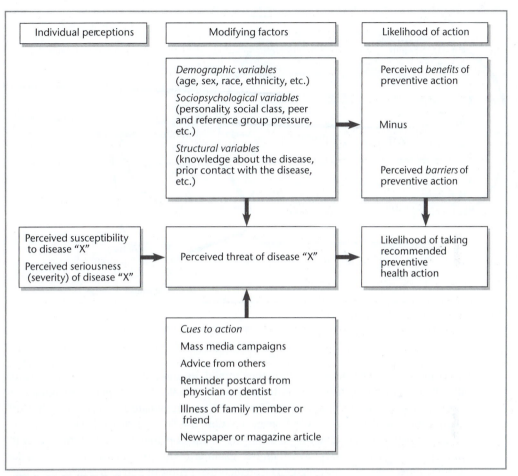

▲ Figure 4.2 Health Belief Model as a predictor of preventive health behavior

Source: Becker, M. H., et al., from "A new approach to explaining sick-role behavior in low income populations," *American Journal of Public Health* 64, March 1974: 205–216, Fig 1. Used by permission of Sheridan Press.

recommended that self-efficacy be added to the HBM (Rosenstock, Strecher, & Becker, 1988). According to the HBM, if people are going to be successful in changing a behavior, they must feel threatened by their current behavior (i.e., perceived susceptibility and severity), feel that a change in the behavior will result in an outcome they value (perceived benefit), and believe that they are competent (self-efficacy) to overcome perceived barriers (perceived cost) to engage in the new behavior (Champion & Skinner, 2008). Because dieting has a high failure rate, support groups such as Weight Watchers can increase a person's self-efficacy because it can help them feel competent in adopting a new lifestyle (Mann, et al., 2007).

THEORY OF PLANNED BEHAVIOR (TPB)

The **Theory of Planned Behavior (TPB)** (see **Figure 4.3**) is an extension of the Theory of Reasoned Action (Fishbein & Ajzen, 1975). According to the TPB, individuals' intention to perform a given behavior is a function of their attitude toward performing the behavior, their

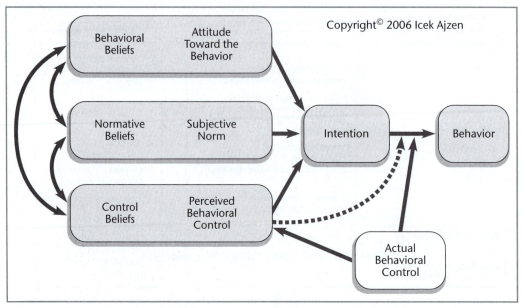

▲ **Figure 4.3** Theory of Planned Behavior (TPB)

Source: "Theory of Planned Behavior Diagram" (TPB Diagram) by Dr. Icek Ajzen, http://www.people.umass.edu/aizen/tpb.diag.html. Reprinted by permission.

beliefs about what relevant others think they should do, and their perception of the ease or difficulty of performing the behavior. **Intention** "is an indication of a person's readiness to perform a given behavior, and it is considered to be the immediate antecedent of behavior" (Ajzen, 2006). Unlike the Theory of Reasoned Action, the TPB was developed to explain not just health behavior but all volitional behaviors ("behaviors that can be performed at will" [Luszczynski & Sutton, 2005, p. 73]). Using the example of the use of marijuana as a behavior not fully under volitional control, the TPB predicts that people intend to give up its use if they

- have a positive attitude toward quitting (**attitude toward the behavior**),
- think that others whom they value believe it would be good for them to quit (**subjective norm**) (see **Figure 4.4**),
- perceive that they have control over whether or not they quit (**perceived behavioral control**), and
- have the skills, resources, and other prerequisites needed to quit (**actual behavioral control**).

ELABORATION LIKELIHOOD MODEL OF PERSUASION (ELM)

The Elaboration Likelihood Model of Persuasion (**ELM**) or the Elaboration Likelihood Model for short, was initially developed to help explain inconsistencies in research results from the study of attitudes (Petty, Barden, & Wheeler, 2009). Specifically, the ELM was designed to help explain how persuasion messages (communication), aimed at changing attitudes, are received and processed by people. Though not created specifically for health communication, the ELM has been used to interpret and predict the impact of health messages.

▶ **Figure 4.4** Subjective norm is an important construct to be considered when planning programs for adolescents and young adults.

The ELM does three things. First, it proposes that attitudes can be formed via two different types of routes to persuasion: peripheral routes and central routes (Petty et al., 2009). The distinction between the two routes is the amount of elaboration. **Elaboration** refers to the amount of cognitive processing (i.e., thought) that a person puts into receiving messages. Peripheral route processing involves minimal thought and relies on superficial cues, or mental shortcuts (called *heuristics*), about issue-relevant information as the primary means for attitude change (Petty et al., 2009). For example, people may form an attitude after hearing a persuasive message simply because the person delivering the message is someone they admire.

On the other hand, central route processing involves thoughtful consideration (or effortful cognitive elaboration) of issue-relevant information and one's own cognitive responses as the primary basis for attitude change: "Two conditions are necessary for effortful processing to occur—the recipient of the message must be both *motivated* and *able* to think carefully" (Petty et al., 2009, p. 188). An example of central route processing is a motorcyclist's formation of an attitude about wearing a helmet. Processing is based on thoughtful consideration of a message about the pros and cons of helmet use, recalling knowledge learned in a motorcycle safety class, and possibly the outcomes of a motorcycle crash in which a relative was involved.

Second, when using the ELM, the results of the two routes can be similar. However, the two routes usually lead to attitudes with different consequences. "Attitudes changed through central route processing are more enduring and have different effects on behavior than attitude change achieved through more peripheral processing, which is less resilient to counterarguments" (Simons-Morton et al., 2012, p. 285).

Third, "the model specifies how variables have an impact on persuasion" (Petty et al., 2009, p. 197). The variable can have an influence on people's motivation to think or ability to think, as well as the valence of people's thought or the confidence in the thoughts generated (Petty et al., 2009). For example, variables that have an impact on how a message is processed include the source of the message (e.g., friend, expert), the message itself (e.g., funny, serious), the context (e.g., delivered person-to-person, on the Internet), and various characteristics of the recipient (e.g., intelligence, age, attentiveness).

Utilizing the routes to processing that the ELM provides, health education specialists can create health messages that are more meaningful to a priority population, and in turn, can be more successful in reaching program goals. **Figure 4.5** provides a diagram of the ELM as presented by Petty and colleagues (2009).

INFORMATION-MOTIVATION-BEHAVIORAL SKILLS MODEL (IMB)

The Information-Motivation-Behavioral Skills Model (IMB) (see **Figure 4.6**) was initially created to address the critical need for a strong theoretical basis for HIV/AIDS prevention efforts (Fisher & Fisher, 1992). Because of its success in dealing with HIV/AIDS prevention behavior, the IMB model has been applied to a number of other risk reduction behaviors (Fisher, Fisher, & Shuper, 2009). According to this model, the constructs of information, motivation, and behavioral skills are the fundamental determinants of preventive behavior. The information provided needs to be relevant, easily enacted based on the specific circumstances, and serve as a guide to personal preventive behavior. "In addition to facts that are easy to translate into behavior, the IMB model recognizes additional cognitive processes and content categories that significantly influence performance of preventive behavior" (Fisher et al., 2009, p. 27). An example is the following guideline that someone may use to make a decision: "If my best friend is willing to ride a motorcycle without a helmet, it must be okay."

Even though people are well informed about a particular health issue, they may not be motivated to act. According to the IMB model, prevention motivation includes both personal motivation to act (i.e., one's attitude toward a specific behavior) and social motivation to act (social support for the preventive behavior) (Fisher et al., 2009). Both types of motivation are necessary to act.

In addition to being well informed and motivated to act, the IMB model also indicates that people must possess behavioral skills to engage in the preventive behavior. The behavioral skills component of the IMB model includes an individual's objective ability and his or her perceived self-efficacy to perform the preventive behavior.

When applying the IMB model, health education specialists cannot just use their own judgment to determine what information to provide, how best to motivate, and what behavioral skills to teach to a given population. The process should begin by eliciting information from a subsample of the priority population to identify deficits in their health-relevant information, motivation, and behavioral skills. Next, health education specialists need to design and implement "*conceptually-based, empirically-targeted, population-specific*" (p. 29) interventions, constructed on the basis of the elicited findings (Fisher et al., 2009). Then, after the implementation of the intervention, health education specialists must evaluate the intervention to determine if it had significant and sustained effects on the information, motivation, and behavioral skill determinants of the preventive behavior and on the preventive behavior itself (Fisher et al., 2009).

TRANSTHEORETICAL MODEL OF CHANGE (TMC)

The **Transtheoretical Model of Change (TMC)** proposes that intentional behavior change "occurs in stages. As people attempt to change their behavior, they move through a variety of stages using different processes to help them get from one stage to the next until a desired

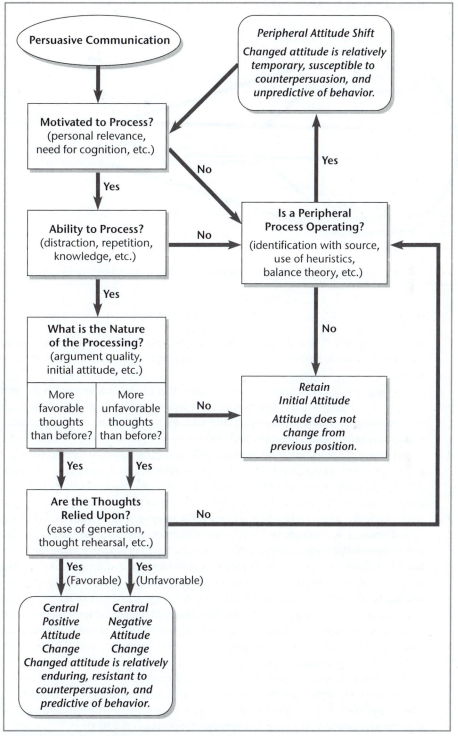

▲ **Figure 4.5** The Elaboration Likelihood Model of Persuasion (ELM)

Source: From Petty, R. E., Barden J., & Wheeler, S. C., "The Elaboration Likelihood Model of Persuasion: Developing health promotions for sustained behavioral change" in *Emerging theories in health promotion practice and research*, 2nd ed.; DiClemente, R. J., Crosby, R. A., & Kegler, M. (Eds.), p. 196. Copyright © 2009 John Wiley & Sons, Inc. Reproduced with permission of John Wiley & Sons, Inc.

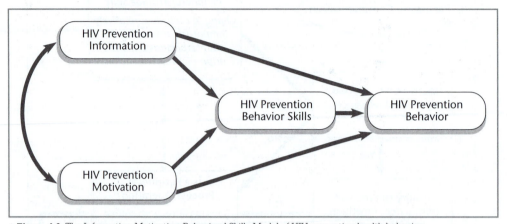

▲ **Figure 4.6** The Information-Motivation-Behavioral Skills Model of HIV prevention health behavior

Source: From Fisher, J. D., & Fisher, W. A., "Changing AIDS risk behavior," *Psychological Bulletin 111* (3), 455–474, 1992. Published by American Psychological Association (APA). Reprinted by permission.

behavior is attained" (Hayden, 2014, pp. 138–139). The TMC draws from the constructs of a number of theories, "hence the name 'Transtheoretical'" (Prochaska, Johnson, & Lee, 1998, p. 59).

Although each TMC construct is important, this model is best known for its stages of change. TMC suggests that "people move from *precontemplation*, not intending to change, to *contemplation*, intending to change within 6 months, to *preparation*, actively planning change, to *action*, overtly making changes, and into *maintenance*, taking steps to sustain change and resist temptation to relapse" (Prochaska, Redding, Harlow, Rossi, & Velicer, 1994, p. 473).

TMC was first used in psychotherapy. It was developed by Prochaska (1979) after he completed a comparative analysis of various therapy systems and many therapy studies. Since then, program planners have used TMC with a wide variety of topics ranging from alcohol abuse to weight control (Prochaska, Redding, & Evers, 2008; Spencer, Adams, Malone, Roy, & Yost, 2006).

Following is an example of TMC's stage construct applied to smoking cessation. In the **precontemplation stage**, smokers "have no intention to take action in the foreseeable future (usually defined as within the next 6 months)" (DiClemente, Redding, Crosby, & Salazar, 2013, p. 109). There are a number of reasons why people are in this stage. It may be that they are discouraged from previous unsuccessful attempts at changing, or it may be that they are either uninformed or under-informed about the consequences of their behavior (Prochaska et al., 2008).

In the **contemplation stage**, smokers know that smoking is bad for them and consider quitting. They "are intending to take action in the next six months" (Prochaska, 2005, p. 111). In the **preparation stage**, the smokers have combined intention and behavioral criteria. Often, during the past year, they have already taken a step toward changing their behavior. For example, they may have enrolled in an organized class to help them change, had a conversation with a physician or counselor, or purchased a self-help book or app for their smartphone to help guide their change (Prochaska et al., 2008).

In the **action stage**, smokers have overtly made changes in their behavior, experiences, or environment to stop smoking in the past six months. "Not all modifications of behavior count as action in this model" (Prochaska et al., 2008, p. 100). To be considered in this stage, people need to meet a level of behavior that scientists and professionals agree is sufficient to reduce the risk of disease. In our example, reducing the number of cigarettes smoked per day does not meet the necessary level for action; only total abstinence qualifies (Prochaska et al., 2008). As the smokers make these changes, they are moving toward the next stage, maintenance.

The focus of the **maintenance stage** is to prevent relapse. Thus, individuals who have quit smoking are working to not smoke again. People in this stage have changed their problem behavior for at least six months and are increasingly more confident that they can continue their change (Prochaska et al., 1998; Redding, Rossi, Rossi, Velicer, & Prochaska, 1999). In other words, their change is more of a habit, and their chance of relapse is lower, but their new behavior still requires some attention (Redding et al., 1999).

The final stage is **termination**. This stage is defined as the time when individuals who made a change now have zero temptation to return to their old behavior. They have 100 percent self-efficacy (a lifetime of maintenance). In our example, smokers have become non-smokers. No matter what their mood, they will not return to their old behavior (Prochaska et al., 2008). This is a stage that few people reach with certain behaviors (e.g., alcoholism).

PRECAUTION ADOPTION PROCESS MODEL (PAPM)

The Precaution Adoption Process Model (PAPM) tries to explain how people get to the point of making a decision about taking action and how they apply their decision to taking action (Weinstein et al., 2008). Although the previously discussed TMC and the PAPM are both stage models that appear similar, they are applied quite differently. The PAPM is most applicable for the adoption of a new precaution (e.g., getting a mammogram or a hepatitis B vaccination), or the abandonment of a risky behavior that requires a deliberate action (e.g., not wearing a safety belt). It can also be used to explain why and how people make deliberate changes in habitual patterns (e.g., flossing one's teeth two times a day instead of one). The PAPM is not applicable for actions that require the gradual development of habitual patterns of behavior, such as exercise and diet (Weinstein et al., 2008).

In the following example, the seven stages of the PAPM (see **Figure 4.7**) are applied to participating in a colon cancer screening program. In Stage 1, Unaware of Issue, people are totally

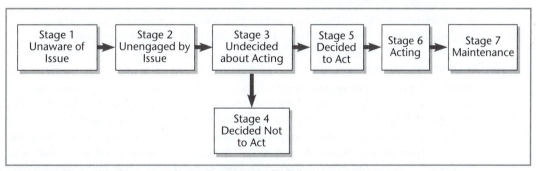

▲ **Figure 4.7** Stages of the Precaution Adoption Process Model (PAPM)

Source: From Weinstein, N. D., Sandman, P. M., & Blalock, S. J., "The Precaution Adoption Process Model" in *Health behavior and health education: Theory, research, and practice*, 4th ed., K. Glanz, B. K. Rimer, and K. Viswanath, (Eds.), p. 127. Copyright © 2008 John Wiley & Sons, Inc. Reproduced with permission of John Wiley & Sons, Inc.

unaware of the need to be screened. When people first learn something about the screening, they are no longer unaware, but they are not necessarily engaged by it, either. This is Stage 2, Unengaged.

In Stage 3, Undecided about Acting, people have become engaged in thinking about the screening, and they are considering participation. Once people have reached this stage, one of three things happen: (1) they suspend judgment and stay in this Stage, (2) they decide to act and move to Stages 5-7, or (3) they decide not to act (Stage 4) (Weinstein et al., 2008).

Once the people participate in the screening, they have initiated the behavior, and they are in Stage 6, Acting. Finally, if the people participate in the screening at the medically recommended intervals, they are in Stage 7, Maintenance. Note that this last stage of the PAPM is not applicable to some decision-making processes, for example, actions required only once in a lifetime, such as a vaccination that immunizes a person for life (Weinstein et al., 2008).

Interpersonal Theories

The category of interpersonal theories contains theories that "assume individuals exist within, and are influenced by, a social environment. The opinions, thoughts, behavior, advice, and support of the people surrounding an individual influence his or her feelings and behavior, and the individual has a reciprocal effect on those people" (Rimer & Glanz, 2005, p. 19). Research shows that social relationships can be a powerful influence on health and health behaviors (Heaney & Israel, 2008). As such, a number of theories have been created to explain concepts such as

- *Social norms*—*"what are perceived to be true and acceptable"* (Simons-Morton et al., 2012, p. 158)
- *Social learning*—learning that occurs in a social context
- *Social power*—ability to influence others or resist activities of others
- *Social integration*—structure and quality of relationships
- *Social networks*—"person-centered webs of social relationships" (Sharma & Romas, 2012, p. 283)
- *Social support*—"help obtained through social relationships and interpersonal exchanges" (Sharma & Romas, 2012, p. 284)
- *Social capital*—"the relationships and structures within a community, such as civic participation, networks, norms of reciprocity, and trust, that promote cooperation of mutual benefit" (Putnam, 1995, p. 66)
- *Interpersonal communication*

Because of space limitations, only three interpersonal theories are overviewed in this chapter, one that is well-established (Social Cognitive Theory) and two newer theories (Social Network Theory and Social Capital Theory). The latter two may be theories in name only. As stated previously in this chapter, some theories have the term *model* in their title because that is the way they were initially identified. Even though there is now empirical evidence to call them theories, the model title has remained. The social network and social capital theories may have been called theories prematurely; they are probably more in the model stage. However, you should be aware of the main concepts in each one.

SOCIAL COGNITIVE THEORY (SCT)

The Social Cognitive Theory (SCT) (Bandura, 1986) dates back to the 1950s (Bandura, 1977; Rotter, 1954), when it was known as the Social Learning Theory (SLT). When studying about theories, you may yet hear a reference to SLT. In brief, the SCT asserts "that the social environment, the personal characteristics of the individual, and behavior interact and influence each other" (Crosby, Salazar, & DiClemente, 2013b, p. 164). Those who advocate for the SCT believe that reinforcement contributes to learning. However, the combination of reinforcement with an individual's expectations of the behavior's consequences is what determines the behavior. The SCT explains learning through its constructs. Unlike the other theories presented so far in this chapter, there is no diagram for the SCT nor is the interrelationship of its constructs specific in nature. Those constructs most often used in health education/promotion are presented in **Table 4.2**, along with an example of each.

SOCIAL NETWORK THEORY (SNT)

The term **social network** refers to the "person-centered web of social relationships" (Sharma & Romas, 2012, p. 283). Barnes, a sociologist who studied Norwegian villages (Barnes, 1954), created the term in the 1950s. He used it to describe villagers' social relationships and characteristics that were not traditional social units like families (Edberg, 2007; Heaney & Israel, 2008). Since that time, sociologists and professionals in various disciplines, including health education/promotion, have continued to study and use the social network concept.

Social epidemiological observational studies clearly document the beneficial effects of supportive networks on health status (Heaney & Israel, 2008). But some people question whether there is enough evidence to suggest a Social Network Theory (SNT). Heaney and Israel (2008) feel that the social network concept, and the closely related one of social support, are really not theories but rather are concepts that describe social relationships. They feel that intervention studies are "needed to identify the most potent causal agents and critical time periods for social network enhancement" (p. 197). For example, it is not known how much social networking is needed to enhance health, or how much is too much. Also unknown are the characteristics of "good networks" that result in positive health behavior (i.e., regular exercise) versus characteristics of "bad networks" that lead to negative health behavior (i.e., smoking). We do know, however, that people who are part of social networks are healthier, as a whole, than those who are not involved in social networks.

Edberg (2007) described different types of social networks such as ego-centered networks and full relational networks (see **Figure 4.8**). He indicated that the key component to SNT is the relationships between and among individuals, including how those relationships influence beliefs and behaviors. He further stated that those using SNT need to consider the following items when assessing a network's role on the health behavior of individuals who are part of the network (Edberg, 2007):

- Centrality versus marginality of individuals in the network: How involved is the person in the network?
- Reciprocity of relationships: Are relationships one-way or two-way?
- Complexity or intensity of relationships in the network: Do the relationships exist between two people, or are they multiplexed?
- Homogeneity or diversity of people in the network: Do all members of the network have similar characteristics, or are they different from one another?

TABLE 4.2 **Often-used constructs of the Social Cognitive Theory and examples of their application**

Construct	Definition	Example
Behavioral capability	Knowledge and skills necessary to perform a behavior	If a woman is going to perform a breast self-exam (BSE), she needs to know the proper way to do it.
Expectations	Beliefs about the likely outcomes of certain behaviors	If a woman performs BSE or receives a mammogram, she expects the process to find cancer at an early vs. late stage.
Expectancies	Values people place on expected outcomes	Does the woman value early detection?
Locus of control	Perception of the center of control over reinforcement	Women who feel they have control over reinforcement are said to have internal locus of control and feel participating in screening provides them the ability to detect cancer early. Those who perceive reinforcement under the control of an external force are said to have external locus of control. These women feel practicing BSE or having a mammogram won't help because if they are going to get cancer; it is their fate.
Reciprocal determinism	"Environmental factors influence individuals and groups, but individuals and groups can also influence their environments and regulate their own behavior" (McAlister, Perry, & Parcel, 2008, p. 171)	If women are not utilizing mammograms because of time off from work, employers can schedule a mobile mammogram unit to come to the worksite.
Observational learning	Learning by watching others	Provide women with the opportunity to watch others (in person or on a video) properly performing BSE on a breast model.
Reinforcement (directly, vicariously, self-management)	Responses to behaviors that increase the chances of recurrence	Giving verbal encouragement to those women who have completed their mammogram or correctly performed BSE.
Self-control, or self-regulation	Gaining control over own behavior through monitoring and adjusting it	If want to increase BSE, have women track how often they perform it.
Self-efficacy	People's confidence in their ability to perform a certain desired task or function	If women are going to properly perform BSE, they must feel they can do it.
Collective efficacy	Beliefs about the ability of the group to perform concerted actions that bring desired outcomes (McAlister et al., 2008, p. 171)	If a group of women is going to work to change a community's culture toward mammograms, they must feel that they can do it.
Emotional-coping response	For people to learn, they must be able to deal with the sources of anxiety that surround a behavior.	Fear is an emotion that can be involved in learning, and people would have to deal with it before they could learn a behavior. If the women feel scared they will find a lump, or if they do, it is fatal, that fear can prevent them from doing screenings.

Sources: Created from Baranowski, T., Perry, C. L., & Parcel, G. S., (2002). "How individuals, environments, and health behavior interact: Social Cognitive Theory." In K. Glanz, B. K. Rimer, & F. M. Lewis (Eds.), *Health behavior and health education: Theory, research, and practice*, 3rd ed., 165–184); McAlister, A. L., Perry, C. L., & Parcel, G. S. (2008). "How individuals, environments, and health behavior interact: social cognitive theory." In K. Glanz, B. K. Rimer, & K. Viswanath (Eds.), *Health behavior and health education: Theory, research, and practice*, 4th ed., 169–188, San Francisco, CA: Jossey-Bass; McKenzie, J. F., Neiger, B. L. & Thackery, R. (2013). *Planning, implementing, and evaluating health promotion programs: A primer*, 6th ed., Pearson, Boston, MA; Simons-Morton, B. G., McLeroy, K. R., & Wendel, M. L. (2012). *Behavior theory in health promotion practice and research*. Burlington, MA: Jones & Bartlett Learning.

▲ **Figure 4.8** A simple sociogram, centered on a "focus individual" or ego

Source: From Edberg, M., *Essentials of health behavior: Social and Behavioral Theory in public health,* 1st ed., Fig. 5-1, p. 56. Copyright © 2007, Jones and Bartlett Publishers, Sudbury, MA. http://www.jblearning.com. Reprinted by permission.

- Subgroups, cliques, and linkages: Are there concentrations of interactions among some members? If so, do they interact with others, or are they isolated from others?
- Communication patterns in the network: How does information pass between the members in the network?

In summary, we know that social networks can impact health, but the specifics of who is most affected and how best to set up and use social networks are unknown. Even so, health education specialists who are planning interventions need to consider whether social networks should be a part of their strategy to bring about change. With the power of the Internet, the impact of social networks in the work of health education specialists will continue to grow.

SOCIAL CAPITAL THEORY

The term **social capital** got its start in political science and has been used in health education/promotion since the mid-1990s. An often-quoted definition is "the relationships and structures within a community, such as civic participation, networks, norms of reciprocity, and trust that promote cooperation of mutual benefit" (Putnam, 1995, p. 66). "Social capital is a collective asset, a feature of communities rather than the property of individuals. As such, individuals both contribute to it and use it, but they cannot own it" (Warren, Thompson, & Saegert, 2001, p. 1).

"The influence of social capital is well documented" (Crosby et al., 2009). There are epidemiological studies that show that greater social capital is linked to several different positive outcomes (i.e., reduced mortality). There are also correlational studies that show a lack of social capital is related to poorer health outcomes (e.g., Kawachi, Kennedy, Lochner, & Prothrow, 1997). But as with social networks, a cause-effect relationship has not been established between social capital and better health. "Social capital does not provide theories of change,

▶ **Figure 4.9** Social capital

Source: From Hayden, J., *Introduction to Health Behavior Theory*, 1st ed., Fig 9-3, p. 125. Copyright © 2009, Jones and Bartlett Publishers, Sudbury, MA. http://www.jblearning.com. Reprinted by permission.

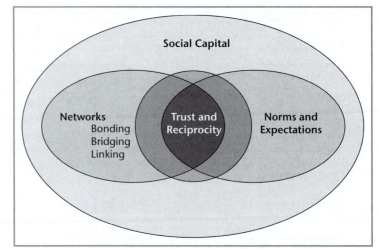

tools, or time lines for change; nor does it necessarily guarantee improved outcomes if social capital is improved" (Minkler & Wallerstein, 2005, p. 38). However, it does seem to have an impact on health.

Figure 4.9 provides a graphic representation of social capital. This particular figure includes the key concepts of Putman's (1995) definition of social capital and three different types of network resources: bonding, bridging, and linking social capital. These three types are differentiated based on the strength of the relationships between/among those people in the social network (Hayden, 2014). Originally, *bonding social capital*, sometimes referred to as exclusive social capital, was defined as "the type that brings closer together people who already know each other" (Gittell & Vidal, 1998, p. 15). More recently, this concept was expanded to include people who are similar or people who are members of the same group. Examples of bonding social capital include those who may be members in a service organization (e.g., Lions, Elks, and American Legion) or religious community.

Bridging social capital, sometimes referred to as inclusive social capital, was originally defined as "the type that brings together people or groups who previously did not know each other" (Gittell & Vidal, 1998, p. 15). Bridging social capital is now seen more as the resources people obtain from their interaction with others outside their group, who often are people with different demographic characteristics. An example is people from different parts of a community who come together to create a community park.

The most recently recognized and weakest (Hayden, 2014) network resource is *linking social capital*. This type of network resource comes from relationships between or among "individuals and groups in different social strata in a hierarchy where power, social status, and wealth are accessed by different groups" (U.K. Office of National Statistics, 2001, p. 11). An example may be when a boss and an employee are working together on a project.

As with social networks, it is important that health education specialists think about the concept of social capital when planning interventions. Although it is not an intervention in itself, it is a concept that needs to be considered and monitored.

Community Theories

This group of theories includes three categories of factors from the socio-ecological approach—organizational, community, and public policy. Organizational factors include rules, regulations, and policies of an organization that can impact health behavior. Community factors include social norms (e.g., what is deemed a desirable behavior within a particular community) whereas public policy includes legislation that can impact health behavior such as antismoking laws or motorcycle helmet laws. Theories associated with these three factors include theories of community organizing and community building (see Chapter 1), organizational change, the Diffusion Theory, and the Community Readiness Model (a stage model). The latter two are described in the following sections.

DIFFUSION OF INNOVATIONS THEORY (DIF)

The **Diffusion Theory (DIF)** provides an explanation for how new products, ideas, techniques, behaviors, or services (known as innovations) are adopted within populations. When people become "consumers" of an innovation, they are referred to as adopters. Rogers (2003) categorized adopters on the basis of when they adopt innovations. These categories include innovators, early adopters, early or late majority, and laggards. The percentage at which people become adopters over time can be represented by continuum in **Figure 4.10**.

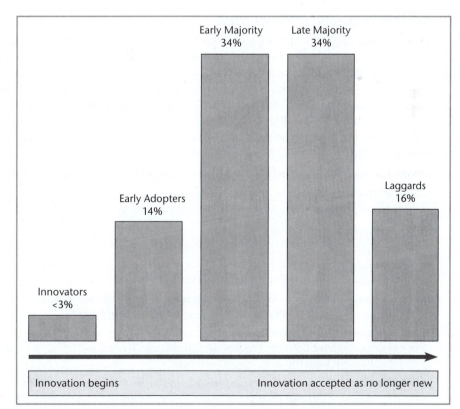

▲ **Figure 4.10** Bar chart depicting percentages of persons adopting an innovation over time.

Innovators are the first to adopt an innovation. They are venturesome, independent, risky, and daring. They want to be the first to do something. **Early adopters** are very interested in innovation, but they do not want to be the first involved. Early adopters are respected by others in the social system and looked at as opinion leaders.

Following the early adopters is the **early majority**. This group of people may be interested in the innovation but need some external motivation to get involved. These people, along with those in the late majority, make up the largest groups. The **late majority** comprises people who are skeptical. They will not adopt an innovation until most people in the social system have done so. The **laggards** are the last ones to get involved in an innovation, if they get involved at all.

Following is an application of the Diffusion Theory. The health education staff at the Family Medicine Residency (FMR) is beginning a new series of classes designed to assist adults in patient families making healthier choices when shopping for food. About 3 percent of the patients (the innovators) will sign up and attend the classes as soon as they hear about the series. Shortly thereafter, another 14 percent (early adopters) will probably get involved, possibly after reading about the program's merits. At this point, the health education staff must work harder to attract others to the program. It will take constant reminders to get the early majority (~34 percent) involved. Buddy, peer, or mentoring programs might be needed to get the late majority (~34 percent) involved. The laggards (~16 percent) probably will not attend the food shopping sessions at all.

COMMUNITY READINESS MODEL (CRM)

The Community Readiness Model (CRM) is a stage theory for communities. Communities, like individuals, are in various stages of readiness for change. Yet, the stages of change for communities are not the same as for individuals. "The stages of readiness in a community have to deal with group processes and group organization, characteristics that are not relevant to personal readiness" (Edwards, Jumper-Thurman, Plested, Oetting, & Swanson, 2000, pp. 296–297). Although the CRM was developed initially to deal with alcohol and drug abuse, it also has been used in a variety of health and nutrition areas, environmental issues, and social programs (Edwards et al., 2000). The CRM has nine stages (Edwards et al., 2000):

1. *No Awareness.* The problem is not generally recognized by the community or leaders.

2. *Denial.* There is little or no recognition in the community that there is a problem. If recognition exists, there is a feeling that nothing can be done about the problem.

3. *Vague Awareness.* Some people in the community feel there is a problem and something should be done, but there is no motivation or leadership to do so.

4. *Preplanning.* There is a clear recognition by some that a problem exists and something should be done. There are leaders, but no focused or detailed planning.

5. *Preparation.* Planning is taking place but it is not based on collected data. There is leadership and modest support for efforts. Resources are being sought.

6. *Initiation.* Information is available to justify and begin efforts. Staff is either in training or has just completed training. Leaders are enthusiastic. There is usually little resistance and involvement from the community members.

7. *Stabilization.* The program is running, staffed, and supported by the community and decision makers. The program is perceived as stable with no need for change. This stage may include routine tracking, but no in-depth evaluation.

TABLE 4.3 **Community readiness stages and goals**

Stage	Goal
(1) *No Awareness*	Raise awareness of the issue.
(2) *Denial*	Raise awareness that the problem or issue exists in the community.
(3) *Vague Awareness*	Raise awareness that the community can do something.
(4) *Preplanning*	Raise awareness with concrete ideas to combat condition.
(5) *Preparation*	Gather existing information to help plan strategies.
(6) *Initiation*	Provide community specific information.
(7) *Stabilization*	Stabilize efforts/programs.
(8) *Confirmation/Expansion*	Expand and enhance service.
(9) *Professionalism*	Maintain momentum and continue growth.

Source: Created from Edwards, R. W., Jumper-Thurman, P., Plested, B. A., Oetting, E. R., & Swanson, L. (2000). "Community readiness: Research to practice." *Journal of Community Psychology, 28* (3), 291–307.

8. *Confirmation/Expansion.* Standard efforts are in place, which are supported by the community and decision makers. The program has been evaluated and modified, and efforts are in place to seek resources for new efforts. There is ongoing data collection to link risk factors and problems.

9. *Professionalism.* Much is known about prevalence, risk factors, and cause of problems. Highly trained staff members run effective programs aimed at the general population and appropriate subgroups. Programs have been evaluated and modified. The community is supportive but should hold programs accountable.

A community's readiness can be assessed through interviews with key informants. As with other stage theories, once the stage of readiness is known, there are suggested processes for moving a community from one stage to the next. **Table 4.3** presents the nine stages and the goal for each stage.

▷ Planning Models

Good health education/promotion programs are not created by chance. "A systematic process is important in these endeavors" (Bartholomew, Parcel, Kok, Gottlieb, & Fernández, 2011). Well-thought-out and well-conceived models provide health education specialists with "frames" on which to build plans (see **Box 4.2**). Although many planning models have similar principles and common elements, those elements may have different labels. In fact, "there are important differences in sequence, emphasis, and the conceptualization of the major components that make certain models more appealing than others to individual practitioners" (Simons-Morton, Greene, & Gottlieb, 1995, pp. 126–127).

The following sections provide an overview of seven models used for planning health education/promotion programs. Although many more models exist, these seven have been used successfully, and they represent a wide range of planning approaches. **Box 4.3** lists other planning models that may be just as sound from a theoretical perspective, but currently they are not used as frequently in health promotion research. For more detailed explanations, see the original publications of the models.

THEORIES AND PLANNING MODELS Trevor W. Newby

CURRENT POSITION/TITLE: Public Health Advisor / Project Officer

EMPLOYER: Centers for Disease Control and Prevention (CDC)

MAJOR: Health Promotion

DEGREES: Master of Health Science in Health Promotion and Bachelor of Science in Health Promotion

INSTITUTION: Boise State University

How I obtained my job: Obtaining my current job started in college with my graduate assistantships, where I was able to align myself with supervisors and professors at Boise State University, which made me more marketable upon graduation. Following a lead from a professor, I applied for a position as a Health Education Specialist with the Idaho State Respiratory Health Program. This experience allowed me to work with a number of statewide programs and a variety of different organizations while taking part in a number of collaboration efforts related to that position. Most notably, I was able to work with our project officer, as well as others from CDC, who mentored me with technical assistance and programmatic directives related to the grant I was working on. This not only increased my knowledge in public health, but also allowed me to gain the networking I needed to take the next step in my professional career.

How I use theory in my job: At CDC, I have the opportunity to provide technical assistance for tobacco prevention and control efforts taking place on a nationwide level. This involves knowing a wide variety of theories, including stages of change, that are commonly used to assist smokers with quitting tobacco from the pre-contemplation stage through the maintenance stage of their behavior change process. Social norm changes are implemented with policies from the local and state levels, which are supported by CDC providing written testimony, evidence-based science, and supporting data. In addition to this, public health–related theories are also commonly used and supported by CDC to maintain and enhance programmatic and

policy-driven efforts. These include states collaborating with partners to implement clean indoor air laws, point of sale restrictions to prevent minors from purchasing tobacco, and other environmental change strategies that promote smoking cessation and decrease exposure to secondhand smoke.

Programmatic efforts are organized using logic models, work plans, and budgets that are implemented and evaluated at the state level. These plans are approved by CDC project officers. In addition to this, monthly technical assistance calls are used to verify the progression and challenges being faced concerning work plan efforts. Evaluation efforts are also monitored on a monthly basis, and data collected from the states are used to formulate state-specific data, as well as comparisons on a nationwide basis in relation to tobacco.

Recommendations for health education specialists: First, secure internship opportunities. Internship settings will not only provide valuable work experience that will put you ahead of other potential job seekers but will also allow you to apply classroom learning while offering networking opportunities at the same time. The more internships you secure, the more diverse and enticing your portfolio will become for potential employers. Never base your internships on a lack of knowledge or the amount of pay it offers, if any. Second, be proficient in grant writing and managing a budget. These are valuable skills that are necessary in the public health profession. Third, take a number of marketing classes. Marketing plays an imperative role in public health. A public health program could have the most dynamic program or resource available, but it won't provide any benefit unless it is effectively marketed to its intended audience. Fourth, be your own advocate. Take every opportunity to network within a wide variety of public health topics. Don't limit your networking opportunities to the public health topic

BOX 4.2

continued

you are currently assigned. Knowledge is important, but knowing the individuals that can help you open doors to career opportunities or new innovative ideas is paramount to your success. Networking will play a vital role in helping you achieve these goals. Lastly, don't be afraid to learn. Public health is a constantly evolving field with a wide variety of topics. In order to be a proficient educator, constant research and information gathering are critical.

Future of the health education/promotion profession: I consider the future of health education specialists in public health to be very positive. It has taken many years for businesses, lawmakers, and policy makers to realize the worth of proper prevention methods provided by public health professionals, but now the dynamic is changing. Prevention practices have already been proven to be effective with research surrounding tobacco. Prevention strategies, such as those found in CDC's *Best Practices*, have saved millions of dollars in healthcare costs to taxpayers in relation to tobacco use and have begun to change the social norm of tobacco use as a whole. I am certain prevention practices will play a vital role in the Affordable Care Act with tobacco cessation being a utilized strategy, along with a host of other prevention strategies pertaining to public health. As more emphasis is placed on prevention practices, the government, as well as businesses, will save millions of dollars on secondary and tertiary clinical care by implementing effective prevention practices provided by public health professionals. This will provide many jobs to health education specialists in an increasingly changing and meaningful profession.

BOX 4.3

Other Planning Models

- *Comprehensive Health Education Model* (Sullivan, 1973)
- *Model for Health Education Planning* (Ross & Mico, 1980)
- *Model for Health Education Planning and Resource Development* (Bates & Winder, 1984)
- *Planned Approach To Community Health (PATCH)* (CDC & USDHHS, n.d.)
- *Generic Health/Fitness Delivery System* (Patton, Corry, Gettman, & Graff, 1986)
- *Community Health Assessment aNd Group Evaluation: The Change Tool* (CDC, 2010)
- *Assessment Protocol for Excellence in Public Health* (APEX/PH) (National Association of County and City Health Officials [NACCHO], 1991)
- *Logic Model* (W.K. Kellogg Foundation, 2004 and Weiss, C., & Wholey, J., n.d.). More information on this process can be found in the Weblinks section of this chapter.
- *Healthy Plan-It* (CDC, 2000)
- *Healthy People in Healthy Communities* (U.S. Department of Health and Human Services [USDHHS], 2001)
- *The Health Communication Model* (National Cancer Institute [NCI], 2002)
- *The Planning, Program Development, and Evaluation Model* (Timmreck, 2003)
- *MAP-IT* (USDHHS, 2011)
- *SWOT* (Strengths, Weaknesses, Opportunities, Threats) *Analysis*

PRECEDE-PROCEED

Currently, the best known planning model is **PRECEDE-PROCEED**. As its name implies, this model has two components. PRECEDE is an acronym that stands for *p*redisposing, *r*einforcing, and *e*nabling *c*onstructs in *e*ducational/*e*cological *d*iagnosis and *e*valuation. PROCEED stands for *p*olicy, *r*egulatory, and *o*rganizational *c*onstructs in *e*ducational and *e*nvironmental *d*evelopment (Green & Kreuter, 2005).

The PRECEDE-PROCEED model was developed over a period of 15 to 20 years. The PRE-CEDE framework was conceived in the early 1970s, whereas the PROCEED portion was developed in the early to mid-1980s. As shown in **Figure 4.11**, PRECEDE-PROCEED has eight phases. The first four phases, which make up the PRECEDE portion of the model, consist "of a series of planned assessments that generate information that will be used to guide subsequent decisions" (Green & Kreuter, 2005, p. 8). PROCEED also has four phases and "is marked by the strategic implementation of multiple actions based on what was learned from the assessments in the initial phase" (Green & Kreuter, 2005, p. 9).

At first glance, the PRECEDE-PROCEED model appears overly complicated. However, there is a logical sequence to the eight phases that outlines the health promotion planning process. The underlying approach of this model begins by identifying the desired outcome, then determines what causes it, and finally designs an intervention aimed at reaching the desired outcome. In other words, PRECEDE-PROCEED starts with the final consequences and works backward to the causes (McKenzie et al., 2013). **Table 4.4** provides an overview of the eight phases of this model.

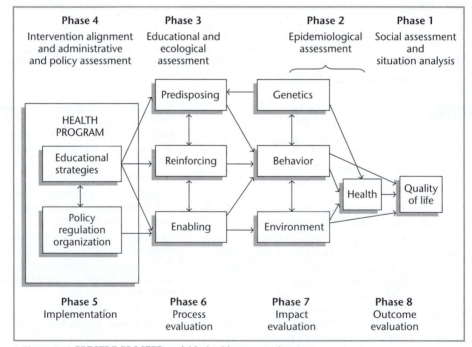

▲ **Figure 4.11** PRECEDE-PROCEED model for health program planning

Source: From Green, L. W., & Kreuter, M. W., *Health program planning: An educational and ecological approach*, 4th ed., p. 17, Fig 1.5. Copyright © 2005 The McGraw-Hill Companies, Inc. Reprinted by permission.

TABLE 4.4 **The eight phases of the PRECEDE-PROCEED model**

Phase 1	**Social assessment** is "the assessment in both objective and subjective terms of high-priority problems or aspirations for the common good, defined for a population by economic and social indicators and by individuals in terms of their quality of life" (p. G-8). **Situational analysis** is "the combination of social and epidemiological assessments of conditions, trends, and priorities with a preliminary scan of determinants, relevant policies, resources, organizational support, and regulations that might anticipate or permit action in advance of a more complete assessment of behavioral, environmental, educational, ecological, and administrative factors" (pp. G-7–8).
Phase 2	**Epidemiological assessment** is "the delineation of the extent, distribution, and causes of a health problem in a defined population" (p. G-3).
Phase 3	**Educational assessment** is "the delineation of factors that predispose, enable, and reinforce a specific behavior, or through behavior, environmental changes" (p. G-3), and **ecological assessment** is "a systematic assessment of factors in the social and physical environment that interact with behavior to produce health effects or quality-of-life outcomes" (p. G-3).
Phase 4a	**Intervention alignment** is matching appropriate strategies and interventions with projected changes and outcomes identified in earlier phases.
Phase 4b	**Administrative and policy assessment** is "an analysis of the policies, resources, and circumstances prevailing in an organizational situation to facilitate or hinder the development of the health program" (p. G-1).
Phase 5	**Implementation** is "the act of converting program objectives into actions through policy changes, regulation, and organization" (p. G-5).
Phase 6	**Process evaluation** is "the assessment of policies, materials, personnel, performance, quality of practice or services, and other inputs and implementation experiences" (p. G-6).
Phase 7	**Impact evaluation** is "the assessment of program effects on intermediate objectives including changes in predisposing, enabling, and reinforcing factors, as well as behavioral and environmental changes, and possibly health and social outcomes" (p. G-5).
Phase 8	**Outcome evaluation** is an "assessment of the effects of a program on its ultimate objectives, including changes in health and social benefits or quality of life" (p. G-6).

Source: From Green, L. W., & Kreuter, M. W., *Health program planning: An educational and ecological approach,* 4th ed. Copyright © 2005 The McGraw-Hill Companies, Inc. Reprinted by permission.

MATCH

MATCH is an acronym for Multilevel Approach To Community Health. This planning model (see **Figure 4.12**) was developed in the late 1980s (Simons-Morton, Simons-Morton, Parcel, & Bunker, 1988). Like the PRECEDE-PROCEED model, MATCH has also been used in a variety of settings. For example, several intervention handbooks created by the Centers for Disease Control and Prevention (CDC) used MATCH (Simons-Morton et al., 1995).

MATCH is a socio-ecological planning approach. It recognizes that intervention activities can and should be aimed at a variety of objectives and individuals. This approach is illustrated in Figure 4.12 by the various levels of influence.

The MATCH framework is recognized for emphasizing program implementation (Simons-Morton et al., 1995). "MATCH is designed to be applied when behavioral and environmental

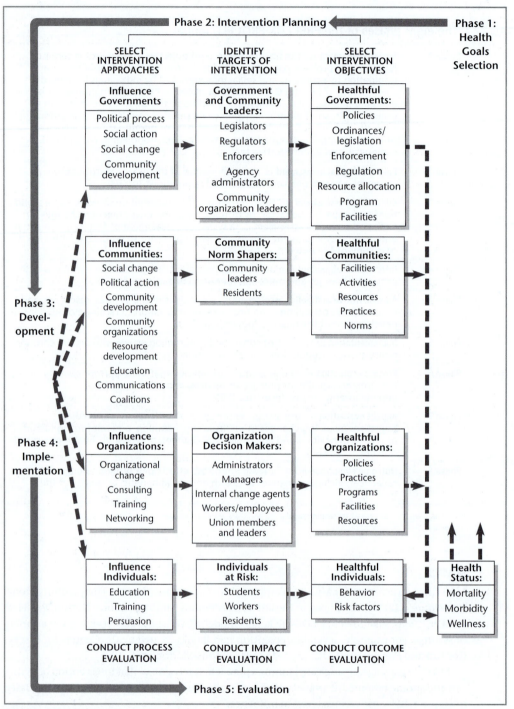

▲ **Figure 4.12** MATCH: Multilevel Approach To Community Health risk and protective factors for disease or injury are generally known and when general priorities for action have been determined, thus providing a convenient way to turn the corner from needs assessment and priority setting to the development of effective programs" (Simons-Morton et al., 1995, p. 155).

INTERVENTION MAPPING

Intervention mapping focuses on planning programs that are based on theory and evidence (Bartholomew et al., 2011). It also draws on multiple principles used in the PRECEDE-PROCEED and MATCH models.

Intervention mapping has six steps. The first step, *needs assessment*, includes two major components: (1) scientific, epidemiological, behavioral, and social analysis of a priority population or community; and (2) an effort to get to know and understand the character of the priority population (Bartholomew et al., 2011).

Step 2, *matrices of change objectives*, specifies who and what will change as a result of the intervention (Bartholomew et al., 2011). Although the identification of goals and objectives is included in all planning models, intervention mapping makes a unique contribution in how this is carried out. In this step, planners create a matrix of change objectives for the intervention. By doing so, planners can more clearly see who and what will change as a result of the intervention.

In Step 3, *theory-based methods and practical applications*, planners work to identify theory-based methods and practical applications that hold the greatest promise to change the health behavior(s) of individuals in the priority population. Although planners seek theory-based methods, they also ensure that practical applications are selected and that final applications match the change objectives from the matrices.

In Step 4, *program production*, planners create the intervention details and materials and protocol needed for the program's implementation. This step is based on the methods and applications identified in Step 3.

Step 5, *adoption and implementation*, is like Step 2 in that it includes the development of matrices. However, these matrices focus on adoption and implementation performance objectives (Bartholomew et al., 2011). In other words, instead of concentrating on who and what will change within the priority population, the focus is on what will be done by whom among planners or program partners.

The sixth, and last, step of this model is *evaluation planning*. In this step, planners decide if determinants were well specified, if strategies were appropriately matched to methods, what proportion of the priority population was reached, and whether or not implementation was complete and executed as planned (Bartholomew et al., 2011).

CDCynergy

CDCynergy, or **Cynergy** for short, is a health communication planning model developed in 1997 by the Office of Communication at the CDC. It was first issued in 1998 (Parvanta & Freimuth, 2000). Cynergy was developed primarily for the CDC public health professionals who had responsibilities for health communication. However, because of widespread interest in the model, the CDC made it available to other health professionals in a variety of health education/promotion settings. Currently, CDCynergy is considered public domain, which means restrictions are not placed on copying or general use.

The basic edition of Cynergy presents a general methodology for health communication planning, a step-by-step guide, a reference library, and links to templates that allow tailored plans to be created (CDC & USDHHS, 2003). Cynergy uses six phases involving multiple steps to help planners: acquire a thorough understanding of a health problem and whom it affects; explore a wide range of possible intervention strategies for influencing the problem; systematically select the intervention strategies that show the most promise; understand the role communication can play in planning, implementing, and evaluating selected strategies; and develop a comprehensive communication plan (CDC & USDHHS, 2003). **Table 4.5** displays the six sequential, yet interrelated, phases, which are designed to build on the previous phases and prepare program planners for subsequent phases. Completion of these phases will lead to a strategic communication plan that is both science and audience based.

In addition to the basic edition of Cynergy, which is available in a Web version, CDC and its partners have produced content-specific editions of Cynergy to meet the particular needs of health education specialists addressing various health problems. There are content-specific editions for American Indian/Alaska Native Diabetes, Cardiovascular Disease, Diabetes, Emergency Risk Communication, Immunizations, Micronutrients, Social Marketing, STD Prevention, and Tobacco Prevention and Control (see Weblinks at the end of this chapter).

TABLE 4.5 *CDCynergy lite* **(an abridged version of the CDCynergy health communication model)**

Phase 1: Describe Problem

- Identify and define health problem(s) that may be addressed by your program interventions.
- Examine and/or conduct necessary research to describe the problem(s).
- Assess factors and variables that can affect the project's direction, including strengths, weaknesses, opportunities, and threats (SWOT).

Phase 2: Analyze Problem

- List causes of each problem you plan to address.
- Develop goals for each problem.
- Consider strengths, weaknesses, opportunities, threats, and ethics of health (1) engineering, (2) communication/education, (3) policy/enforcement, and (4) community service intervention options.
- Select the types of intervention(s) that should be used to address the problem(s).

Phase 3: Plan Intervention

- Decide whether communication is needed as a dominant intervention or as support for other intervention(s).
- If communication is used as a dominant intervention, list possible audiences.
  - If communication is to be used to support Community Services, Engineering, and/or Policy/Enforcement interventions, list possible audiences to be reached in support of each selected intervention.
- Conduct necessary audience research to segment intended audiences.
- Select audience segment(s) and write communication objectives for each audience segment.
- Write a creative brief to provide guidance in selecting appropriate concepts or messages, settings, activities, and materials.

TABLE 4.5 *continued*

Phase 4: Develop Intervention

- Develop and test concepts, messages, settings, channel-specific activities, and materials with intended audiences.
- Finalize and briefly summarize a communication implementation plan. The plan should include
  - Background and justification, including SWOT and ethics analyses
  - Audiences
  - Communication objectives
  - Messages
  - Settings and channels for conveying your messages
  - Activities (including tactics, materials, and other methods)
  - Available partners and resources
  - Tasks and timeline (including persons responsible for each task, date for completion of each task, resources required to deliver each task, and points at which progress will be checked)
  - Internal and external communication plan
  - Budget
- Produce materials for dissemination.

Phase 5: Plan Evaluation

- Determine stakeholder information needs.
- Decide which types of evaluation (e.g., implementation, reach, effects) are needed to satisfy stakeholder information needs.
- Identify sources of information and select data collection methods.
- Formulate an evaluation design that illustrates how methods will be applied to gather credible information.
- Develop a data analysis and reporting plan.
- Finalize and briefly summarize an evaluation implementation plan. The plan should include
  - Stakeholder questions
  - Intervention standards
  - Evaluation methods and design
  - Data analysis and reporting
  - Tasks and timeline (including persons responsible for each task, date for completion of each task, resources required to deliver each task, and points at which progress will be checked)
  - Internal and external communication plan
  - Budget

Phase 6: Implement Plan

- Integrate, execute, and manage communication and evaluation plans.
- Document feedback and lessons learned.
- Modify program components based on feedback.
- Disseminate lessons learned and evaluation findings.

Source: Centers for Disease Control and Prevention (CDC), U.S. Department of Health and Human Services (USDHHS). 2003. *CDCynergy 3.0: Your guide to effective health communication (CD-ROM Version 3.0)*. Atlanta: Author.

SMART

Social marketing has been defined as "the application of commercial marketing technologies to the analysis, planning, execution, and evaluation of programs designed to influence the voluntary behavior of target audiences in order to improve their personal welfare and that of their society" (Andreasen, 1995, p. 7). This process offers benefits the audience wants, reduces barriers the audience faces, and uses persuasion to influence intentions to act favorably (Albrecht, 1997). The concept of social marketing is more than 30 years old, but its application to health education/promotion is much more recent (McDermott, 2000).

Even though the use of social marketing is relatively new in health education/promotion, several different authors (Andreasen, 1995; Bryant, 1998; Walsh, Rudd, Moeykens, & Moloney, 1993) have presented planning processes, models, or frameworks based on social marketing. The Social Marketing Assessment and Response Tool **(SMART)** is a social marketing planning framework developed by Neiger and Thackeray (1998) and influenced primarily by Walsh and colleagues (1993). It is presented here because it provides a composite of other social marketing models and because it has been used from start to finish on multiple occasions in several social marketing interventions (Neiger & Thackeray, 2002).

SMART is composed of seven phases (see **Table 4.6**). "Like other social marketing planning frameworks, the central focus of SMART is consumers. The heart of this model, composed of Phases 2 through 4, pertains to acquiring a broad understanding of the consumers who will be the recipients of a program and its interventions. These three phases seek to understand consumers before interventions are even developed or implemented. Though these phases (2–4) are displayed in linear fashion . . . they are typically performed simultaneously with members of the priority population" (McKenzie et al., 2013, p. 60).

MAPP

MAPP is an acronym for Mobilizing for Action through Planning and Partnerships. It is a relatively new planning model created by the National Association of County and City Health Officials (NACCHO) to assist local health departments (LHDs) at the city or county level with planning. This model blends many of the strengths of the five planning models already presented in this chapter. The MAPP approach is designed to improve health and quality of life by mobilizing partnerships and taking strategic action (NACCHO, 2001).

MAPP is composed of multiple steps within six phases (see **Figure 4.13**). In the first phase of MAPP, Organize for Success and Partnership Development, planners assess whether or not the MAPP process is timely, appropriate, and even possible. This involves assessing resources, including funding, personnel, and general interest of community members. If resources are not in place, the process is delayed. If resources are sufficient, the following work groups are created: (1) a core support team, which prepares most, if not all, of the material needed for the process; (2) the MAPP Committee, composed of key sponsors from the community who provide legitimacy and resources, and stakeholders who guide and oversee the process; and (3) the community itself, which provides input, representation, and decision making.

In Phase 2, Visioning, the community is guided through a process that results in a shared vision—what the ideal future looks like—and common values—principles and beliefs that will guide the remainder of the planning process (NACCHO, 2001). This phase is usually handled by a facilitator and involves anywhere from 50 to 100 participants, including the advisory committee, the MAPP committee, and key community leaders.

TABLE 4.6 **The SMART model**

Phase 1: Preliminary Planning

- Identify a health problem and name it in terms of behavior.
- Develop general goals.
- Outline preliminary plans for evaluation.
- Project program costs.

Phase 2: Consumer Analysis

- Segment and identify the priority population.
- Identify formative research methods.
- Identify consumer wants, needs, and preferences.
- Develop preliminary ideas for preferred interventions.

Phase 3: Market Analysis

- Establish and define the market mix (4Ps).
- Assess the market to identify competitors (behaviors, messages, programs, etc.), allies (support systems, resources, etc.), and partners.

Phase 4: Channel Analysis

- Identify appropriate communication messages, strategies, and channels.
- Determine how channels should be used.
- Assess options for program distribution.
- Identify communication roles for program partners.

Phase 5: Develop Interventions, Materials, and Pretest

- Develop program interventions and materials using information collected in consumer, market, and channel analyses.
- Interpret the marketing mix into a strategy that represents exchange and societal good.
- Pretest and refine the program.

Phase 6: Implementation

- Communicate with partners and clarify involvement.
- Activate communication and distribution strategies.
- Document procedures and compare progress to timelines.
- Refine the program.

Phase 7: Evaluation

- Assess the degree to which the priority population is receiving the program.
- Assess the immediate impact on the priority population and refine the program as necessary.
- Ensure that program delivery is consistent with established protocol.
- Analyze changes in the priority population.

Source: Adapted from Walsh, R. E., et al. (1993). "Social marketing for public health," *Health Affairs 12* (2), 104–119; and adapted from Neiger, B. L., & Thackeray, R. (1998). "Social marketing: Making public health sense." Paper presented at the annual meeting of the Utah Public Health Association, Provo, UT.

The strength and defining characteristic of MAPP is found in Phase 3, the Four MAPP Assessments. The four assessments include (1) the community themes and strengths assessment (community or consumer opinion), (2) the local public health system assessment (general capacity of the local public health system), (3) the community health status assessment (measurement of the health of the community by use of epidemiological data), and (4) the

▶ **Figure 4.13** Mobilizing for Action through Planning and Partnerships (MAPP) model

Source: National Association of County and City Health Officials, "Mobilizing for Action through Planning and Partnerships (MAPP) Model" from http://www.naccho.org/topics/infrastructure/mapp/upload/MAPP_Handbook_fnl.pdf. Reprinted by permission.

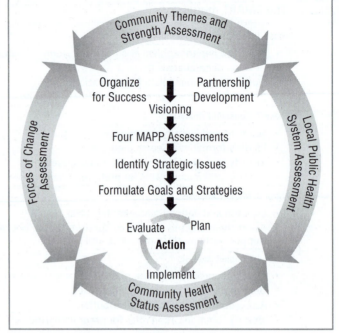

forces of change assessment (forces such as legislation, technology, and other environmental or social phenomena that do or will impact the community) (McKenzie et al., 2013). The four assessments help identify the gaps that exist between current status in the community and the vision identified in Phase 2, as well as the strategic direction for goals and strategies (NACCHO, 2001).

In Phase 4, Identify Strategic Issues, a prioritized list of the issues facing the health of the community is developed. Only issues that jeopardize the vision and values of the community are considered. Important tasks in this phase include considering what would happen if certain issues are not addressed, understanding why an issue is strategic, consolidating overlapping issues, and identifying a prioritized list (McKenzie et al., 2013).

In Phase 5, Formulate Goals and Strategies, the goals and strategies to reach the vision are created. Finally, Phase 6, The Action Cycle, is similar to implementation and evaluation phases in other planning models. In this phase, implementation details are considered, evaluation plans are developed, and plans for disseminating results are made (NACCHO, 2001).

Generalized Model (GM)

As seen in the planning models presented so far, there are various approaches and frameworks on which to develop a program. Each model seems to have its own characteristics, whether it is the terminology used (e.g., predisposing, enabling, and reinforcing or analyzing a problem or consumer analysis), the number of components (e.g., eight phases versus six steps), or the progression through the phases or steps (e.g., circular, linear, or starting with the desired end and working backward). In other words, there are many ways to get

▲ **Figure 4.14** Generalized Model

Source: From McKenzie, J. F., Neiger, B. L., & Thackery, R., *Planning, implementing and evaluating health promotion programs: A primer*, 6th ed., p. 45, Fig. 3.1. Copyright © 2013. Reproduced by permission of Pearson, Boston, MA.

from point A to point B. However, each of the models previously presented revolves around the five primary tasks incorporated in the **Generalized Model** (McKenzie et al., 2013). These five tasks are

1. Assessing needs
2. Setting goals and objectives
3. Developing interventions
4. Implementing interventions
5. Evaluating results (see **Figure 4.14**)

"In addition, pre-planning is a quasi-step in the model but is not included formally since it involves actions that occur before planning technically begins" (McKenzie et al., 2013, p. 44). These tasks plus the quasi-step of pre-planning define planning and evaluation at its core.

To better understand the planning process in health education/promotion and the various models presented, consider the following scenario. A health education specialist was hired to develop health education/promotion programs in a corporate setting. She began her work with the quasi-step of pre-planning by trying to find out as much as possible about the "community" of this corporate setting and get those in the priority population involved in the program planning process. She did this by reading all the material she could find about the company. She also spent time talking with various individuals and subgroups in the company (i.e., new employees, longtime employees, management, clerical staff, labor representatives, etc.) to find out what they wanted from a health education/promotion program. In addition, she reviewed old documents of the company (i.e., health insurance records, labor agreements, written history of the company, etc.). As part of this background work, she formed a program planning committee with representation from the various subgroups of the workforce.

With the help of the planning committee, the health education/promotion specialist was ready to assess the needs of the priority population. She did this by reviewing the relevant literature, examining company health insurance claims, conducting a survey of employees, and holding focus groups with selected employees. As a result of the needs assessment, she was able to identify a target health problem. In this company, the problem was a higher than expected number of breast cancer cases in the priority population. This was a result in part of (1) the limited knowledge of employees about breast cancer, (2) the limited number of employees conducting breast self-examination (BSE), and (3) the low number of employees having mammograms on a regular basis.

With an understanding of the needs of the priority population, the health education specialist created specific objectives to increase the (1) employees' knowledge of breast cancer from baseline to after program participation, (2) number of women receiving mammograms by 30 percent, and (3) number of women reporting monthly BSE by 50 percent. Using these objectives, she planned multiple intervention activities:

1. An information sheet on the importance of BSE and mammography, for distribution with employee paychecks
2. A mobile mammography van on site every other month
3. Plastic BSE reminder cards, suitable for hanging from a showerhead, for distribution to all female employees
4. An article in the company newsletter covering the company's high rate of breast cancer and the new program to help women reduce their risk
5. Posters and pamphlets from the American Cancer Society in the company's lunchroom

Next, all of the listed intervention activities were carried out. Finally, the health education specialist completed an evaluation to determine if there was an increase in knowledge, mammograms, and monthly BSE. As can be seen from this scenario, health education/ promotion involves careful, systematic planning to achieve successful programs.

▶ Summary

Health education/promotion is a multidisciplinary profession that has evolved from the theory and practice of other biological, behavioral, sociological, and health science disciplines. Many of the theories and models used in health education/promotion also have evolved from these other disciplines. This chapter presented an overview of the theoretical foundations and planning models of health education/promotion. Readers were introduced to the definitions of *theory, concept, construct, variable*, and *model*. A rationale was also provided to explain why it is important that health education specialists use theory in their work. Readers were then introduced to eleven of the behavior change theories that health education specialists use in their work. These theories were presented within the socio-ecological approach, which incorporates the seven levels of influence. There was also a distinction made between continuum theories and stage theories. And finally, overviews of seven planning models were provided.

Review Questions

1. Define each of the following and explain how they relate to each other.
   - *Theory*
   - *Concept*
   - *Construct*
   - *Variable*
   - *Model*

2. Why is it important to use theory in the practice of health education/promotion?

3. What are behavior change theories?

4. What are the seven levels of influence within the socio-ecological approach? How do they relate to behavior change theories?

5. Identify the eleven theories presented in this chapter that focus on health behavior change. Briefly describe each of the theories and name their components.

6. What is the difference between continuum theories and stage theories?

7. Why is it important that health education specialists have a good understanding of stage models?

8. What are three advantages to using a planning model when preparing to conduct a health promotion intervention?

9. Name the seven planning models presented in this chapter and list one distinguishing characteristic of each.

10. Of the seven planning models presented in this chapter, which one is best known? Name the phases of this model.

 # Case Study

Sally graduated a year ago with a bachelor's degree in health education. She felt very fortunate to "beat out" 10 interviewees for the health education specialist position at the Ada County Health Department. Though the health department has a good reputation throughout the state, it turns out that Sally is the only person on the staff hired to do health education.

Sally's supervisor, Rick Shaw, is the Environmental Health Coordinator for the health department. Shaw has worked for the department for about 35 years. He holds a bachelor's degree from the same university Sally graduated from. However, Shaw received his general studies degree in health and fitness before the university formed new departments and implemented new majors including the current community/public health education major.

Throughout Sally's tenure with the health department, she and Rick have had a good working relationship. However, when asked to plan a tobacco cessation program for a group of teenagers in the county, Sally ran into a situation that caused her some concern. After conducting a needs assessment and writing the program goals and objectives, she could not decide which behavior change theory to use to plan her intervention so she decided to seek her supervisor's advice. When she asked Shaw what theory or model he would recommend, he responded rather dramatically, "Theory-shmeary, you don't need to use that stuff; just skip the theory part and get to work planning the intervention. Remember, this program needs to be up and running by the end of the month."

Based on this short conversation with her supervisor, Sally was left unsure as to how to proceed. During her undergraduate preparation at the university, Sally was told time and time again to "never plan an intervention that was not based on theory." Sally does not want to upset her supervisor, but she also knows that her program should be grounded in theory. What are Sally's options at this point? How should she proceed? What process would you use to address this dilemma?

 ## Critical Thinking Questions

1. This chapter presented a number of different theories focusing on health behavior change. If you were trying to help a friend stop smoking, at the friend's request, what behavior change theory would you use to develop the intervention to help your friend? Defend why you selected this theory and explain how you would apply each of the constructs.

2. You have been invited by the Nelson Corporation to interview for a newly created position in the company as a health education specialist. The position has been described as one that will focus on helping employees become more healthy by modifying or changing selected health behaviors. As a part of the interview, the director of human resources asks you this question: "Of all the theories related to health education/ promotion you studied in your college courses, which one do you think will have the greatest application to your work here at the Nelson Corporation?" Defend your response.

3. What would you say to a person who asked you, "Tell me how the socio-ecological approach applies to changing health behavior?"

Activities

1. Interview a practicing health education specialist, asking about the theories and models the person has used in planning and implementing health education/promotion programs. Ask why those theories and models were used. Also, find out if the health education specialist has run into any problems trying to use the theories and models. Summarize the interview in a one-page paper.

2. Choosing and selecting from the components found in the planning models, create your own model. Draw a diagram of your model and, in two paragraphs, explain why you have included the components you did.

3. Choose a health behavior. Conduct a literature search to determine if the behavior you chose has been researched using one of the behavior change theories in the chapter.

Weblinks

1. http://www.naccho.org

   National Association of County and City Health Officials

   At this Web site, the MAPP model is comprehensively presented and explained (search for "MAPP" on the homepage). To get access to the specifics, you have to register. There is no cost to do so.

2. http://www.healthypeople.gov/2020

   Healthy People

   Choose 'Social Determinants of Health Interventions and Resources' under the 'Tools on Healthy People.gov' category. This links the user to tools and strategies to help communities reach their health objectives.

3. http://www.cdc.gov

   CDCynergy

   Search the CDC homepage for "CDCynergy Health Communication" for an overview of *CDCynergy*, news and updates, information on all editions, current campaigns, practice areas, and resources. It also provides a link to the Web version of the original edition.

4. http://www.uri.edu

   Cancer Prevention Research Center (CPRC), University of Rhode Island

   Search the university's homepage for the Cancer Prevention Research Center, which is the home of the Transtheoretical Model of Change. Information about the model as well as measures that can be used to "stage" a person can be found at this site.

5. http://people.umass.edu/aizen/tpb.html

   Theory of Planned Behavior

   This is a Web page of Icek Ajzen, creator of the Theory of Planned Behavior. Information about the theory as well as example measures that can be used to measure the constructs of the theory can be found at this site.

6. http://www.cancer.gov

   National Cancer Institute (NCI)

   The National Cancer Institute presents the primer *Theory at a Glance: A Guide for Health Promotion Practice*. This volume explains why theories and models are important. It also describes how to use theory. Explanations of several behavior change theories, as well as a couple of program planning models, are included. (Find it by searching at the NCI's homepage.)

7. http://www.cancer.gov/publications/health-communication/pink-book.pdf

   National Cancer Institute (NCI)

   This is the site where the entire 2002 edition of *Making Health Communication Programs Work*, also called the Pink Book, can be downloaded.

8. http://www.smartgivers.org/uploads/logicmodelguidepdf.pdf

   W.K. Kellogg Foundation

   This site provides an excellent tutorial workbook for creating "logic models" as a part of a health promotion program plan. Examples are included. The workbook can be downloaded.

▷

References

Ajzen, I. (2006). *Theory of Planned Behavior Diagram.* Retrieved May 19, 2013, from http://www.people.umass.edu/aizen/index.html.

Albrecht, T. L. (1997). Defining social marketing: Twenty five years later. *Social Marketing Quarterly, 3,* 21–23.

Andreasen, A. (1995). *Marketing sound change: Changing behavior to promote health, social development, and the environment.* San Francisco: Jossey-Bass.

Bandura, A. (1977). *Social learning theory.* Englewood Cliffs, NJ: Prentice-Hall.

Bandura, A. (1986). *Social foundations of thought and action.* Englewood Cliffs, NJ: Prentice-Hall.

Barnes, J. A. (1954). Class and committees in a Norwegian island parish. *Human Relations, 7,* 39–58.

Bartholomew, L. K., Parcel, G. S., Kok, G., Gottlieb, N. H., & Fernández, M. E. (2011). *Planning health promotion programs: An intervention mapping approach* (3rd ed.). San Francisco: Jossey-Bass.

Bates, I. J., & Winder, A. E. (1984). *Introduction to health education.* Palo Alto, CA: Mayfield.

Bronfenbrenner, U. (1974). Developmental research, public policy, and the ecology of childhood. (1974). *Child Development, 45* (1), 1–5.

Bronfenbrenner, U. (1979). *The ecology of human development: Experiments by nature and design.* Cambridge, MA: Harvard University Press.

Bryant, C. (1998). *Social marketing: A tool for excellence.* Eighth annual conference on social marketing in public health. Clearwater Beach, FL.

Centers for Disease Control and Prevention (CDC). (2000). *Healthy plan-it: A tool for planning and managing public health programs. Sustainable Management Development Program.* Atlanta, GA: Author.

Centers for Disease Control and Prevention (CDC). (2010). Community Assessment aNd Group Evaluation: the CHANGE Tool. Retrieved on May 5, 2016, from http://www.cdc.gov/nccdphp/dch/programs/healthycommunitiesprogram/tools/change.htm

Centers for Disease Control and Prevention (CDC), U.S. Department of Health and Human Services (USDHHS). (2003). *CDCynergy 3.0: Your guide to effective health communication* (CD-ROM Version 3.0). Atlanta, GA: Author.

Centers for Disease Control and Prevention (CDC), U.S. Department of Health and Human Services (USDHHS). (n.d.). *Planned approach to community health: Guide for local coordinators.* Atlanta, GA: Author.

Champion, V. L., & Skinner, C. S. (2008). The health belief model. In K. Glanz, B. K. Rimer, & K. Viswanath (Eds.), *Health behavior and health education: Theory, research, and practice* (4th ed., pp. 45–65). San Francisco: Jossey-Bass.

Chaplin, J. P., & Krawiec, T. S. (1979). *Systems and theories of psychology* (4th ed.). New York: Holt, Rinehart & Winston.

Crosby, R. A., Kegler, M. C., & DiClemente, R. J. (2009). Theory in health promotion practice and research. In R. J. DiClemente, R. A. Crosby, & M. C. Kegler (Eds.), *Emerging theories in health promotion practice and research* (2nd ed., pp. 4–17). San Francisco: Jossey-Bass.

Crosby, R. A., Salazar, L. F., & DiClemente, R. J. (2013a). How theory informs health promotion and public health practice. In R. J. DiClemente, L. F. Salazar, & R. A. Crosby, *Health behavior theory for public health: Principles, foundations, and application* (pp. 27–44). Burlington, MA: Jones & Bartlett Learning.

Crosby, R. A., Salazar, L. F., & DiClemente, R. J. (2013b). Social cognitive theory applied to health behavior. In R. J. DiClemente, L. F. Salazar, & R. A. Crosby, *Health behavior theory for public health: Principles, foundations, and application* (pp. 163–185). Burlington, MA: Jones & Bartlett Learning.

Demerritt, P. (2013). Cigarette culture changing in America and on campus. *The Signal at Georgia State University,* May. Retrieved on May 3, 2016, from http://georgiastatesignal.com/cigarette-culture-changing-in-america-and-on-campus/

DiClemente, R. J., Crosby, R. A., & Kegler, M. (2009). *Emerging theories in health promotion practice and research* (2nd ed.). San Francisco: Jossey-Bass.

DiClemente, R. J., Redding, C. A., Crosby, R. A., & Salazar, L. F. (2013). Stage models for health promotion. In R. J. DiClemente, L. F. Salazar, & R. A. Crosby, *Health behavior theory for public health: Principles, foundations, and application* (pp. 105–129). Burlington, MA: Jones & Bartlett Learning.

DiClemente, R. J., Salazar, L. F., & Crosby, R. A. (2013). *Health behavior theory for public health: Principles, foundations, and applications.* Burlington, MA: Jones & Bartlett Learning.

Edberg, M. (2007). *Essentials of health behavior: Social and behavioral theory in public health.* Sudbury, MA: Jones & Bartlett.

Edberg, M. (2015). *Essentials of health behavior: Social and behavioral theory in public health* (2nd ed.). Burlington, MA: Jones & Bartlett Learning.

Edwards, R. W., Jumper-Thurman, P., Plested, B. A., Oetting, E. R., & Swanson, L. (2000). Community readiness: Research to practice. *Journal of Community Psychology, 28* (3), 291–307.

Fishbein, M., & Ajzen, I. (1975). *Belief, attitude, intention and behavior: An introduction to theory and research.* Reading, MA: Addison-Wesley.

Fisher, J. D., & Fisher, W. A. (1992). Changing AIDS risk behavior. *Psychological Bulletin, 111*, 455–474.

Fisher, J. D., Fisher, W. A., & Shuper, P. A. (2009). The informational-motivation-behavioral skills model of HIV preventive behavior. In R. J. DiClemente, R. A. Crosby, & M. C. Kegler (Eds.). *Emerging theories in health promotion practice and research* (2nd ed., pp. 21–63). San Francisco: Jossey-Bass.

Gittell, R., & Vidal, A. (1998). *Community organizing: Building social capital as a development strategy.* Thousand Oaks, CA: Sage.

Glanz, K., & Rimer, B. K. (1995). *Theory at a glance: A guide for health promotion practice* (NIH publication no. 95–3896). Bethesda, MD: National Institutes of Health, National Cancer Institute.

Glanz, K., Rimer, B. K., & Viswanath, K. (Eds.). (2008a). *Health behavior and health education: Theory, research, and practice* (4th ed.). San Francisco: Jossey-Bass.

Glanz, K., Rimer, B. K., & Viswanath, K. (2008b). Theory, research, and practice in health behavior and health education. In K. Glanz, B. K. Rimer, & K. Viswanath (Eds.), *Health behavior and health education: Theory, research, and practice* (4th ed., pp. 23–40). San Francisco: Jossey-Bass.

Goodson, P. (2010). *Theory in health promotion research and practice: Thinking outside the box.* Sudbury, MA: Jones & Bartlett.

Gore, T. D., & Bracker, C. C. (2005). Testing the theoretical design of a health risk message: Re-examining major tenants of the Extended Parallel Processing Model. *Health Education & Behavior, 32* (1), 27–41.

Green, L. W., Glanz, K., Hochbaum, G. M., Kok, G., Kreuter, M. W., et al. (1994). Can we build on, or must we replace, the theories and models in health education? *Health Education Research, 9* (3), 397–404.

Green, L. W., & Kreuter, M. W. (2005). *Health program planning: An educational and ecological approach* (4th ed.). Boston, MA: McGraw-Hill.

Hayden, J. (2009). *Introduction to health behavior theory.* Sudbury, MA: Jones & Bartlett.

Hayden, J. (2014). *Introduction to health behavior theory* (2nd ed.). Burlington, MA: Jones & Bartlett Learning.

Heaney, C. A., & Israel, B. A. (2008). Social networks and social support. In K. Glanz, B. K. Rimer, & K. Viswanath (Eds.), *Health behavior and health education: Theory, research, and practice* (4th ed., pp. 189–210). San Francisco: Jossey-Bass.

Institute of Medicine (IOM). (2001). *Health and behavior: The interplay of biological, behavioral, and societal influences.* Washington, DC: National Academy of Sciences.

Kawachi, I., Kennedy, B. P., Lochner, K., & Prothrow-Stith, D. (1997). Social capital, income, equality, and mortality. *American Journal of Public Health, 87* (9), 1491–1497.

Kerlinger, F. N. (1986). *Foundations of behavioral research* (3rd ed.). Austin: Holt, Rinehart & Winston.

Luszczynska, A., & Sutton, S. (2005). Attitudes and expectations. In J. Kerr, R. Weikunat, & M. Moretti (Eds.), *ABC of behavior change: A guide to successful disease prevention and health promotion* (pp. 71–84). Edinburgh: Elsevier.

Mann, T. Tomiyama, A. J., Westling. E., Lew. A., Samuels, B., & Chatman, J. (2007). Medicare's search for effective obesity treatments: Diets are not the answer. *American Psychologist, 62* (3), 220–233.

McAlister, A. L., Perry, C. L., & Parcel, G. S. (2008). How individual, environments, and health behaviors interact: Social cognitive theory. In K. Glanz, B. K. Rimer, & K. Viswanath (Eds.), *Health behavior and health education: Theory, research, and practice* (4th ed., pp. 169–188). San Francisco: Jossey-Bass.

McDermott, R. J. (2000). Social marketing: A tool for health education. *American Journal of Health Behavior, 24* (1), 6–10.

McKenzie, J. F., Neiger, B. L., & Thackeray, R. (2013). *Planning, implementing, and evaluating health promotion programs: A primer* (6th ed.). Boston: Pearson.

McLeroy, K. R., Bibeau, D., Steckler, A., & Glanz, K. (1988). An ecological perspective for health promotion programs. *Health Education Quarterly, 15* (4), 351–378.

Minkler, M., Thompson, M., Bell, J. & Rose, K. (2001). Contributions of community involvement to organizational level empowerment: The federal Healthy Start experience. *Health Education & Behavior, 28* (6), 283–307.

Minkler, M., & Wallerstein, N. (2005). Improving health through community organization and community building: A health education perspective. In M. Minkler (Ed.), *Community organizing and community building for health* (2nd ed., pp. 26–50). New Brunswick, NJ: Rutgers University Press.

National Association of County and City Health Officials (NACCHO). (1991). *APEX/PH, Assessment protocol for excellence in public health.* Washington, DC: Author.

National Association of County and City Health Officials (NACCHO). (2001). *Mobilizing for Action through Planning and Partnerships (MAPP).* Washington, DC: Author.

National Cancer Institute (NCI). (2002). *Making health communication programs work* (NIH Publication No. 02-5145). Washington, DC: U.S. Department of Health and Human Services (USDHHS).

Neiger, B. L., & Thackeray R. (1998). *Social marketing: Making public health sense.* Paper presented at the annual meeting of the Utah Public Health Association. Provo, UT.

Neiger, B. L., & Thackeray, R. (2002). Application of the SMART model in two successful social marketing campaigns. *American Journal of Health Education, 33,* 291–293.

Parvanta, C. F., & Freimuth, V. (2000). Health communication at the Centers for Disease Control and Prevention. *American Journal of Health Behavior, 24* (1), 18–25.

Patton, R. P., Corry, J. M., Gettman, L. R., & Graff, J. S. (1986). *Implementing health/ fitness programs.* Champaign, IL: Human Kinetics.

Petty, R. E., Barden, J., & Wheeler, S. C. (2009). The elaboration likelihood model of persuasion: Developing health promotions for sustained behavioral change. In R. J. DiClemente, R. A. Crosby, & M. C. Kegler (Eds.), *Emerging theories in health promotion practice and research* (2nd ed., pp. 185–214). San Francisco: Jossey-Bass.

Petty, R. E., & Cacioppo, J. T. (1986). The elaboration likelihood model of persuasion. In L. Berkowitz (Ed.). *Advances in experimental social psychology* (Vol. 19, pp. 123–205). New York: Academic Press.

Prochaska, J. (2005). Stages of change, readiness, and motivation. In J. Kerr, R. Weitkunat, & M. Moretti (Eds.), *ABC of behavior change: A guide to successful disease prevention and health promotion* (pp. 111–123). Edinburgh: Elsevier.

Prochaska, J. O. (1979). *Systems of psychotherapy: A transtheoretical analysis.* Homewood, IL: Dorsey Press.

Prochaska, J. O., & DiClemente, C. C. (1983). Stages and processes of self-change of smoking: Toward an integrative model of change. *Journal of Consulting and Clinical Psychology, 51* (3), 390–395.

Prochaska, J. O., Johnson, S., & Lee, P. (1998). The transtheoretical model of behavior change. In S. A. Shumaker, E. B. Schron, J. K. Ockene, & W. L. McBee (Eds.), *The handbook of health behavior change* (2nd ed., pp. 59–84). New York: Springer Publishing Company.

Prochaska, J. O, Redding, C. A., & Evers, K. E. (2008). The transtheoretical model and stages of change. In K. Glanz, B. K. Rimer, & K. Viswanath (Eds.), *Health behavior and health education: Theory, research, and practice* (4th ed., pp. 97–121). San Francisco: Jossey-Bass.

Prochaska, J. O., Redding, C. A., Harlow, L. L., Rossi, J. S., & Velicer, W. F. (1994). The transtheoretical model of change and HIV prevention: A review. *Health Education Quarterly, 24* (4), 471–486.

Putman, R. D. (1995). Bowling alone: America's declining social capital. *Journal of Democracy, 6* (1), 65–78.

Redding, C. A., Rossi, J. S., Rossi, S. R., Velicer, W. F., & Prochaska, J. O. (1999). Health behavior models. In G. C. Hyner, K. W. Peterson, J. W. Travis, J. E. Dewey, J. J. Foerster, & E. M. Framer (Eds.), *SPM handbook of health assessment tools* (pp. 83–93). Pittsburgh: The Society of Prospective Medicine.

Rimer, B. K., & Glanz, K. (2005). *Theory at a glance: A guide for health promotion practice* (2nd ed.). [NIH Pub. No. 05-3896]. Washington, DC: National Cancer Institute.

Rogers, E. M. (2003). *Diffusion of innovations* (5th ed.). New York: Free Press.

Rogers, R. W. (1983). Cognitive and physiological processes in fear-based attitude change: A revised theory of protection motivation. In J. Caccioppo & R. Petty (Eds.), *Social psychophysiology: A sourcebook* (pp. 153–176). New York: Guilford.

Rogers, R. W. (1975). A protection motivation theory of fear appeals and attitude change. *Journal of Psychology, 91,* 93–114.

Rosenstock, I. M. (1966). Why people use health services. *Milbank Memorial Fund Quarterly, 44,* 94–124.

Rosenstock, I. M., Strecher, V. J., & Becker, M. H. (1988). Social learning theory and the health belief model. *Health Education Quarterly, 15* (2), 175–183.

Ross, H. S., & Mico, P. R. (1980). *Theory and practice in health education.* San Francisco: Mayfield.

Rotter, J. B. (1954). *Social learning and clinical psychology.* New York: Prentice-Hall.

Salazar, L. F., Crosby, R. A., & DiClemente, R. J. (2013). Health behavior in context of the "new" public health. In R. J. DiClemente, L. F. Salazar, & R. A. Crosby. *Health behavior theory for public health: Principles, foundations, and applications* (pp. 3–26). Burlington, MA: Jones & Bartlett Learning.

Sharma, M., & Romas, J. A. (2012). *Theoretical foundations of health education and health promotion* (2nd ed.). Sudbury, MA: Jones & Bartlett.

Simons-Morton, B. G., Greene, W. H., & Gottlieb, N. H. (1995). *Introduction to health education and health promotion* (2nd ed.). Prospect Hts., IL: Waveland Press, Inc.

Simons-Morton, B. G., McLeroy, K. R., & Wendel, M. L. (2012). *Behavior theory in health promotion practice and research.* Burlington, MA: Jones & Bartlett Learning.

Simons-Morton, D. G., Simons-Morton, B. G., Parcel, G. S., & Bunker, J. F. (1988). Influencing personal and environmental conditions for community health: A multilevel intervention model. *Family and Community Health, 1* (2), 25–35.

Spencer, L., Adams, T. B., Malone, S., Roy, L., & Yost, E. (2006). Applying the transtheoretical model to exercise: A systematic and comprehensive review of the literature. *Health Promotion Practice, 7* (4), 428–443.

Street, D. A., Hopkins, K. & Olson, S. (2002). From discovery to delivery: Injury prevention at CDC. *Health Promotion Practice, 4* (2), 98–103.

Sullivan, D. (1973). Model for comprehensive, systematic program development in health education. *Health Education Report, 1* (1), (November/December), 4–5.

Timmreck, T. C. (2003). *Planning, program development, and evaluation* (2nd ed.). Boston: Jones & Bartlett.

Timmreck, T. C., Cole, G. E., James, G., & Butterworth, D. D. (2010). Health education and health promotion: A look at the jungle of supportive fields, philosophies, and theoretical foundations. In J. M. Black, S. Furney, H. M. Graf, & A. E. Nolt (Eds.), *Philosophical foundations of health education* (pp. 67–78). San Francisco: Jossey-Bass.

U.K. Office of National Statistics, Social Analysis and Reporting Division. (2001). Social capital: A review of the literature. Newport, South Wales: Author.

Ungar, M. (2008). Putting resilience theory into action: Five principles for intervention. In L. Liebenberg & M. Ungar (Eds), *Resilience in action* (pp. 17–38). Toronto: University of Toronto Press.

U.S. Department of Health and Human Services (USDHHS). (2001). *Healthy people in healthy communities: A community planning guide using Healthy People 2010.* Washington, DC: Author.

U.S. Department of Health and Human Services (USDHHS). (2011). *MAP-IT: A guide to using Healthy People in your community.* Retrieved May 23, 2013, from http://www.healthypeople.gov/2020/implementing/default.aspx.

W.K. Kellogg Foundation. (2004). *Logical model development guide.* Retreived May 5, 2016, from http://www.smartgivers.org/uploads/logicmodelguidepdf.pdf

Walsh, D. C., Rudd, R. E., Moeykens, B. A., & Moloney, T. W. (1993). Social marketing for public health. *Health Affairs, 12,* 104–119.

Warren, M. R., Thompson, J. P., & Saegert, S. (2001). The role of social capital in combating poverty. In S. Saegert, J. P. Thompson, & M. R. Warren (Eds.), *Social capital and poor communities* (pp. 1–28). New York: Sage Foundation.

Weinstein, N. D., Rothman, A. J., & Sutton, S. R. (1998). Stage theories of health behavior: Conceptual and methodological issues. *Health Psychology, 17,* 290–299.

Weinstein, N. D., & Sandman, P. M. (2002). The precaution adoption process model and its application. In R. J. DiClemente, R. A. Crosby, & M. C. Kegler (Eds.), *Emerging theories in health promotion practice and research: Strategies for improving public health* (pp. 16–39). San Francisco: Jossey-Bass.

Weinstein, N. D., Sandman, P. M., & Blalock, S. J. (2008). The precaution adoption process model. In K. Glanz, B. K. Rimer, & K. Viswanath (Eds.), *Health behavior and health education: Theory, research, and practice* (4th ed., pp. 123–147). San Francisco: Jossey-Bass.

Ethics and Health Education/Promotion

Chapter Objectives

After reading this chapter and answering the questions at the end, you should be able to:

- Identify and define the three major areas of philosophy.
- Define *ethics*.
- Explain the difference between ethics and morality.
- Explain why it is important to act ethically.
- Define *professional ethics*.
- Explain and briefly describe the two major categories of ethical theories.
- Identify principles that create a common ground for all ethical theories.
- Outline a guide for making ethical decisions.
- Identify ethical issues associated with the profession of health education/promotion.
- Explain how a profession can ensure that its professionals will act ethically.
- Define *code of ethics* and identify the source of the code available for health education specialists.

In recent years, there has been an increasing interest in ethical questions in all walks of life. The interest has become so great that it is difficult to avoid the topic of ethics in everyday living. Newspapers and television networks are constantly covering stories that involve ethical issues, many of which are related to health. Examples include genetic engineering, allocating donor organs, end of life issues, the reduction of welfare benefits, health research, appropriate sexual behavior, and professional behavior, to name a few.

How do we determine what is ethical or unethical? By whose standards do we make such judgments? To answer these questions requires some background and perspective. In this chapter, we will provide the background and perspective to understand how ethics relates to the profession of health education/promotion. First, we will present key terms that relate to the study of ethics and examine the origin of ethics. Next, we look at reasons why people should work from an ethical base. We will then briefly look at the theories used to create ethical "yardsticks" and how these theories can be used to make ethical decisions. Within this context, a sampling of ethical issues facing health education specialists today will be presented. Finally, we conclude with a discussion on how a profession can ensure that its professionals will act ethically.

▷ Key Terms and Origin

Ethics, the study of morality (Morrison, 2006), is one of the three major areas of philosophy. The other two are **epistemology**, the study of knowledge, and **metaphysics**, the study of the nature of reality (Thiroux, 1995). Ethics, or **moral philosophy** as it is often stated, dates back two thousand plus years to the Greek philosopher Socrates (470–399 B.C.E.), "who spent his days in the Athenian marketplace challenging people to think about how they lived" (White, 1988, p. 7). Though philosophers do not sit in the marketplace (or malls) today to challenge people, the behavior, actions, and values of people are constantly being examined for their appropriateness.

You will note that the word *ethics* was described using the words *moral* and *morality*. The reason for this is that both words, *ethics* and *morals,* have ancient Greek and Latin roots in the words *ethos* and *mores* and both mean *character*. Thus, most associate *good character* with ethical behavior (White, 1988). Sperry (2007) has made a distinction between morality and ethics saying that morality "is the activity of making choices and of deciding, judging, justifying, and defending those actions or behaviors called moral," whereas ethics is "the science of how choices are made or should be made" (p. 38). Pigg (2010) has stated that "*ethics* defines acceptable and unacceptable behavior within the norms of a particular group" (pp. 11–12), whereas "*morality* sets standards for right and wrong in human behavior" (p. 12). Nevertheless, to avoid confusion throughout the rest of this chapter, we will use **ethical** and **moral** to mean the same thing. "The important thing to remember here is that moral, ethical, immoral, and unethical, essentially mean, good, right, bad, and wrong, often depending on whether one is referring to people themselves or to their actions" (Thiroux, 1995, p. 3).

White (1988) refers to the words *good, right, bad*, and *wrong* as the labels people use when making ethical judgments about human actions. Some authors have used these words to define ethics. Feeney and Freeman (1999) state, "Ethics is the study of right and wrong, duty and obligation" (p. 5). In the end, factual knowledge is not the concern of ethics but rather the virtues and values that drive human conduct (Pozgar, 2013).

▷ Why Should People Act Ethically?

Because ethics is one of the three major areas of philosophy, a philosophical answer to the question of why people should act ethically is that to act ethically brings meaning or purpose to the life of an individual (McGrath, 1994). It provides a standard by which to live. Ethical living, in turn, provides for a better society for all. It is the right thing to do for society and self.

Personally, observation has shown "that those who are ethical tend to lead healthier, more emotionally satisfying lives" (McGrath, 1994, p. 131). Professionally, those who implement community interventions, including health education specialists, have much to gain from ethical behavior. Rabinowitz (2015) has noted that ethical practices make programs more effective, promote a sense of trust in an organization, contribute to moral credibility and leadership, and assure good standing legally and professionally. In short, ethics help guide our decision making and assist us in making better choices.

Professional Ethics

Whereas personal values and morality may guide us in our everyday living, it is important to note that they may not be sufficient to guide our professional behavior. People come to their work with different personal experiences. Because of these different experiences, they do not hold the same values nor have they learned the same moral lessons. Even those who hold the same beliefs may not apply them in the same way in a professional setting (Feeney & Freeman, 1999). Thus, in a work setting, individuals are guided by professional ethics. **Professional ethics** focuses on the "actions that are right and wrong in the workplace and are of public matter. Professional moral principles are not statements of taste or preference; they tell practitioners what they ought to do and what they ought not do" (Feeney & Freeman, 1999, p. 6). Coming to an understanding of what behaviors are appropriate in a professional role is referred to as *professional socialization* (Morrison & Furlong, 2014).

Ethical behavior is expected from professionals. "'Ethics' delineates what we consider acceptable and unacceptable conduct regarding professional practice in Health Science education. Ethical conduct is particularly important to professional health educators, since we belong to a profession with a mission to serve the individual" (Pigg, 1994, p. iii). Health education/promotion is a profession with much human interaction. Dorman (1994) adds, "As writers, reviewers, and scientists we must insist on the highest of ethical practices in publication and research. As practitioners, we must seek to actively practice ethical behavior in our service and teaching. Individually, we must aspire for a reputation which reflects a life of personal integrity. The wisdom of King Solomon probably puts it best: '*A good name is more desirable than great riches; to be esteemed is better than silver or gold*'" (p. 4). Or, as Pigg (2006) stated when he summarized the lesson on integrity he learned from observing his father throughout life, "When fame and fortune fade, only our reputations remain as important but fragile reflections of our true nature" (p. 41).

Within the larger realm of *professional ethics* there may be some subsets of ethical behavior that are specific to certain tasks of the professional. For example, among the seven responsibilities of health education specialists is Responsibility IV "Conduct Evaluation and Research Related to Health Education/Promotion" (National Commission for Health Education Credentialing [NCHEC], 2015) (see the discussion of the responsibilities in Chapter 6). To conduct evaluation and research, health education specialists need to be aware not only of appropriate general professional ethics but also of ethical behavior as it relates to the evaluation and research processes. Such behavior falls under the area of *research ethics*. **Research ethics** "comprises principles and standards that, along with underlying values, guide appropriate conduct relevant to research decisions" (Kimmel, 2007, p. 6). An ethical principle associated with the research process is the concept of voluntary participation. That is, potential research participants should not be forced or coerced into participating in a research study, but rather should do so on a voluntary basis (see **Box 5.1** for other issues related to research process).

Examples of Ethical Issues Related to Research

The research process includes a number of steps that could have ethical ramifications. Examples of such issues are presented based on whether it is a consideration before the research begins, during the research process, or after the research is complete.

Before the research begins

- Selecting a research topic; must weigh risk (harm) to benefit (positive value)
- Recruiting participants: equitable opportunity to participate; voluntary participation; concern for vulnerable groups
- Institutional Review Board approval of research protocol

During the research process

- Obtaining participant consent and/or assent
- Using deception (active or passive) as part of the intervention

- Participant privacy: anonymity or confidentiality
- Using an untreated comparison or control group
- Data analysis: careless use of data; manipulation of data; selective use or elimination of data; over-analysis of data

After the research is complete

- Reporting results: what to report; protecting confidentiality; declaring conflict of interest; disclosing sponsorship
- Sharing results with participants; debriefing experimental, control, and comparison groups
- Publication/presentation of results: determining authorship and order of authors; avoiding duplication of published works, fragmentation into several publications, and plagiarism

▷ Ethical Theories

Philosophers do not speak with a common voice about the standards of morality. Depending on the ethical theory espoused, one philosopher may see a certain behavior as moral or ethical, whereas another may see the same behavior as immoral or unethical. For example, one philosopher may see capital punishment as a moral action to punish a person for murder, and the other sees the taking of another life, for whatever reason, as immoral. The purpose of this section is to categorize and summarize the better-known theories (see **Table 5.1**) and to suggest ways by which their content can be applied to health education/promotion practice.

TABLE 5.1 **Summary of ethical theories**

Category	Primary Reasoning	Examples of Such Theories
Deontology (also known as formalism or nonconsequentialism)	The end does not justify the means.	Natural law morality, deontological ethics, existentialism
Teleology (also known as consequentialism)	The end does justify the means.	Contractarian ethics, utilitarianism, pragmatism

Ethical theories provide frameworks whereby health education specialists and others are able to evaluate whether human actions are acceptable (Shive & Marks, 2006). The primary means by which ethical theories have been categorized has been to place them in the category of deontology (also referred to as **formalism**, or **nonconsequentialism**) or teleology, (commonly called **consequentialism**). **Deontological theories** (from Greek *deontos*, "of the obligatory" or *deon* meaning duty) "are those that claim that certain actions are inherently right or wrong, or good or bad, without regard for their consequences" (Reamer, 2006, p. 65). For example, a deontologist would argue that lying to a client or patient is wrong even if it is done to help that person. According to this theory, the mere act of lying is wrong, regardless of the benefits it may bring. Deontology theories involve making decisions based on a moral code or rules (Pozgar, 2013)—that is to say, the end (the consequences) *does not* justify the means (the act).

Teleological theories (from Greek *teleios*, "brought to its end purpose"), on the other hand, evaluate the moral status of an act by the goodness of the consequences (Reamer, 2006). If the act produces good or happiness, it is morally okay; if it does not, it is immoral. Using the same example of lying to a patient or client, if the consequences turned out okay, the consequentialist would see this act as morally okay. In short, this category of ethical theories states that the end *does* justify the means.

As can be seen from these descriptions of formalism and consequentialism, the primary point of contention is whether or not the means justify the end. Most people would say that neither category of ethical theory can answer all moral questions in their lives. In fact, Summers (2014) has stated, "humans have yet to develop an ethical theory that will satisfactorily handle all issues" (p. 62). There are times when deontology provides guidance for the ethical way to act, whereas teleology is best in other situations. What this means is that each person must carefully study the ethical theory options, combine what is compatible and resolve what is inconsistent in those options, and attempt to work out a moral consensus for herself and society (Mellert, 1995). This is not an easy process. Many times, philosophical questions and problems are abstract or conceptual in nature. For example, is there ever a time when it is okay for a health education specialist to lie to his supervisor? Such questions are answered through philosophical thought, using reason, logic, and argument. Thus, the most important tool people can use to find these answers is the mind.

When analyzing an ethical problem, people need to depend more on thinking than feeling—using their minds and not their hearts (White, 1988). For example, if a person says, "I feel that abortion, no matter when it occurs, is morally wrong," that person is really saying there is something about abortion that makes her uneasy, unhappy, or distressed. This person is expressing a feeling, not a moral position. This person's feelings would be better stated if she were to say, "Abortion makes me feel upset." However, if a person states that abortion is immoral, then she should be prepared to provide specific reasons for holding this belief (White, 1988). For example, she may hold the belief that life begins at conception and having an abortion is ending the life of another human being. It is for these reasons that answering ethical questions is a thinking, not a feeling, process. Or, as Penland and Beyrer (1981) have stated, "If ethics is to have personal meaning it demands thoughtful examination. The answers to ethical questions are found by looking within, examining our personal belief systems and values, and using our intelligence to integrate what we have learned and what we have experienced with what we believe and value" (p. 6).

▷ Basic Principles for Common Moral Ground

As was shown in the previous section, deontoloists and teleologists are not in agreement when it comes to the rationale to be used in making moral decisions. No single ethical theory can answer every ethical question to the satisfaction of all, yet, to live in a moral society, all must be able to work from a common moral ground. "We must search for a larger meeting ground in which the best of all these theories and systems can operate meaningfully with a minimum of conflict and opposition" (Thiroux, 1995, p. 172).

To help us with this common ground, Thiroux (1995) has identified five basic principles that can apply to human morality, regardless of the embraced theory. The principles do not provide the answers to how one should behave, but rather help to provide a foundation for making ethical decisions. The first is the **value of life** principle. This is the most basic of principles. Without living human beings, there can be no ethics. Thiroux (1995) has specifically stated this principle as "human beings should revere life and accept death" (p. 180). This means that no life should be ended without strong justification. This, for example, is why topics such as abortion, suicide, euthanasia, and capital punishment raise a number of ethical questions.

The second is the principle of **goodness (rightness)**. "Good" and "right" are at the core of every ethical theory. Theorists may disagree on what is good and bad and right and wrong, but they all strive for goodness and rightness. "'Good' should not only be in abstract, but it should be seen in relation to (other) human beings. As an example, a person who is suicidal may no longer value his or her life as 'good,' but that person's mother may have a very different concept of the value of her child's life" (Tschudin, 2003, p. 56).

The principle of goodness includes two parallel principles of ethics: (1) the principle of **nonmaleficence** and (2) the principle of **beneficence**, or **benevolence**. "Briefly, nonmaleficence refers to the non-infliction of harm to others" (Balog, Shirreffs, Gutierrez, & Balog, 1985, p. 91). Further, nonmaleficence can "be broken into three components: not inflicting harm, preventing harm, and removing harm when it is present" (Greenberg, 2001, p. 3). Though the concepts presented in this explanation of nonmaleficence are seemingly straightforward, the application of the concepts can be difficult. For example, what is meant by harm? Are there degrees of harm like "a little harm" and "a lot of harm"? Must an action produce no harm to be acceptable from an ethical point of view? These are difficult questions to answer and make some situations difficult to respond to in an ethical way.

"Beneficence implies more than just avoiding doing harm" (Summers, 2014, p. 49). It "describes the principle of doing good, demonstrating kindness, showing compassion, and helping others" (Pozgar, 2013, p. 9). In the bioethical realm, nonmaleficence and beneficence make up the "benefit-harm ratio" in which, ideally, benefits outweigh costs and in which the "minimization of harm" rather than the "maximation of good" is more strongly emphasized (Fox & Swazey, 1997).

Thiroux's third principle is the principle of **justice (fairness)**. This principle deals with people treating other people fairly and justly in distributing goodness (benefits) and badness (burdens) (Summers, 2014; Thiroux, 1995). Justice can be examined in two ways—(1) *procedural* and (2) *distributive* (Summers, 2014). **Procedural justice** deals with whether or not fair procedures were in place and whether those procedures were followed, while **distributive justice** deals with the allocation of resources (Summers, 2014). Does this mean that all people will always get their fair share of goodness and badness? No, but it does mean everyone will have an equal chance at obtaining the good (Thiroux, 1995). "The bottom line is that one has indeed acted justly toward a person when that person has been given what she or he is due or owed" (Balog et al., 1985, p. 90). For example, should only those who are able to pay for them receive health education/promotion services?

The fourth principle of this common moral ground is that of **truth telling (honesty)**. At the heart of any moral relationship is communication. A necessary component of any meaningful communication is telling the truth, being honest. This may be the most difficult principle to live by. This is not to say that people will never lie or that lying might be justified, but there is a need for a strong attempt to be truthful. In the end, morality depends on what people say and do (Thiroux, 1995). Health education specialists working in a clinical setting may be faced with this principle when caught in a situation in which an ill child (and a minor by law) asks about his or her health problem, but the child's parent or guardian has strictly forbidden such communication.

The fifth principle is that of **individual freedom (equality principle or principle of autonomy)** (See **Figure 5.1**). "The word *autonomy* comes from the Greek words *autos* ("self") and *nomos* ("rule," "governance," or "law") and originally referred to as self-governance in Greek city-states" (Greenberg, 2001, p. 3). "This principle means that people, being individuals with individual differences, must have the freedom to choose their own ways and means of being moral within the framework of the first four basic principles" (Thiroux, 1995, p. 187). This is to say that individual freedom is limited by the other four principles. Underlying the principle "of autonomy is the idea that we are to respect others for who they are" (Summers, 2014, p. 50). This is a principle that health education specialists deal with on a regular basis, specifically as it relates to helping others engage in enhancing health behavior. Health education specialists need to respect the rights of others to deliberate, choose, and act (Balog et al., 1985).

With the grounding of the ethical theories and the establishment of these basic principles, let us examine the process of making ethical decisions.

▲ **Figure 5.1** Individual freedom is an important principle of human morality.

▷ Making Ethical Decisions

"Ethical decision making in health education, as in other areas, involves determining right and wrong within situations where clear demarcations do not exist or are not clearly apparent to the decision maker ... . To be considered a professional health educator, one must possess requisite skill and knowledge in making individual decisions. And, in making decisions it is imperative that one has analyzed his or her decisions in terms of standards of right and wrong, good and bad" (Balog et al., 1985, p. 88). To decide and, in turn, act in an ethical manner, people must rely on their values, principles, and ethical thinking. To assist in this process, a number of authors (e.g., Balog et al., 1985; Fisher, 2003; Mellert, 1995; Melnick, 2015; Nelson, 2005; Reamer, 2006; Remley & Herlihy, 2007; Svara, 2007; Thompson, Melia, & Boyd, 2000) have presented guides for applying the concepts presented previously in this chapter to everyday ethical decision making. Though the number of steps and labels used to identify the steps are different from guide to guide, they are similar in that they provide a framework for making an ethical decision. Because of the limitation of space, we are presenting a single approach (see **Figure 5.2**) to ethical decision making that blends the ideas and is representative of these guides.

The ethical decision-making process should begin long before any ethical problems surface. The process begins when a person develops and sustains a professional commitment to doing what is right (Fisher, 2003). Such a commitment will go a long way toward creating a work environment that can prevent many ethical problems. This is not to say that all ethical problems will be avoided. Ethical problems can arise in situations in which two or more ethical principles appear to be in conflict, in unforeseen reactions from those with whom a

▲ **Figure 5.2** Steps in ethical decision making

Sources: Adapted from: Balog et al., (1985); Mellert (1995); Nelson (2005); Reamer (2006); Remley & Herlihy (2007); Svara, (2007).

health education specialist may work, or in unexpected events (Fisher, 2003). However, having a commitment to doing what is right becomes a form of "primary prevention" for many ethical problems.

Aligned with a commitment to doing what is right is familiarity with what the health education/promotion profession expects of practicing professionals. Stated differently, what are the expected norms for those who practice health education/promotion? Such expectations can be found in the profession's code of ethics. With a commitment to doing what is right and knowing what is expected of them, practicing health education specialists are enhancing their *moral sensitivity*. Rest, Narvaes, Bebeau, and Thoma (1999) explained **moral sensitivity** as being aware that an ethical problem exists and having an understanding of what impact different courses of action may have on the people involved.

The first step to take when confronted with an ethical decision is to define the problem/concern, identify the ethical issue(s), clarify the facts, and seek answers to relevant questions (Mellert, 1995; Melnick, 2015; Nelson, 2005; Reamer, 2006; Remley & Herlihy, 2007; Svara, 2007). This first step is one of clarification and gathering relevant information. Several questions need to be answered. What is the problem/concern that makes you believe there is an ethical decision to be made? Is there a legal question that needs to be answered? What do you know? What do you need to find out? Does a decision have to be made? If so, by when, and in what context? Are these decisions within the realm of your authority, or does someone else with other responsibilities/authority/resources determine them?

Second, identify the individuals, groups, and organizations that are likely to be affected by this ethical decision (Nelson, 2005; Reamer, 2006) and what stakes they have in the outcome (Svara, 2007). When making an ethical decision, it is important to understand all who will be impacted because one solution may create additional ethical problems for others.

Third, "contemplate the ultimate goals and ideals for which you as a moral person are striving. What are the most noble human aspirations that pertain to this concrete situation?" (Mellert, 1995, p. 156). How should you as an ethical person want to act in this situation? Consider the ethical theory you embrace and the principles for common ethical ground. How do these goals and ideals apply to this decision? Ultimate goals and ideals do not always apply to every decision and sometimes may not be appropriate, but, to the extent that they do apply, let them help with the decision.

Fourth, identify all the possible alternatives to solving the problem (viable courses of action), the people involved in each, and the potential benefits and risks of each (Reamer, 2006). It is important to brainstorm the various alternatives to help organize subsequent analysis (Reamer, 2006). Consider ethical and health theories, a code of ethics (Melnick, 2015), and consult with colleagues and, if necessary, experts. Be aware that there may not be a "best alternative;" you may have to deal with an ethical dilemma. An **ethical dilemma** is

> a situation that forces a decision that involves breaking some ethical norm or contradicting
> some ethical value. It involves making a decision between two or more possible actions in
> which any one of the actions can be justified as being right decision, but whatever action is
> taken, there always remains some doubt as to whether the correct course of action was chosen.
> The effect of an action may put others at risk, harm others, or violate the rights of others.
> (Pozgar, 2013, pp. 534–535)

Fifth, "consider the probable consequences of each alternative" (Mellert, 1995, p. 157). Look at both the short- and long-term consequences of each alternative. How will these consequences affect you, others, and the environment? In other words, weigh the strengths and weaknesses of the alternatives based on the consequences (Balog et al., 1985). Maybe the consequences are different, or maybe they are not and thus, may not be important in the final decision.

Sixth, "consider the nature of the alternatives" (Mellert, 1995, p. 157). Consider the deontologist approach to the decision-making process in selecting an alternative. Does the alternative lead to an act or a behavior that is wrong? Would you be violating anyone's basic rights? Does it go against basic human ideals and intrinsic moral values? If you answer *yes* to any of these questions, you do not necessarily need to eliminate the alternative from further consideration but should give greater consideration to alternatives that do not violate this portion of your reflection.

Seventh, "reflect on yourself" (Mellert, 1995, p. 157). What impact will a proposed course of action have on you as a moral person? Will it enhance or detract from your moral stature? If it detracts, then maybe other alternatives should be considered. If you cannot accept a course of action "as part of your inner self and as data for your own moral growth, then there must be something morally questionable about it" (Mellert, 1995, pp. 157–158). Although you may be striving to be objective as you work toward a decision, be aware that your emotions will also play a part. Your emotions will influence your judgment and may help guide you in your decision making (Remley & Herlihy, 2007).

Eighth, "reflect on your society and your environment" (Mellert, 1995, p. 158). Will your action mesh with that of society and the environment? Moral acts are unselfish acts in that they do not prefer one's own interests at the expense of the interests of others (Mellert, 1995). Will society in general see your action as morally correct? (See **Figure 5.3**.)

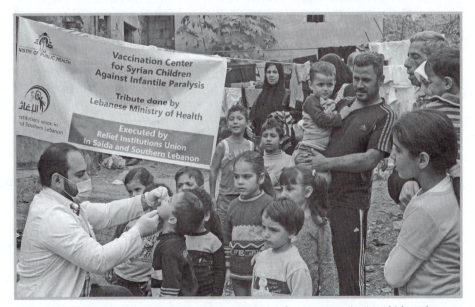

▲ **Figure 5.3** Many vaccine-related ethical debates center around access to vaccination which can be influenced by socioeconomic and racial ethnic minority status causing to question whether or not all lives are of equal value.

Ninth, "apply the categorical imperative" (Mellert, 1995, p. 158). Would you want your course of action to be a role model for others? If others were faced with the same decision, is this how you would want them to act?

Tenth, choose the best alternative, provide a reasoned justification for the choice (Svara, 2007), "act courageously and decisively" (Mellert, 1995, p. 158), monitor and evaluate the results, and if necessary make adjustments (Svara, 2007). "Choosing among conflicting options is difficult, but at least one can feel confident that the choice did not ignore an important alternative" (Svara, 2007, p. 109). Having said this, you still may not feel comfortable after the choice has been made.

Context of Ethical Decision Making

In considering the components in this decision-making process, it is important to note that moral decision making does not occur in a vacuum (Mellert, 1995). If it did, every decision would be resolved with the "right" alternative for all. Each decision is surrounded by the context in which it must be made. Mellert feels that, when working through the process, a person must consider and be aware of the context. When making ethical decisions, people must have a sense of the following:

1. **Place.**   Be aware of the appropriateness of an action in a particular environment. One action may be appropriate in one setting but not in another.

2. **Time.**   Be aware of the history leading up to the decision and other similar decisions. Learn from past decisions.

3. **Identity.**   Who am I? How does this moral decision relate to me?

4. **Social relationships.**   Be aware that making moral decisions will impact social relationships. There is a good chance that not everyone will agree with your decision and action.

5. **The ideal.**   When making a moral decision, aim for the most noble ideals of humanity.

6. **The concrete.**   Never lose sight of the fact that choices arise from concrete events.

7. **Seriousness.**   When making a moral decision, do so with an attitude that is appropriate to the situation.

▷ Applying the Ethical Decision-Making Process

Now let us see if we can apply this decision-making process to the profession of health education/promotion. A health education specialist, let's call her Anne, is employed by an organization and is in charge of the organization's employee health promotion program. Based on the results of the health risk assessments (HRA) taken by employees, Anne is aware that one employee, "high up in the organization" (e.g., school principal or department manager), is a consistent abuser of alcohol. The person's supervisor is aware of the situation but has ignored it. The employee in question is well liked within the organization and is a good employee. To the best of Anne's knowledge, alcohol has not impacted this person's work performance, but she feels it has the potential to do so. Anne is not sure if the alcohol has impacted the employee's personal life. What should Anne do with this information? Let's look at how we might analyze this situation using the 10-step process presented on the previous pages.

Step 1. Define the problem, identify the ethical issue, and gather relevant information.

The problem is that the employee is abusing a substance, and the health education special-ist knows it, as does the employee's supervisor. Is it an ethical problem? Anne knows that an alcohol-impaired person can harm himself or herself and others, either intentionally or unintentionally, and thus has an obligation to protect their health (see Article I, Section 4, of Appendix A). Anne also knows she has an obligation to protect the privacy of the employees (see Article I, Section 6, of Appendix A). This appears to be an ethical situation to Anne be-cause of the two competing issues. Anne has decided to get more information before acting. She decides to look at the employee handbook to see if anything like this appears there. She also decides to ask her own supervisor for guidance and check with the Human Resources (HR) Department for information. And, last, she looks to see when the employee is scheduled for his or her HRA feedback appointment.

Step 2. Identify who will be affected.

Anne is aware that, depending on what actions are taken, the parties impacted by those ac-tions are the employee, his or her supervisor, the organization and its reputation, family members of the employee, and even Anne herself and her supervisor.

Step 3. Contemplate the ultimate goals and ideals.

Anne wants to do what is ethically right. From a theoretical point of view, Anne embraces the deontological viewpoint of dealing with ethical situations. In other words, she believes that the ends do not justify the means. She is trying to make sense of how that applies to this situation.

Step 4. Identify the alternatives (viable courses of action).

Anne sees the following as viable courses of action: (1) Approach the employee's supervisor and ask him or her to handle it; (2) Talk to the employee about it at his or her scheduled HRA feedback appointment; (3) Turn the information over to the HR Department to let someone there deal with the problem; (4) Turn the information over to her supervisor so that it can be dealt with at the managers' level; (5) Do nothing until something happens because of the employee's alcohol use; or (6) Do nothing at all.

Step 5. Consider the consequences of the alternatives.

Here are the consequences Anne sees with each of the alternatives she identified in Step 4: Alternative 1—The supervisor may do nothing or may now be forced to act because someone else is aware of the situation. This may lead to the employee's dismissal, or the employee may get the help he or she needs, or the supervisor may decide not to act on the information. Alter-native 2—This alternative would protect the employee's privacy, bring the problem to the at-tention of the employee, and let the employee act without others knowing about it. Anne also knows that the employee may not take the feedback session well and may "blow up" at Anne. Alternative 3—This alternative places the situation in the hands of those trained to deal with them effectively. Depending on the organization's policy, it may also lead to the employee's dismissal, or the employee may get the help he or she needs. Alternative 4—Similar to Alterna-tives 2 and 4, it places the problem in someone else's hands and would probably have much the same consequences as those two alternatives. Alternative 5—Nothing may ever come of the employee's alcohol abuse, or some serious harm may come to the employee or someone around him or her. Or Alternative 6—Doing nothing at all, which would change nothing. The employee possibly will continue as a good employee with no problem for himself or herself or others, or harm could come to the employee, his or her coworkers, or members of the employee's family.

Step 6. Consider the nature of the alternatives.

Anne does not feel that by acting she would be violating any human ideals or intrinsic moral rules or values. She does feel, however, that she cannot do "nothing." She does not like the alternatives, but she feels an ethical obligation to act. Anne may be facing an ethical dilemma.

Step 7. Reflect on yourself.

Anne knows that if she does nothing, she will not be able to live with herself because she sees herself as a moral person. But she is concerned about being seen as the "goody-goody" employee or even a "tattle tale" or an employee who cannot be trusted with confidential information.

Step 8. Reflect on society and the environment.

Anne had a hard time reasoning through this step of the process. Because a large percentage of U.S. adults consume alcohol, she feels that society in general may see the employee's situation as "none of her business." But she still sees a need to act.

Step 9. Apply the categorical imperative.

Anne feels she needs to act because it is her duty. She wonders what kind of health education specialist she would be if she were not concerned about the health of a coworker and the possible harm that coworker could bring to self or others. She feels that she needs to be a role model for others.

Step 10. Choose an alternative, provide a rationale, act, and monitor the results.

Anne decided to act by talking to the employee about the alcohol abuse at his or her scheduled HRA feedback appointment. She chose this approach not only because it does not violate the employee's privacy, but it also tries to protect both the employee's health and that of those around him or her. If this approach does not induce the employee to change, Anne feels that she may need to take further action.

 As you can see, moral decisions are not easy to make. They are not to be taken lightly, and responsible action is important. Remember, this decision will not occur in a vacuum; the "ideal" decision may not be the best decision. What do you think about Anne's actions?

▷ Ethical Issues and Health Education/Promotion

As previously noted, ethical concerns interface with all aspects of our lives. That includes our professional lives too. "Ethical issues permeate almost every decision and action undertaken in health education" (Goldsmith, 2006, p. 33). Although some of the ethical issues faced by health education specialists are specific to the profession, such as the ethical issues surrounding getting clients to begin a health-enhancing behavior, using interventions to protect and promote at the population level, and dealing with the potential pervasiveness of most things in life impacting peoples' health (Dawson & Verweij, 2007), the majority of concerns affecting most professions are similar (Hiller, 1987). Here are some situations that are specific to preventive care and public health programs.

Bayles (1989) has organized the substantive obligations of professions and professionals, regardless of the profession, from which most professional ethical situations arise. The following is a list of these obligations, with several questions that relate the obligations to the practice of health education/promotion. [Note: These obligations closely align with the *Code of Ethics for the Health Education Profession* (Coalition of National Health Education Organizations [CNHEO], 2011).]

1. **Obligations and availability of services.** The primary issue related to this obligation is the equality of opportunity for making professional services available to all citizens. Examples of ethical issues associated with this obligation include the right to legal counsel, access to health care, and refusal to accept clients for lack of ability to pay. (Who should receive health education/promotion? What about clients who are hard to reach? In what settings should it be offered? Should clients have to pay for health education/promotion, or should health education/promotion be denied if a person cannot pay? Should health education specialists ever terminate an intervention before it is complete? Is there ever a time when a health education specialist should use an intervention in which the possible outcomes are questionable?)

2. **Obligations between professionals and clients.** Once the services of a professional have been secured, a number of ethical issues can arise from the professional–client relationship. (See **Figure 5.4.**) "The fiduciary model presents the best ethical ideal for the professional-client relationship" (Bayles, 1989, p. 100). In such a model, the professional is honest, candid, competent, loyal, fair, and discreet. At the same time, the client keeps commitments to the professional, is truthful to the professional, and does not request unethical acts from the professional. (Is there ever a time when health education specialists should not be candid or honest with their clients? How should health education specialists respond when their clients ask them about their personal behavior? Is there ever a time when health education specialists should not obtain informed consent before proceeding with an intervention?) (See **Box 5.2.**)

▶ **Figure 5.4** The professional–client relationship is an obligation that is often encountered by health education specialists.

BOX

5.2

Informed Consent: An Ethical Obligation

The term **informed consent** is often associated with medical procedures or research projects, but it is also important in health education/promotion. The concept behind informed consent is that people—whether patients, research participants, or participants in a health education/promotion program—should be given sufficient information from which to make informed choices about whether or not they want a certain medical procedure, or to participate in a research project or health education/promotion program. From an ethical standpoint, it is based on the common ground principle of individual freedom. That is, freedom to choose after being well informed on the consequences of participation.

Though receiving a medical procedure or participating in a clinical trial often carries more risks than participating in a health

education/promotion program, individuals should not be allowed to participate in any health education/promotion program without giving their informed consent (McKenzie, Neiger, & Thackeray, 2013). In practice, the informed consent process should include (1) the health education specialist discussing the details of the program (i.e., purpose of the program, description of the intervention, risks and benefits associated with participation, alternative programs that will accomplish the same thing, and the freedom to discontinue participation at any time) with the prospective participant; (2) the participant having an opportunity to ask questions about the program; (3) the participant understanding what he or she has been told; and (4) the participant signing a written informed consent document (Cottrell & McKenzie, 2011).

---

3. **Obligations to third parties.** This obligation revolves around what others need to know about the professional–client relationship. Often professionals are confronted with the issue of whether or not to share client information with family members of the client, people in a supervisory capacity (e.g., teachers, employers), legal authorities (e.g., police, lawyers), or peers (e.g., professional colleagues). (What duty does a health education specialist have to share information with a student's parents when the student has shared the information with the health education specialist in confidence? Is there ever a time when a health education specialist can share confidential information? How about with the insurance company of a client? With the client's employer?) (See **Box 5.3**.)

4. **Obligations between professionals and employers.** Employed professionals have obligations to employers that are similar to the obligation they have to their clients (see #2). "However, the obligation to obey employers is stronger than an obligation to clients. It includes acting as, and only as, authorized" (Bayles, 1989, p. 158). On the other hand, "employers' obligations to professional employees are universal, role related, and contractual" (Bayles, 1989, p. 159). Ethical issues related to this obligation often involve due process, confidentiality, and professional support. (Should health education specialists always implement "company" policy when they know it is wrong or could bring harm to a client? What if a health education specialist has a conflict of interest between his personal life and what his employer says he must do? Is there ever a time when health education specialists should publicly speak against their employers?)

5. **Obligations to the profession.** "These obligations rest on the responsibilities of a profession as a whole to further social values" (Bayles, 1989, p. 179). Issues associated with this obligation include conducting research, reforming the profession, and

BOX 5.3 Privacy, HIPAA, and GINA

One of the most basic concepts associated with providing a service (e.g., health education) to other people is that of privacy. **Privacy** has been defined as "the claim of individuals, groups, or institutions to determine for themselves when, how, and to what extent information about them is communicated to others" (Westin, 1968, p. 7). Thus, when people have agreed to participate in a health education/promotion program, it becomes the duty of the health education specialist to protect the information provided by participants.

The importance of privacy for health education specialists, and all others associated with health care, was further emphasized with the enactment of the Health Insurance Portability and Accountability Act of 1996 (officially known as Public Law 104-191 and referred to as HIPAA) and the Genetic Information Nondiscrimination Act of 2008 (officially known as Public Law 110-233 and referred to as GINA). The HIPAA and GINA regulations apply to protected health information (PHI), whether transmitted orally, in writing, or electronically, that is generated by an employer, a health plan, a health clearinghouse, or a healthcare provider, or in connection with financial or administrative activities related to health care (Fisher, 2003). Failure to implement the standards can lead to civil and criminal penalties (U.S. Department of Health and Human Services [USDHHS], n.d.). The two techniques that are used to protect the privacy of program participants are anonymity and confidentiality. **Anonymity** exists when no one, including those conducting the program, can relate a participant's identity to any information pertaining to the program. In applying this concept, health education specialists would need to ensure that collected information had no identifying marks attached to it such as the participant's name, social security number, or any other less common information. In practice, because of the nature (the need to know about the participants) of most health education/promotion programs, anonymity is not often used. Its most common application in health education/promotion is in conducting research projects.

Conversely, the concept of confidentiality is common in health education/promotion programs. **Confidentiality** exists when only those responsible for conducting a program can link information about a participant with the individual and do not reveal such information to others. Thus, health education specialists need to take every precaution to protect participants' information. Often this means keeping the information "under lock and key" while the program is being conducted, then destroying (e.g., shredding) the information when it is no longer needed.

maintaining respect for the profession. (Is there ever a reason why health education specialists should not behave in a professional manner? What duty does a health education specialist have to report the inappropriate behavior of a colleague? What obligations do health education specialists have to keep up-to-date on the content of their fields?)

Having identified problems that may cut across all professions, let us examine those that are more specific to health education/promotion. First, Penland and Beyrer (1981) state that ethical issues are defined by two criteria. "First they must be 'issues'; that is, there must be controversy related to the problem or topic. There must be 'two sides,' supported by people with two different viewpoints" (p. 6). Issues, by definition, are controversial. For example, the need for youth to know sexual information is not an issue; however, from whom and when such information should be provided may be an issue.

"The second criterion for an ethical issue in health education is that it must involve a question of right and wrong" (Penland & Beyrer, 1981, p. 6). "Can health education/promotion programs in the worksite change health behavior?" may be a controversial issue, but it does not deal with rightness and wrongness. Thus, it is not an ethical issue, but "does an employer have the right to make all employees attend the health education/promotion program?" is an ethical issue.

Now that we know what constitutes an ethical issue, let us look at some of the ethical issues health education specialists are likely to face. The literature is abundant with examples of ethical issues in health education/promotion. Issues cited include abstinence-only and abstinence-plus sexuality education (Wiley, 2002), community organization and community participation (Bromly, Mikesell, Jones, & Khodyakov, 2015; Minkler, Pies, & Hyde, 2012), ethics instruction (Modell & Citrin, 2002), global health (Stapleton, Schröder-Bäck, Laaser, Meerschoek, & Popa, 2014), health education research (Bastida, Tseng, McKeever, & Jack, 2010; Buchanan et al., 2002; Minkler et al., 2002; Minkler, Vasquez, Tajik, & Petersen, 2008; Paul & Brooks, 2015), health disparities (Shaw-Ridley & Ridley, 2010), health literacy (Marks, 2009), health promotion evaluation (Thurston, Vollman, & Burgess, 2003), health risk appraisals (The Society of Prospective Medicine Board of Directors [SPM], 1999), health screenings (Melnick, 2015), practice of health education/practice (Kahan, 2012; Shive & Marks, 2006), research/scientific inquiry/publishing (Margolis, 2000; McKenzie, Seabert, Hayden, & Cottrell, 2009; Pigg, 1994, 2006; Price & Dake 2002; Price, Dake, & Islam 2001), service by health education specialists (Price, Dake, & Telljohann, 2001; Young & Valois, 2010), social marketing (Rothschild, 2000; Siegel & Lotenberg, 2007), the teaching of health (Telljohann, Price, & Dake, 2001), topical areas (Eve, Marty, McDermott, Klasko, & Sanberg, 2008; Knight et al, 2014), and the teaching of ethics (Goldsmith, 2006). McLeroy, Bibeau, and McConnell (1993) have identified other areas of ethical concern, which reflect the inclusion of health education as a component of health promotion. The major categories of issues raised by McLeroy and colleagues (1993) include

1. "Assigning individual responsibility to the victim for becoming ill due to personal failures" (p. 314)—for example, becoming ill because one does not exercise or continues to use tobacco products.

2. "Attempting to change individuals and their subsequent behaviors rather than the social environment that supports and maintains unhealthy lifestyles" (p. 314)—for example, telling employees to manage their stress when it is environmental stressors causing the stress.

3. Using "system interventions to promote health behaviors" (p. 315)—for example, public policy strategies or coercive strategies to modify unhealthy actions.

4. Overemphasizing behavior change as a program outcome instead of focusing more on changes in the social and physical environment.

5. Overemphasizing the importance of health, forgetting that health is a means to an end, not an end in itself.

6. Educating the public on the concept of risk and how to properly use risk factor information.

7. Underemphasizing professional behavior, regardless of the health education/promotion setting—for example, keeping up-to-date, serving as a role model, and providing ethics education for the next generation of health education specialists.

As you can see, there are a number of ethical issues that can arise in the process of carrying out the work of a health education specialist. Rabinowitz (2015) has provided several issues that need to be considered when planning, implementing, and evaluating community interventions. They are presented in **Box 5.4**.

BOX

5.4

Ethical Issues that Need to Be Considered with Community Interventions

1. **Confidentiality.** Probably the most familiar of ethical issues—perhaps because it's the one most often violated—is the expectation that communications and information from participants in the course of a community intervention or program (including conversations, written or taped records, notes, test results, etc.) will be kept confidential.

2. **Consent.** There are really three faces of consent: program participants giving program staff consent to share their records or information with others for purposes of service provision; participants giving informed consent to submit to particular medical or other services, treatment, research, or program conditions; and community members consenting to the location or operation of an intervention in their neighborhood.

3. **Disclosure.** Like consent, disclosure in this context has more than one meaning: disclosure to participants of the conditions of the program they're in; disclosure of participant information to other individuals, agencies, etc.; and disclosure—by the program and by the affected individuals—of any conflict of interest that the program represents to any staff or board members.

4. **Competence.** By offering services of any kind, an organization is essentially making a contract with participants to do the job it says it will do. Implied in that contract is that those actually doing the work, and the organization as a whole, are competent to accomplish their goals under reasonable circumstances.

5. **Conflict of interest.** A conflict of interest is a situation in which someone's personal (financial, political, professional, social, sexual, family, etc.) interests could influence his or her judgment or actions in a financial or other decision, in carrying out his or her job, or in his or her relationships with participants. In community interventions, conflicts of interest may change—to the community's disadvantage—how a program is run or how its money is spent.

6. **Grossly unethical behavior.** This is behavior far beyond the bounds of the normally accepted ethical standards of society. In some cases, grossly unethical behavior may stem from taking advantage of a conflict of interest situation. In others, it may be a simple case of dishonesty or lack of moral scruples. Both individuals and organizations can be guilty of some instances of it, and in both cases it is often a result of someone managing to justify the unjustifiable. Community programs need to be clear about their own ethical standards, and to hold individuals to them and to any other standards their professions demand. In most cases, staff members guilty of grossly unethical behavior should be dismissed as quickly as possible, and prosecuted where that is appropriate.

7. **General ethical responsibilities.** Ethical behavior for a community intervention is more than simply following particular professional codes and keeping your nose clean. It means actively striving to do what is right for participants and for the community, and treating everyone—participants, staff members, funders, the community at large—in an ethical way.

Source: From Rabinowitz, P., edited by Berkowitz and Brownlee. (2015). "Ethical issues in community interventions," *The community tool box: Ethical issues in common interventions*. Reproduced by permission of the Work Group for Community Health and Development, The Community Tool Box: http://ctb.ku.edu.

▷ Ensuring Ethical Behavior

The majority of this chapter has been used to examine ethical theory, identify and deal with ethical issues, and discuss why it is important to act ethically. What we have yet to discuss is the answer to the question "how the profession can ensure that professionals will behave ethically?" The answer is it cannot. Professionals who act unethically usually do so (1) for personal financial gain and reputation and (2) for the benefit of clients or employers without considering the effects on others (Bayles, 1989). However, a profession can put procedures into place to work toward ethical behavior by all.

Certain professional procedures or practices are limited to those who are in professional preparation programs and those who have already been admitted to the profession. Traditional ways of doing this have been through (1) selective admissions into academic programs, (2) retention standards to remain in academic programs, (3) graduation from academic programs, (4) completion of internships, (5) the process of becoming credentialed (i.e., certified or licensed to practice), and (6) continual updating to retain the credential. While proceeding through these steps, individuals may have to provide evidence of good moral character.

Upon entering the field, professionals are expected to behave according to a system of norms. As noted previously in this chapter, this system of norms (or professional moral consensus, as some refer to it) is often placed in writing and referred to as a code of ethics. More specifically, a **code of ethics** is a "document that maps the dimensions of the profession's collective social responsibility and acknowledges the obligations individual practitioners share in meeting the profession's responsibilities" (Feeney & Freeman, 1999, p. 6). Such a document is useful not only for the professional but also for those who use the services of the professional. An ethical code's principal function is to "organize in a systematic way basic ethical standards, rules, and principles of professional conduct" (Pritchard, 2006, p. 85). In other words, "codes serve to *constrain* and set limits by identifying behaviors that should be avoided. They *guide* or instruct by identifying obligations and desirable qualities" (Svara, 2007, p. 75). And, "they can *inspire* and set forth the broad goals that the adherents are supposed to promote" (Svara, 2007, p. 76). They also provide the consumers of health education/promotion services with an understanding of what they should expect from the provider.

Svara (2007) has noted that most codes of ethics have four different types of statements in them. **Box 5.5** lists these four different types of statements and references to where they may be found in the *Code of Ethics for the Health Education Profession* (CNHEO, 2011).

In addition to a code of ethics, a profession should also have a means by which to deal with (discipline) professionals who violate the code of ethics. "A wide range of enforcement mechanisms are possible" (Taub, Kreuter, Parcel, & Vitello, 1987, p. 82). Such mechanisms may range from self-monitoring (also referred to as self-regulating) to a more formal process in which a committee of peers reviews ethics cases. When self-monitoring is used, charges of the ethical violation "might be conveyed directly to the professional charged with the violation. That person would then be responsible for resolving the situation. This procedure works well when there is peer pressure for professionals to behave consistent with a clearly identifiable set of standards and rules of professional conduct" (Gold & Greenberg, 1992, p. 143). When ethical violations are reviewed by an ethics committee of the profession or as part of a professional organization, the "committees usually have the authority to recommend sanctions

BOX 5.5

Types of Ethical Statements and Examples Found in the *Code of Ethics for the Health Education Profession*

"Don't" statements

Ex. There are no "Don't" statements in the *Code of Ethics for the Health Education Profession* (CNHEO, 2011), but they are assumed. All statements are made in the positive of what health education specialists will do, not what they shouldn't do. For example, instead of saying that health education specialists should never violate one's right to privacy, Article I, Section 6 states, "Health Educators are ethically bound to respect, assure, and protect the privacy, confidentiality, and dignity of individuals" (CNHEO, 2011, p. 2).

Obligations and Responsibilities

Ex. Article IV, Section 6—"Health Educators communicate the potential outcomes of proposed services, strategies, and pending decisions to all individuals who will be affected" (CNHEO, 2011, p. 4).

Virtues, Personal Qualities, and/or Values

Ex. Article I, Section 8—"Health Educators respect and acknowledge the rights of others to hold diverse values, attitudes, and opinions" (CNHEO, 2011, p. 2).

Aspirations

Ex. Article VI, Section 2—"Health Educators strive to make the educational environment and culture conducive to the health of all involved, and free from all forms of discrimination and harassment" (CNHEO, 2011, p. 6).

against members who are judged to behave unethically" (Gold & Greenberg, 1992, p. 143). First or minor violations of ethical behavior often carry disciplinary measures of "warnings." Repeated or major violations can lead to more serious penalties like limitations on the ability to practice and "even outright expulsion from the profession (that is, decertification or rescinding the member's license to practice)" (Gold & Greenberg, 1992, p. 145). In determining the sanctions, review committees may base their decision on a variety of factors including but not limited to (1) the type of violation (e.g., violation of privacy vs. sexual misconduct), (2) number of prior violations by the professional, (3) the willfulness of the violation, and (4) the level of responsibility of the professional (Svara, 2007).

Ensuring Ethical Behavior in the Health Education/Promotion Profession

Previously, we identified a number of steps that a profession can take to try to ensure ethical behavior from its professionals. Let's look at how the health education/promotion profession has dealt with this, starting with admission into a health education professional preparation program at a college or university.

Currently, the admission procedure into the profession of health education/promotion is not clear. Some colleges and universities preparing health education specialists have selective admission standards, but most have open admissions, meaning that students can enter the health education/promotion program if admitted to the institution. Once in the program, all academic institutions have varied retention standards, minimum grade point averages, and graduation requirements. In regard to the amount of education required in the profession, a bachelor's degree is required to sit for the certified health education specialist (CHES) examination (see Chapter 6); however, there is no consensus in the profession that a bachelor's degree should be the standard. Many feel a master's degree is more appropriate. Regardless of whether a bachelor's or master's degree is required to take the credentialing examination, the earned credentials (CHES or MCHES) are not universally accepted, either in or out of the profession, as necessary to practice health education/promotion.

A professional code of ethics has existed for decades within the field. The first was created in 1976 by the Society for Public Health Education (SOPHE) while another was later written by the American Association for Health Education in 1994. In 1995 the National Commission for Health Education Credentialing, Inc. (NCHEC) (see Chapter 6 for more on NCHEC) and the Coalition of National Health Education Organizations (CNHEO) (see Chapter 8 for more on CNHEO) cosponsored a conference, "The Health Education Profession in the Twenty-First Century: Setting the Stage," at which it was recommended that efforts be expanded to develop a profession-wide code of ethics. Soon after that conference the CNHEO began work on such a code. After several years of work, in 1999 the *Code of Ethics for the Health Education Profession* was created and approved by all members of CNHEO, thus replacing the earlier codes developed by SOPHE and AAHE. That code was updated in 2011(see Appendix A for a copy of the code and more information on its development). However, like the codes before it, this code does not include a formal procedure for enforcement. So currently, the profession has informal enforcement via "the subtle influences colleagues exert on one another" (Iammarino, O'Rourke, Pigg, & Weinberg, 1989, p. 104). "One of the true weaknesses of our present code of ethics is no accountability to its standards" (Goldsmith, 2006, p. 36).

Although moving in the right direction, the health education/promotion profession has much opportunity to refine its ethical foundations.

▶ Summary

Ethical questions impact all aspects of life. Individuals on both a personal and professional level are constantly being confronted with ethical situations. To deal with these situations, people must have a basic understanding of how to make an ethical decision. To prepare readers for this task, this chapter presented key terms, such as philosophy, ethics, and morals; the philosophical, practical, and professional viewpoints of why people and professionals should work from an ethical base; the two major categories of theories (deontology and teleology) used to create ethical "yardsticks" for making ethical decisions; a set of principles and a guide for ethical decision making; a sampling of the ethical issues facing health education specialists today; and a discussion about how a profession can ensure that its professionals will act ethically.

▶ Review Questions

1. What are the three major areas of philosophy? What does each of them mean?
2. In your own words, how do you define *ethics?*

3. What do the definitions of *ethics* and *morals* share? How are they different?

4. Why is it important to act ethically and who determines what qualifies as ethical?

5. What is meant by the term *professional ethics?* What is *research ethics?* In general terms, why are professional ethics important to you? How might that change over the course of your career?

6. Summarize the difference between the two major categories of ethical theories (deontology and teleology)?

7. Outline Thiroux's five principles that create a common ground for all ethical theories?

8. What should be included in a process for making ethical decisions? Are there things that should not be included in ethical decision making?

9. What is meant by the term *moral sensitivity?* Do you feel this should have a legitimate place in the health field?

10. Name five ethical issues currently facing the profession of health education/promotion. Can an issue be seen as ethical by one person, while seen as unethical by another? Give an example of a health-related issue that might create this dynamic.

11. What does the profession currently do to ensure its professionals act ethically? What, if anything, might the profession change/improve to encourage more of their own to act ethically?

12. Define *code of ethics.* Should ethics play a role in all health-related decisions? Can you describe a situation in which ethics would not play a role?

Case Study

Emily accepted a position as a patient educator with the Hamilton Township Hospital after graduating with her bachelor's degree last spring. She is one of five health education specialists employed by the patient education department. About three months after Emily was hired, she observed Robert, the most experienced patient educator in the department, engage in what she believed was unethical behavior. Emily observed Robert accepting a really nice windbreaker (worth about $80) from a pharmaceutical company representative. In return, the pharmaceutical rep asked Robert to recommend the pharmaceutical company's glucometer during the diabetes education sessions he ran. Robert said that "that would be no problem." Do you agree with Emily—do you think this is unethical behavior? On what ethical principles do you base your response? Is there something in the *Code of Ethics for the Health Education Profession* (Appendix A) that supports your position? Say you agree with Emily; what would be your course of action? Do you think Robert's supervisor should be involved? Why or why not? Do you think Robert should be sanctioned by the profession? If so, how could it be enforced?

Critical Thinking Questions

1. Ethical dilemmas are rarely crystal clear and there are often more than one point of view to any given situation. How would you handle a co-worker behaving in an unethical manner? Would your response change if you knew it was an isolated event? That it would

continue? That it might result in a co-worker being fired? That you might be viewed negatively for "whistle blowing"?

2. Do you think it is ethical to use disincentives to change people's health behavior? For example, charging smokers more for life insurance, or fining a person for not wearing a safety belt or motorcycle helmet. Provide a rationale for your response.

3. If you were asked by one of your professors to help design a professional ethics course for health education/promotion majors or minors at your college/university, what would you suggest be included in the course? Why?

4. Several professions (e.g., medicine and law) have procedures for dealing with members' unethical behavior. In fact, if the offense is extreme enough a lawyer can be disbarred and a physician could lose his or her license to practice medicine. Do you think the profession of health education/promotion should create a similar process to review unethical behavior and if necessary take away the certification of certified health education specialists (CHES or MCHES)? Defend your response.

5. Do you think that all health education/promotion majors/minors should be required to take an ethics course while in college? Why or why not? If you responded yes to the question, do you think that a general ethics course open to all university students would be sufficient, or do you think the course should be specific to the profession? Why?

▷ Activities

Directions for activities 1–4. You will find four scenarios that include an ethical issue. Using the 10-step decision-making process put forth in this chapter, write a response to one of the scenarios. In your response, include a response for each of the 10 components. Your responses to the 10 components should state your course of action.

1. You have been hired to work for the city health department to complete a project that was begun by your predecessor and funded with money from a local foundation. The grant requires the health department to develop X number of programs on the topic of hepatitis and then to present these programs to X number of people representing specific priority groups in the community. After being hired, you discover that the administrator of the grant, your supervisor, has not adhered to the grant guidelines. Only half the number of programs have been developed as the grant required. Further, the number of presentations is less than required, and presentations have been given to people not in the identified priority groups. In addition, your supervisor has taken some of the travel funds allocated to pay for your travel to and from presentations and has diverted them into his personal travel fund to attend a national conference in Las Vegas. It is now time for you to develop your year-end report, which will be sent directly to the local foundation office. Your supervisor has provided you with a copy of the original grant proposal and says to make sure your figures agree with those in the proposal. In other words, he expects you to "fudge" the data. What will you do?

2. As the health and fitness director of a large corporate wellness program, you have been asked to provide data to your supervisor that supports the effectiveness of your program. The trend in the company has been to cut programs that do not "carry their weight." The "bottom line" is important. In your review of the data related to your program, it is obvious that the data are not strong. However, in fairness to you, the program has been in operation for only two years, and it is too early to see the type of results management is

looking for. You are the only one who has access to the data, and no one will know if the data you submit are accurate. How will you handle this situation?

3. You are a high school health teacher. The school board has just adopted a policy that prohibits the teaching or discussing of information related to contraceptives or abortion in the district. The only approach that can be mentioned in the classroom is abstinence. You have read research that indicates that the abstinence approach is not as effective as some may think. After class one day, one of your students approaches you and informs you that she is pregnant. She requests your help and asks for the name and location of an abortion clinic. She also asks that you not tell anyone else about this. What will you do?

4. You are the health education specialist for a large city hospital. Your supervisor has asked you to develop a program on "safer sex" practices for the LGBT population. The program is to be made available to lesbian and gay groups in the community. Because of your strong religious convictions, your personal values and beliefs are opposed to the gay/lesbian lifestyle and the "safer sex" approach. In addition, you feel uncomfortable dealing with homosexuals in general and especially with anyone who is HIV-positive. How will you handle this situation?

5. Read thoroughly the *Code of Ethics for the Health Education Profession* presented in Appendix A, then provide written answers to the following questions.

   - What is your overall opinion of the code? Does it include everything you thought it would? Were there any surprises?
   - Do you think it should include any "Don't" statements? (Refer back to Box 5.5.) If yes, which ones? If no, why not?
   - Is there anything in the code you feel should not be there? If so, what and why?
   - If you could add something else to the code, what would it be?
   - Do you think the profession should incorporate a means of enforcement in the code? Why or why not?

6. Select one of the ethical theories presented in Table 5.1 to study further. Find and read from other sources explaining the theory. Then write a three-page paper on the theory's application to the practice of health education/promotion.

7. Make an appointment to meet with one of your professors or with a practicing health education specialist. Inform him or her that you would like to spend about 15 to 20 minutes discussing professional ethics. At the meeting ask if he or she has ever observed a professional situation that involved an ethical issue. If so, ask him or her to describe the situation without revealing the parties who were involved. Then ask how the situation was resolved. After your meeting, summarize the discussion in writing and compare the steps taken in the situation to the components of the 10-step process presented in this chapter. Do you think the situation was handled properly? Why or why not?

▶ Weblinks

1. http://www.cnheo.org

   Coalition of National Health Education Organizations (CNHEO)

   This is the home page for the CNHEO. The coalition has as its primary mission the mobilization of the resources of the health education/promotion profession to expand

and improve health education/promotion, regardless of the setting. At this site you can print out a copy of the *Code of Ethics for the Health Education Profession.*

2. http://www.ethics.org/

Ethics & Compliance Initiative

The Ethics & Compliance Initiative (ECI) is composed of three nonprofit organizations that collaborate to provide ethics and compliance research and best practices.

3. http://www.professionalethics.ca/

Professional Ethics

This is a Canadian Web site that provides a wide variety of resources on various topics related to professional ethics. One special feature of this Web site is the presentation of a number of up-to-date articles on professional ethics. It also has links to several other ethics-related Web sites.

4. http://www.hhs.gov

U.S. Department of Health and Human Services (USDHHS)

Search the USDHHS homepage for "Health Information Privacy"; this will bring you to a page where you can get more information about the National Standards to Protect the Privacy of Personal Health Information.

5. http://appe.indiana.edu/

Association for Practical and Professional Ethics (APPE)

The APPE is a professional organization that works to advance scholarship, education, and practice in practical and professional ethics. It offers both individual and institution memberships.

6. http://www.who.int/ethics/en/

The World Health Organization (WHO)

The Global Health Ethics Unit of the WHO examines ethical issues, supports addressing ethical issues that arise, and challenges healthcare professionals to raise and address questions related to access and allocation of health care.

References

Balog, J. E., Shirreffs, J. H., Gutierrez, R. D., & Balog, L. F. (1985). Ethics and the field of health education. *The Eta Sigma Gamma Monograph Series, 4* (1), 65–110.

Bastida, E. M., Tseng, T-S., McKeever, C., & Jack, Jr., J. (2010). Ethics and community-based participatory research: Perspectives from the field. *Health Promotion Practice, 11* (1), 16–20.

Bayles, M. D. (1989). *Professional ethics* (2nd ed.). Belmont, CA: Wadsworth.

Bromley, E., Mikesell, L., Jones, F., & Khodyakov, D. (2015). From subject to participant: Ethics and the evolving role of community in health research. *American Journal of Public Health, 105* (5), 900–908.

Buchanan, D., Khoshnood, K., Stopka, T., Shaw, S., Santelices, C., & Singer, M. (2002). Ethical dilemmas created by the criminalization of status behaviors: Case examples from ethnographic field research with injection drug users. *Health Education & Behavior, 29* (1), 30–42.

Coalition of National Health Education Organizations (CNHEO). (2011). *Code of ethics for the health education profession.* Retrieved April 4, 2016, from http://cnheo.org/ethics.html.

Cottrell, R. R., & McKenzie, J. F. (2011). *Health promotion and education research methods: Using the five-chapter thesis/dissertation model* (2nd ed.). Sudbury, MA: Jones & Bartlett.

Dawson, A., & Verweij, M. (Eds.). (2007). *Ethics, prevention, and public health.* New York: Oxford University Press, Inc.

Dorman, S. M. (1994). The imperative for ethical conduct in scientific inquiry. In R. M. Pigg (Ed.), Ethical issues of scientific inquiry in health science education. *The Eta Sigma Gamma Monograph Series, 12* (2), 1–5.

Eve, D. J., Marty, P. J., McDermott, R. J., Klasko, S. K., & Sanberg, P. R. (2008). Stem cell research and health education. *American Journal of Health Education, 39* (3), 167–179.

Feeney, S., & Freeman, N. K., (1999). *Ethics and the early childhood educator.* Washington, DC: National Association for the Education of Young Children.

Fisher, C. B. (2003). *Decoding the ethics code: A practical guide for psychologists.* Thousand Oaks, CA: Sage Publications.

Fox, R. C., & Swazey, J. P. (1997). Medical morality is not bioethics: Medical ethics in China and the United States. In N. S. Jecker, A. R. Jonsen, & R. A. Pearlman (Eds.), *Bioethics: An introduction to history, methods and practice* (pp. 237–251). Sudbury, MA: Jones and Bartlett.

Gold, R. S., & Greenberg, J. S. (1992). *The health education ethics book.* Dubuque, IA: Wm. C. Brown Publishers.

Goldsmith, M. (2006). Ethics in health education: Issues, concerns, and future directions. *The Health Education Monograph Series: Foundations of Health Education, 23* (1), 33–37.

Greenberg, J. S. (2001). *The code of ethics for the health education profession: A case study book.* Boston: Jones & Bartlett Publishers.

Hiller, M. D. (1987). Ethics and health education: Issues in theory and practice. In P. M. Lazes, L. Kaplan, & G. A. Gordon (Eds.), *The handbook of health education* (pp. 87–108). Rockville, MD: Aspen.

Iammarino, N. K., O'Rourke, T. W., Pigg, R. M., & Weinberg, A. D. (1989). Ethical issues in research and publication. *Journal of School Health, 59* (3), 101–104.

Kahan, B. (2012). Using a comprehensive best practices approach to strengthen ethical health-related practice. *Health Promotion Practice, 13*, 431–437.

Kimmel, A. J. (2007). *Ethical issues in behavioral research: Basic and applied perspectives* (2nd ed.). Malden, MA: Blackwell Publishing.

Knight, R., Schoveller, J., Greyson, D., Kerr, T., Gilbert, M., & Shannon, K. (2014). Advancing population and public health ethics regarding HIV testing: A scoping review. *Critical Public Health, 24* (3), 238–295.

Margolis, L. (2000). Commentary: Ethical principles for analyzing dilemmas in sex research. *Health Education & Behavior, 27* (1), 24–27.

Marks, R. (2009). Ethics and patient education: Health literacy and cultural dilemmas. *Health Promotion Practice, 10* (3), 328–332.

McGrath, E. Z. (1994). *The art of ethics: A psychology of ethical beliefs.* Chicago: Loyola University Press.

McKenzie, J. F., Neiger, B. L., & Thackeray, R. (2013). *Planning, implementing, and evaluating health promotion programs: A primer* (6th ed.). Boston: Pearson.

McKenzie, J. F., Seabert, D. M., Hayden, J., & Cottrell, R. R. (2009). Textbook writing: A form of professional development. *Health Promotion Practice, 10* (1), 10–14.

McLeroy, K. R., Bibeau, D. L., & McConnell, T. C. (1993). Ethical issues in health education and health promotion: Challenges for the profession. *Journal of Health Education, 24* (5), 313–318.

Mellert, R. B. (1995). *Seven ethical theories.* Dubuque, IA: Kendall/Hunt.

Melnick, A. L. (2015). Case finding: Screening, testing, and contact tracing. In R. Gaare Bernheim, J. F. Childress, R. J. Bonnie, and A. L. Melnick (Eds.), Essentials of public health ethics (pp. 119–143). Burlington, MA: Jones & Bartlett Learning.

Minkler, M., Fadem, P., Perry, M., Blum, K., Moore, L., & Rogers, J. (2002). Ethical dilemmas in participatory action research: A case study from the disability community. *Health Education & Behavior, 29* (1), 14–29.

Minkler, M., Pies, C., & Hyde, C. A. (2012). Ethical issues in community organizing and building. In M. Minkler (Ed.), *Community organizing and community building for health* (3rd ed., pp. 110–129). New Brunswick, NJ: Rutgers University Press.

Minkler, M., Vasquez, V. B., Tajik, M., & Petersen, D. (2008). Promoting environmental justice through community-based participatory research: The role of community and partnership capacity. *Health Education & Behavior, 35* (1), 119–137.

Modell, S. M., & Citrin, T. (2002). Ethics instruction in an issues-oriented course on public health genetics. *Health Education & Behavior, 29* (1), 43–60.

Morrison, E. E. (2006). *Ethics in health administration: A practical approach for decision makers.* Sudbury, MA: Jones & Bartlett.

Morrison, E. E., & Furlong, B. (2014). *Health care ethics: Critical issues for the 21st century* (3rd ed.). Burlington, MA: Jones & Bartlett Learning.

National Commission for Health Education Credentialing, Inc. (2015). *Health educator specialist practice analysis (HESPA) study: Executive summary.* Retrieved April 4, 2016, from http://www.nchec.org/health-educator-job-analysis-projects.

Nelson, W. A. (2005). An organizational ethics decision-making process. *Healthcare Executive, 20* (4), 8–14.

Paul, C., & Brooks, B. (2015). The rationalization of ethical research: Revisionist accounts of the Tuskegee syphilis study and the New Zealand "unfortunate experiment." *American Journal of Public Health, 105* (10), e12–e19.

Penland, L. R., & Beyrer, M. K. (1981). Ethics and health education: Issues and implications. *Health Education, 12* (4), 6–7.

Pigg, R. M. (Ed.). (1994). Ethical issues of scientific inquiry in health science education. *The Eta Sigma Gamma Monograph Series, 12* (2), 1–150.

Pigg, R. M. (2006). Conflict and consensus on ethics in publishing. *The Health Education Monograph Series: Foundations of Health Education, 23* (1), 38–41.

Pigg, R. M., Jr. (2010). Three essential questions in defining a personal philosophy. In J. M. Black, S. Furney, H. M. Graf, & A. E. Nolte (Eds.), *Philosophical foundations of health education* (pp. 11–15). San Francisco: Jossey-Bass.

Pozgar, G. D. (2013). *Legal and ethical issues for health professionals* (3rd ed.). Burlington, MA: Jones & Bartlett Learning.

Price, J. H., & Dake, J. A. (2002). Ethical guidelines for manuscript reviewers and journal editors. *American Journal of Health Education, 33* (4), 194–196.

Price, J. H., Dake, J. A., & Islam, R. (2001). Ethical issues in research and publication: Perceptions of health education faculty. *Health Education & Behavior, 28,* 51–64.

Price, J. H., Dake, J. A., & Telljohann, S. K. (2001). Ethical issues regarding service: Perceptions of health education faculty. *American Journal of Health Education, 32* (4), 208–215.

Pritchard, M. S. (2006). *Professional integrity: Thinking ethically*. Lawrence: University Press of Kansas.

Rabinowitz, P. (2015). *The community health toolbox: Ethical issues in community interventions*. Retrieved April 4, 2016, from http://ctb.ku.edu/en/table-of-contents/analyze/choose-and-adapt-community-interventions/ethical-issues/main.

Reamer, F. G. (2006). *Social work values and ethics* (3rd ed.). New York: Columbia University Press.

Remley, T. P., & Herlihy, B. (2007). *Ethical, legal, and professional issues in counseling* (2nd ed.). Upper Saddle River, NJ: Merrill, Prentice Hall.

Rest, J., Narvaes, D., Bebeau, M. J., & Thoma, S. J. (1999). *Postconventional moral thinking: A neo-Kohlbergian approach*. Mahwah, NJ: L. Erlbaum Associates.

Rothschild, M. L. (2000). Ethical considerations in support of marketing of public health issues. *American Journal of Health Behavior, 24* (1), 26–35.

Shaw-Ridley, M., & Ridley, C. R. (2010). The health disparities industry: Is it an ethical conundrum? *Health Promotion Practice, 11,* 454–464.

Shive, S. E., & Marks, R. (2006). The influence of ethical theories in the practice of health education. *Health Promotion Practice, 7* (3), 287–288.

Siegel, M., & Lotenberg, L. D. (2007). *Marketing public health: Strategies to promote social change* (2nd ed.). Sudbury, MA: Jones & Bartlett.

The Society of Prospective Medicine Board of Directors (SPM). (1999). Ethics guidelines for the development and use of health assessments. In G. C. Hyner, K. W. Peterson, J. W. Travis, J. E. Dewey, J. J. Foerster, & E. M. Framer (Eds.), *SPM handbook of health assessment tools* (pp. xxii–xxvi). Pittsburgh: The Society of Prospective Medicine.

Sperry, L. (2007). *Dictionary of ethical and legal terms and issues: The essential guide for mental health professionals*. New York: Routledge.

Stapleton, G., Schröder-Bäck, P., Laaser, U., Meerschoek, A., & Popa, D. (2014). Global health ethics: An introduction to prominent theories and relevant topics. *Global Health Action, 7,* 1–7.

Summers, J. (2014). Principles of healthcare ethics. In E. E. Morrison & B. Furlong, *Health care ethics: Critical issues for the 21st century* (3rd ed., pp. 47–63). Burlington, MA: Jones & Bartlett Learning.

Svara, J. (2007). *The ethics primer for public administrators in government and nonprofit organizations*. Sudbury, MA: Jones & Bartlett.

Taub, A., Kreuter, M., Parcel, G., & Vitello, E. (1987). Report of the SOPHE/AAHE joint committee on ethics. *Health Education Quarterly, 14* (1), 79–90.

Telljohann, S. K., Price, J. H., & Dake, J. A. (2001). Selected ethical issues in the teaching: Perceptions of health education faculty. *American Journal of Health Education, 32* (2), 66–74.

Thiroux, J. P. (1995). *Ethics: Theory and practice* (5th ed.). Englewood Cliffs, NJ: Prentice-Hall.

Thompson, I., Melia, K., & Boyd, K. (2000). *Nursing ethics* (4th ed.). Edinburgh, Scotland: Churchill Livingstone.

Thurston, W. E., Vollman, A. R., & Burgess, M. M. (2003). Ethical review of health promotion program evaluation proposals. *Health Promotion Practice, 4* (1), 45–50.

Tschudin, V. (2003) *Ethics in nursing: The caring relationship* (3rd ed.). Edinburgh, Scotland: Butterworth Heinemann.

U.S. Department of Health and Human Services (USDHHS). (n.d.). *Health information privacy*. Retrieved April 9, 2016, from http://www.hhs.gov/ocr/privacy.

Westin, A. F. (1968). *Privacy and freedom*. New York: Atheneum.

White, T. I. (1988). *Right and wrong: A brief guide to understanding ethics*. Englewood Cliffs, NJ: Prentice-Hall.

Wiley, D. C. (2002). The ethics of abstinence-only and abstinence-plus sexuality education. *Journal of School Health, 72* (4), 164–167.

Young, M., & Valois, R. F. (2010). Magic, morals, and health: Plus 40 years. *American Journal of Health Education, 41* (1), 18–19.

The Health Education Specialist: Roles, Responsibilities, Certifications, and Advanced Study

---

Chapter Objectives

After reading this chapter and answering the questions at the end, you should be able to:

- Define *credentialing*.
- Discuss the history of role delineation and certification.
- Explain the differences among *certification, licensure*, and *accreditation*.
- List and describe the seven major responsibilities of a health education specialist.
- Discuss the need for advanced study in health education/promotion.
- Outline factors to consider in applying for master's degree programs.

Although education about health has been around since the beginning of human intelligence, health education/promotion as a profession is, relatively speaking, an infant. When any infant begins to mature, it takes on its own identity. This chapter chronicles major historical events that have helped shape the identity of health education/promotion since the 1970s. The current identity of health education/promotion is also presented in terms of roles, responsibilities, certification, and accreditation. The importance of advanced study and continuing education in the health education/promotion profession is also discussed.

▷ Quality Assurance and Credentialing

As a profession matures and grows, it becomes increasingly important that professional preparation become standardized and that individual practitioners perform at a high level of competency. Quality assurance and credentialing often go hand-in-hand and are utilized to help ensure a profession's excellence. It is important to be familiar with these terms as they apply to health education/promotion. In the business world, the term **quality assurance** means "the planned and systematic activities necessary to provide adequate confidence that the product or service will meet given requirements" (Quality Assurance Solutions, 2016). **Credentialing** is one means by which professions such as health education/promotion demonstrate quality assurance. In other words, credentialing would be the "planned and systematic activities" used to increase confidence that the product or service—in this case, health education specialists—is meeting the requirements of the profession. Credentialing is a process whereby an individual, such as a health education specialist, or a professional preparation program demonstrates that established standards are met. When people or programs meet specific standards established by a credentialing body, they are recognized for having done so. We say, "They earned their credentials," which indicates they are meeting their profession's requirements. Credentialing can take the form of accreditation, licensure, or certification.

Accreditation "is the status of public recognition that an accrediting agency grants to an education institution or program that meets the agency's standards or requirements" (National Transition Task Force on Accreditation in Health Education, 2016). Thus, the health education/promotion program at any particular institution may be accredited by one of several outside agencies discussed later in this chapter. For example, the health education/promotion program at Alpha University could be accredited by Beta Accrediting Group. Such a process takes place after the program at Alpha University creates a self-study document that shows how it meets the Beta Accrediting Group's standards. Accrediting procedures may also include an on-campus visit by representatives from Beta. Throughout the process, factors such as student–teacher ratio, curriculum, faculty qualifications, budget, evaluation procedures, and diversity are closely examined.

Licensure is "the process by which an agency or government [usually a state] grants permission to individuals to practice a given profession by certifying that those licensed have attained specific standards of competence" (Cleary, 1995, p. 39). Licensure applies to most medical professionals, such as doctors, nurses, dentists, and physical therapists. The only health education specialists who are licensed in the United States at the present time are school health education specialists in some states.

Certification "is a process by which a professional organization grants recognition to an individual who, upon completion of a competency-based curriculum, can demonstrate a predetermined standard of performance" (Cleary, 1995, p. 39). Note that certification is granted to an individual, not a program, and it is given by the profession or an independent certifying agency, not by a governmental body. Certification is available for all health education specialists, regardless of specialty area. One who is certified is recognized as a **Certified Health Education Specialist (CHES)** and may use the initials **CHES** after one's name and academic degree. In fall 2010, an advanced certification became available. Those who obtain this advanced certification are **Master Certified Health Education Specialists (MCHES)** and may use the initials **MCHES** after their names. See **Figure 6.1** for an overview of quality assurance mechanisms available for health education programs in the United States.

▷ History of Role Delineation and Certification

Certification in health education got its formal start around 1978. At that time, individual certification for health education specialists was not available, except for school health education specialists, who had to be licensed or certified in the state where they taught.

Program accreditation was available only for school health and master's level public health professional preparation programs. Many public health programs outside schools of public health, and all community health education programs, were not accredited nor was accreditation available for these programs. This gave rise to a situation in which there were great

Figure 6.1 Overview of health education credentialing in the United States

Note: CHES, Certified Health Education Specialist; CAEP, Council for the Accreditation of Educator Preparation; CEPH, Council on Education for Public Health; CPH, Certified in Public Health; MCHES, Master Certified Health Education Specialist; NBCT, National Board Certified Teacher.

Source: Modified from Cottrell, R. R., Auld, M. E., Birch, D. A., Taub, A., King, L. R., & Allegrante, J. P. (2012). Progress and directions in professional credentialing for health education in the United States. *Health Education and Behavior. 39* (6). 681–694.

discrepancies in professional preparation. One program might look entirely different from another program, and one health educator might have very different skills than another. To say that an individual was a health educator had little meaning. In describing the situation, Helen Cleary (see **Figure 6.2**), who was president of the Society for Public Health Education (SOPHE) in 1974, wrote the following:

> What I found in my travels [as SOPHE president] was a profession in disarray. Many, many health educators could neither define themselves nor their role. It was clear that the preparation of most was so varied that there was no common core. There was no professional identity, no sense of a profession. Numbers of competent, bright, young professionals were leaving health education for greener pastures. (Cleary, 1995, p. 2)

As a result of this situation, Cleary began to pursue the idea of credentialing health educators and/or health education programs. To undertake such a project, outside expertise and funding were needed. Thomas Hatch, director of the Division of Associated Health Professions in the Bureau of Health Manpower of the Department of Health, Education and Welfare, expressed an interest in the project. Prior to funding the project, however, he needed assurances that members of the profession would work together to create a credentialing system. Hatch wanted to be certain that those who practiced health education in different settings would have enough in common to develop one set of standards.

▶ **Figure 6.2** Helen P. Cleary— the person most responsible for establishing certification for health education specialists

In response to Hatch's concern, a conference, known as the Bethesda Conference on Commonalities and Differences, was held in February 1978 in Bethesda, Maryland. The conference planning committee was made up of representatives from the eight organizations composing the Coalition of Health Education Organizations. This planning committee formulated two questions to be answered at the conference: (1) What are the commonalities and differences in the function of health educators practicing in different settings? and (2) What are the commonalities and differences in the preparation of health educators? (Cleary, 1995, p. 3).

After much discussion, conference attendees concluded that health education was one profession and that a credentialing system was necessary. "It was the consensus of the participants that standards were essential if they were to provide quality service to the public and if they were to survive as a viable profession" (Cleary, 1986, p. 130). Further, the conference planning committee members were asked to continue as a task force to develop the credentialing system. Thus, the **National Task Force on the Preparation and Practice of Health Educators** was born (see **Table 6.1**).

In January 1979, funding became available to embark on the project, and **role delineation** for health educators got under way. Alan Henderson was hired as the project director. Under his leadership, a working committee of the task force began the difficult job of defining the health education specialist's role. In describing this process, Cleary (1995) notes, "For the first time in the profession's history, specialists in school health education and in community health education faced each other across the table and learned that each was dealing with similar concepts, but using different terminology and, as well, applying them in different settings" (p. 5).

Once the initial phase of role delineation was completed, the next step was to verify and refine the role of a health educator. Funding for this became available in March 1980. Health

TABLE 6.1 **Organizations represented on the National Task Force on the Preparation and Practice of Health Educators, 1978**

American College Health Association

American Public Health Association, Public Health Education Section

American Public Health Association, School Health Education and Services Section

American School Health Association

Association for the Advancement of Health Education (AAHE)

Conference of State and Territorial Directors of Public Health Education

Society for Public Health Education, Inc.

Society of State Directors of Health, Physical Education and Recreation

education specialists working in all areas of health education were surveyed to verify the role of a health educator. Survey results were positive; there were no significant differences among practitioners in different settings.

In addition to the survey, a conference for college and university health education faculty members was held in Birmingham, Alabama, in February 1981. The conference provided the opportunity for academics to review the initial role delineation work and discuss its potential impact on the field. The planning committee chairman was Warren E. Schaller from Ball State University, and 238 academics from 125 institutions attended.

Many conference participants were happy with the work and direction of the task force, but others were not. Differences of opinion emerged surrounding the health educator as a content expert versus a process expert and probably reflected the different types of professional preparation programs the faculty represented. Although these differences were real, they were not divisive enough to alter the work of the task force.

The third step in the role delineation process involved creating a curriculum framework based on the verified role of a health educator. Initially, the task force decided to develop a curriculum guide, which is a fairly specific set of rules used to develop a curriculum. Little room is left for interpretation because the curriculum must meet the standards established in the guide. Betty Mathews from the University of Washington and Herb L. Jones from Ball State University were recruited to do the actual writing.

After a draft copy of the curriculum guide was developed, it had to be pretested. Eleven regional workshops were held around the country to obtain feedback on the guide. Again, differences surfaced regarding whether health educators were specialists in content or process. Further, some felt entry-level preparation should be at the bachelor's degree level, whereas others believed it should be at the master's degree level. Feedback was also obtained from professional associations and practitioners in the field.

To deal with some of the criticisms and to make the curriculum guide less rigid, it was ultimately transformed into a curriculum framework. A framework merely provides a frame of reference around which a curriculum can be developed. As Cleary (1995) notes, "It does not tell a faculty what to teach or how to teach it. It simply tells them what the students should know when they have completed the program of studies" (p. 9). Marion Pollock was the individual responsible for transforming the curriculum guide into a curriculum framework.

At this juncture, it was important to check with those in the profession to determine if they wanted to continue with the development of a credentialing system and, if so, what kind of system they wanted. The Second Bethesda Conference was held in February 1986, with 99 attendees. Participants were divided into five groups and asked to answer several predetermined questions. When reports from the groups were analyzed, four of the five were in favor of a certification system for individuals and some form of credentialing for professional preparation programs. They recommended that the task force continue to develop the credentialing system.

Over the next two years, the task force continued to work toward the development of a certification system for individual health education specialists. The Professional Examination Service (PES), which developed certification and licensure exams for many other professions, was contracted to assist with this process. Not only was its experience in test development vital to the process, but it was also willing to provide start-up funds to get the process off the ground.

By June 1988, the National Task Force on the Preparation and Practice of Health Education had functioned for 10 years. With the certification of individual health education specialists about to become a reality, it was time to establish a more permanent structure to manage the certification process. As a result, the **National Commission for Health Education Credentialing, Inc. (NCHEC)** was formed to replace the national task force. Today, NCHEC still oversees and administers the health education certification process. NCHEC's mission "is to enhance the professional practice of Health Education by promoting and sustaining a credentialed body of Health Education Specialists. To meet this mission, NCHEC certifies health education specialists, promotes professional development, and strengthens professional preparation and practice" (NCHEC, 2016c).

▷ Individual Certification

When a new certification program is initiated, charter certification is usually available for a limited time. Charter certification allows qualified individuals to get certified on the basis of their academic training, work experience, and references without taking an exam. After the charter period expires, anyone seeking certification must meet all criteria for certification and pass the examination. The CHES charter certification period began in October 1988 and ended in 1990. After charter certification, when the first exam was held in 1990, 644 candidates passed it to become Certified Health Education Specialists.

The CHES voluntary professional certification program established for the first time a national standard for health education practice. All health education/promotion students are strongly urged to obtain national certification upon graduation (see **Box 6.1**). Certification includes the following benefits:

- Establishes a national standard of practice for all health education specialists.
- Attests to the individual health education specialist's knowledge and skills.
- Assists employers in identifying qualified health education practitioners.
- Develops a sense of pride and accomplishment among certified health education specialists.
- Promotes continued professional development for health education specialists (NCHEC, 2016e).

BOX 6.1

Practitioner's Perspective

HEALTH EDUCATOR Angela Adams

CURRENT POSITION/TITLE: Tobacco Cessation Program Coordinator/Health Educator, Health Promotion and Wellness Department, Naval Hospital, Camp Lejeune, NC.

EMPLOYER: The Arora Group (Contract)

DEGREE/INSTITUTION: B.S., 2014, University of North Carolina Wilmington

MAJOR: Community Health Education

MINOR: Psychology

My job responsibilities: I coordinate all aspects of the Tobacco Cessation Program for the Naval Hospital Camp Lejeune (NHCL). I also am heavily involved in Heart Strong, our heart health program, and present on a variety of health education topics, including sexual responsibility and nutrition. Additionally, I have obtained certification as a Lamaze Certified Childbirth Educator so that I am eligible to teach those classes as the opportunity arises.

How I obtained my job: My internship placement during my last semester at the University of North Carolina Wilmington was with the Health Promotion and Wellness Department Naval Hospital Camp Lejeune. Upon completion of the internship, the site supervisor expressed an interest in hiring me; however, there were no positions available at the time. I kept in contact with the staff and the contract company that hires health educators in the office, making sure they always had a current copy of my resume and knew of my continued interest. One year later, when one of the health educators in the department announced his retirement, I got "the call."

Why I decided to obtain my Certified Health Education Specialist (CHES) credential: The decision to obtain my CHES was a no-brainer. I knew that continuing my education for a master's degree (or beyond) was not an option due to personal circumstances, and I wanted to be credible and competitive in the job market. Knowing the CHES certification would demonstrate my competence as a health educator, I felt it would give me the edge I needed.

How I prepared for the CHES: The study guide offered through National Commission for Health Education Credentialing, Inc. was the best tool for preparation. The first thing I did was read through the guide and make copies of the practice tests. I next took a practice test to see where my strengths and weakness were. I re-read the guide, paying extra attention to areas of responsibility and competencies where my knowledge seemed to be lacking. Additionally, for the questions I missed on the practice exam, I sought out not only the right answer to the question, but the logic behind *why* it was the right answer. I knew the questions on the exam would not be the same as on the practice test, and I really needed a true understanding of the concepts to pass the test and to apply my knowledge in the field. I then re-took practice tests from the copies I made and repeated the process as many times as possible leading up to the exam. Each time I did this, my comprehension increased.

How the CHES credential has helped me: The CHES credential helped me get my job. Without it, I would not have been considered for my position. Beyond the hiring process, the preparation I did in order to pass the exam aided in a deeper understanding of all areas of responsibility of a health educator. The continuing education I do to maintain my certification helps keep me current in the field.

How my work relates to the responsibilities and competencies of a CHES:

Area I: Assess Needs, Assets, and Capacity for Health Education: As a department, we utilize a Health Risk Assessment tool to support Periodic Health Assessments conducted by medical providers, Health Interest Questionnaires, and referrals from medical providers to assess the needs of the active duty,

BOX

6.1

continued

dependents, retirees, and civilian staff served. Based on the findings, our department determines what health issues need to be addressed in terms of education and intervention and what resources are needed for implementation. Additionally, we gauge learning capability, attitudes, and beliefs through a Barriers to Care questionnaire. We develop our programs based on the assessment findings.

Area II: Plan Health Education: My primary focus is tobacco, which is a major problem and very much a part of the military culture. I create and deliver awareness presentations in a variety of settings and tailor according to the target audience, which can be quite diverse.

I use both the Health Belief Model and the Stages of Change Model when planning programs. I identify and analyze the specific factors influencing their behavior, what stage of the change process they are in, what educational and support resources they need, and potential barriers to determine what information and strategies are necessary to successfully meet their goal of becoming tobacco-free. I assist them in the process of developing their individual quit plan using evidence-based strategies. Modifications are made to the program as needed based on resources available in terms of pharmacological therapies, new findings, experience, and (of course) funding.

We market the Tobacco Cessation Program, as well as all other programs, during training for new staff of NHCL, health fairs, emails, newsletters, posters, flyers, all forms of social media, and other base community events.

Area III: Implement Health Education: Whether implementing tobacco awareness education or facilitating tobacco cessation, I incorporate various health education strategies. In an effort to raise awareness for the program, I deliver presentations, participate in community events, and distribute educational materials. I coordinate scheduling and obtain/develop resources for all classes and individual appointments. In addition, I ensure trained program facilitators are in place at off-site NHCL locations.

Area IV: Conduct Evaluation and Research Related to Health Education: To evaluate our Tobacco Cessation Program, I collect baseline data consisting of participant contact information, type of tobacco used, method for quitting, and date of program completion and enter into a database. I follow up with all participants with three- and six-month post program phone calls to determine participant tobacco status and to offer additional assistance in quitting if the participant has not maintained tobacco-free status. I then compile the data in a report and send it up the chain of command.

Area V: Administer and Manage Health Education: Staying on top of professional development opportunities, attendance at meetings with medical providers and other program administrators to gain support and discuss strategies, and familiarizing new hospital staff with our programs and how to submit referrals is a continual part of the job.

Area VI: Serve as a Health Education Resource Person: I am CONSTANTLY reading new findings on tobacco products, their health effects, and cessation strategies, revising and updating my educational materials, and then passing on the information to participants and other instructors.

BOX

6.1

continued

Whether in a classroom, a one-on-one appointment with someone trying to quit, or in discussion with other professionals, I always encourage questions. If I do not know the answer, I will find the answer!

Area VII: Communicate and Advocate for Health and Health Education: The big policy change we are working toward is making NHCL a tobacco-free facility. Currently, we still have designated areas for tobacco use in the hospital. We are using a variety of advocacy strategies that are gradually having an impact and will ultimately result in a tobacco-free facility.

What I like most about my job: The feeling I get when someone calls to thank me for helping them quit smoking is *the* absolute best. Ultimately, their motivation to quit came from within, but the information, strategies, resources, and support I offered made a difference. Making a difference is without a doubt what I like most!

What I like least about my job: The feeling I get when I am not able to help someone is what I like least. Just as I said above, the motivation for change has to come from within. I can provide all the same information, resources, etc. to someone who is not ready or lacks internal motivation for change, and they will not make that change. I just hope that even if the change is not now, the knowledge I provide is enough to facilitate change down the road.

Recommendations for those preparing to become health education specialists: Seek out as much information, and as many additional certifications (especially CHES), as possible. The more knowledge you have, the better you can serve the population with which you are working. Always keep an open mind and develop the ability to think outside the box, whether working with a community as a whole or with an individual.

Currently, eligibility to sit for the CHES exam is based exclusively on academic qualifications. You must "possess a bachelor's, master's or doctoral degree from an accredited institution of higher education; *AND* (1) an official transcript (including course titles) that clearly shows a major in health education, e.g., Health Education, Community Health Education, Public Health Education, School Health Education, etc. Degree/major must explicitly be in a discipline of Health Education/Promotion; *OR* (2) an official transcript that reflects at least 25 semester hours or 37 quarter hours of course work (with a grade 'C' or better) with specific preparation addressing the Seven Areas of Responsibility and Competency for Health Educators" (NCHEC, 2016b).

▷ Graduate Health Education Standards

The roles and responsibilities document, *A Competency-Based Framework for Professional Development of Certified Health Education Specialists* (NCHEC, 1996), defined the skills needed for the entry-level health education/promotion professional. This document provided guidance for professional preparation programs at the bachelor's degree level, but not at the graduate degree level. Although many health education specialists with advanced master's and doctoral degrees had obtained certification, it attested only to the fact that they had entry-level skills. The need existed for an advanced level of certification.

In June 1992, the Joint Committee for Graduate Standards was established. After much work, discussion, and review, the Joint Committee for Graduate Standards developed a draft document that contained additional responsibilities, competencies, and sub-competencies specific to graduate-level preparation (Joint Committee for Graduate Standards, 1996).

In February 1996, 134 health education specialists from more than 100 colleges and universities gathered at the National Congress for Institutions Preparing Graduate Health Educators. At this meeting in Dallas, Texas, the draft document of graduate-level competencies was presented to attendees. After revisions were made, the final version was presented to the AAHE and SOPHE boards of directors, who granted approval in March 1997. These graduate-level competencies served to guide the health education curriculum of professional preparation programs but were not used for individual certification purposes. In fall 2010, an advanced certification became available through NCHEC. Those who obtain this advanced certification are designated Master Certified Health Education Specialists (MCHES). A graduate degree is not required to obtain the MCHES designation; rather, MCHES indicates that an individual is practicing advanced-level competencies.

▷ Competencies Update Project

Since the initial Role Delineation Project began in the 1980s, health education/promotion had evolved and matured. Changes in the profession created a need to re-verify the competencies and sub-competencies of a health education specialist. The **Competencies Update Project (CUP)** began in 1998 and was completed in 2004 (Gilmore, Olsen, Taub, & Connell, 2005). This was the first of three updates that have been completed since the competencies were first developed. The majority of the CUP work was conducted by a three-person steering committee comprising Gary Gilmore, chair; Alyson Taub; and Larry Olsen (see **Figure 6.3**). The profession owes a deep debt of gratitude to these individuals for the time and effort they invested in this project.

▷ NCCA Accreditation and Five-Year Updates

The National Commission for Certifying Agencies (NCCA) accredits professional credentials offered by certifying agencies. Essentially the NCCA accredits the credentials provided by accrediting bodies. The NCHEC and the health education profession thought it important that the CHES and MCHES credentials be accredited by NCCA. To obtain accreditation from NCCA, an accrediting agency must follow recognized best practices. Both the CHES and MCHES credentials have been accredited by the NCCA (NCHEC, 2016d).

One of the best practices required by the NCCA is updating the job analysis and thus the competencies for the agency's field every five years. To meet the five-year update requirement, NCHEC along with AAHE and SOPHE commissioned the 2010 job analysis study (AAHE, NCHEC, & SOPHE, 2010). This study was needed to update the health education competencies, last revised in 2005 by the CUP project. Results of the study were released in 2010, and are referred to as the Health Education Job Analysis 2010 model (*HEJA 2010* model). Again, to

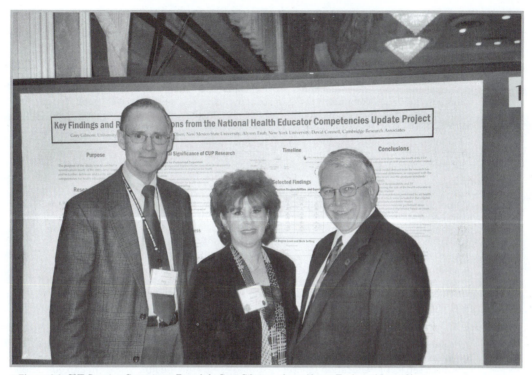

▲ **Figure 6.3** CUP Steering Committee. From left, Gary Gilmore, chair; Alyson Taub; and Larry Olsen.

keep the five-year update requirement, in Spring 2013, NCHEC and its partners SOPHE and ProExam began work for the Health Education Specialist Practice Analysis (HESPA). The 18-month project was completed and results were published in 2015 (National Commission for Health Education Credentialing and Society for Public Health Education, 2015).

The areas of responsibility have remained essentially the same over the three revisions as in the initial entry-level framework with only minor wording changes. This can be seen in **Table 6.2**. That the responsibilities have remained fairly consistent with only minor wording changes helps confirm validity of the Role Delineation Project and subsequent updates.

The important point here is that the health education/promotion profession has and continues to carefully and systematically review and validate the competencies of a health education specialist. The CHES exam is based on these standards, and the health education/ promotion curricula of professional preparation programs should be grounded on them as well.

▷ International Efforts in Quality Assurance

Outside the United States, efforts to ensure quality in health education/promotion have also occurred. According to Allegrante, Barry, Auld, Lamarre, and Taub (2009), Canada, Australia, New Zealand, member states of the European Union and Council of Europe, Spain, Japan,

TABLE 6.2 **Comparison of areas of responsibility (1985–2015)**

Entry-Level Framework (1985)	Graduate-Level Framework (1999)	CUP Model (2006)	HEJA Model (2010)	HESPA Model (2015)
I. Assessing individual and community needs for health education	I. Assessing individual and community needs for health education	I. Assessing individual and community needs for health education	I. Assess needs, assets, and capacity for health education	I. Assess needs, resources, and capacity for health education/ promotion
II. Planning effective health education programs	II. Planning effective health education programs	II. Plan health education strategies, interventions, and programs	II. Plan health education	II. Plan health education/ promotion
III. Implementing health education programs	III. Implementing health education programs	III. Implement health education strategies, interventions, and programs	III. Implement health education	III. Implement health education/ promotion
IV. Evaluating effectiveness of health education programs	IV. Evaluating effectiveness of health education programs	IV. Conduct evaluation and research related to health education	IV. Conduct evaluation and research related to health ed- ucation	IV. Conduct evaluation and research related to health education/ promotion
V. Coordinating provision of health education services	V. Coordinating provision of health education services	V. Administer health education strategies, interventions, and programs	V. Administer and manage health education	V. Administer and manage health education/ promotion
VI. Acting as a resource person in health education	VI. Acting as a resource person in health education	VI. Serve as a health education resource person	VI. Serve as a health education resource person	VI. Serve as a health education/ promotion resource person
VII. Communicating health and health education needs, concerns, and resources	VII. Communicating health and health education needs, concerns, and resources	VII. Communicate and advocate for health and health education	VII. Communicate and advocate for health and health education	VII. Communicate, promote, and advocate for health, health education/ promotion, and the profession
	VIII. Applying appropriate research principles and techniques in health education			
	IX. Administering health education programs			
	X. Advancing the profession of health education			

Source: From National Commission for Health Education Credentialing & Society for Public Health Education. (2015). *A competency-based framework for health education specialists – 2015*. Whitehall, PA: Author. By permission.

Israel, the People's Republic of China, India, and Taiwan have all endeavored to improve health education or health promotion practice.

In an effort to promote international exchange and understanding related to the core competencies of health education/promotion and various credentialing mechanisms, a working group of 26 health education/promotion scholars and leaders from around the world met at the National University of Ireland in the summer of 2008. This meeting, now known as the Galway Consensus Conference, was a first effort to identify and codify agreement around quality assurance and credentialing on an international basis.

At this conference, the Domains of Core Competencies were developed (Allegrante, Barry, Airhihenbuwa et al., 2009). The domains are broader than competencies, but using these broad domains, competencies and credentialing systems can be developed by nations around the world. The Domains of Core Competencies align nicely with the NCHEC Responsibilities of a Health Education Specialist (NCHEC, 2016a). Several of the Domains are exactly the same as the NCHEC responsibilities including assessing, planning, implementing, evaluating, and advocacy. Three Domains, catalyzing change, and leadership and partnerships, are not identified as one of the seven major NCHEC Responsibilities, but would still be considered important skills that would actually be delineated at the competency or sub-competency level by NCHEC.

Since the Galway Consensus Conference, a new round of efforts to enhance professional preparation standards and credentialing has emerged in North America, throughout Europe, and in other regions and countries of the world such as Australia, Canada, Latin America, and New Zealand (Allegrante, Barry, Auld, & Lamarre, 2012). In Europe, professional standards for health promotion have been developed and reviewed (Speller, Parish, Davison, & Zilnyk, 2012).

The International Union for Health Promotion and Education (IUHPE) has established an accreditation system (IUHPE, 2016). The goal of the IUHPE European Health Promotion Accreditation System is, "to promote quality assurance, competence and mobility in Health Promotion practice and education through a Europe-wide accreditation system" (IUHPE, 2016). This accreditation is to provide recognition to individual practitioners as well as education and training courses. The long-term aim is to establish national accrediting organizations (NAOs) in every country. The European Accrediting Organization will then serve to approve the NAOs and accredit full Health Promotion Courses (IUHPE, 2016).

▷ Accreditation Task Forces

"Accreditation is a process by which a recognized professional body evaluates an entire program against predetermined criteria or standards" (Cleary, 1995). In most cases, colleges and universities that train students to enter a given profession are accredited by a recognized professional body that operates independently of the school. If a program does not meet the standards of the recognized professional body, it can be refused accreditation or lose its accreditation status. A nonaccredited program might have difficulty recruiting new students, recruiting quality faculty, placing program graduates in jobs, obtaining grant funds and may be restricted in its participation in the profession. Accreditation helps ensure that all students entering the profession have similar training and preparation. Accreditation has been a major focus for the health education/promotion profession since 2000. In January 2000, the SOPHE and AAHE cosponsored a meeting in Dulles, Virginia, to explore the issue of accreditation. Twenty-four professionals who were broadly representative of health education/promotion professional preparation programs or other stakeholders were invited to attend. Meeting participants reached consensus that a "coordinated accreditation system" was needed.

As a result of this meeting, the SOPHE/AAHE National Task Force on Accreditation in Health Education was established, and Dr. John Allegrante and Dr. Collins Airhihenbuwa agreed to serve as cochairs (Allegrante et al., 2004). The Task Force was charged to (1) "gather background information and refine plans for a comprehensive, coordinated quality assurance system that meets commonly accepted standards of accreditation, and (2) develop processes for ensuring profession-wide involvement in the discussion and design of such a system to foster its adoption and utilization" (SOPHE, 2000, p. 5).

After a comprehensive study of the issue, the task force completed its work in the spring of 2004 and submitted its final report to the AAHE and SOPHE boards of directors (Allegrante et al., 2004). In this report, four principles were given to guide the profession:

1. Health education is a single profession, with common roles and responsibilities.

2. Professional preparation in health education provides the health education specialist with knowledge and skills that form a foundation of common and setting-specific competencies.

3. Accreditation is the primary quality assurance mechanism in higher education.

4. The health education profession is responsible for assuring quality in professional preparation and practice (Allegrante et al., 2004, p. 676).

On the basis of these four principles, the task force developed eight important recommendations that were included within the study's final report. Since the release of the report, many of the recommendations have been implemented. Below is a summary of the eight recommendations, each followed by a comment on the progress that has been made on that recommendation:

1. Accreditation should replace approval as the accepted quality assurance mechanism for health education professional preparation. (This is accomplished. CEPH is now accrediting standalone undergraduate programs. Those health education programs with a current SABPAC approval will maintain that status until their approval expires and then will need to seek CEPH accreditation.)

2. The National Council for the Accreditation of Teacher Education (NCATE) should be the accrediting body for school health education programs, and the Council on Education for Public Health (CEPH) should be the accrediting body for community/public health education programs. (NCATE has evolved into a new organization—CAEP—but it will be the credentialing body for school health education, and CEPH has accepted the responsibility to serve as the accrediting body for undergraduate community/public health education programs. This recommendation has been accomplished.)

3. Future accreditation should be based on the best practices of existing accreditation systems. (This is accomplished with CEPH and CAEP.)

4. Students prepared in health education at the graduate level should meet *all* health education competencies with graduate-level proficiency. (This recommendation has been met. To achieve the MCHES designation, all competencies must be met in addition to additional advanced level competencies.)

5. Separate designations should be developed to identify undergraduate level practitioners from graduate level practitioners. (The NCHEC certification process designates those with entry-level skills [CHES] and those with advanced skills [MCHES]. This recommendation has been met.)

6. Undergraduate and graduate certification of individual health education specialists should be provided by NCHEC. In order to be eligible for CHES and MCHES certification, students must be graduates from schools/programs that are accredited. (This recommendation is in progress. NCHEC is the entity responsible for certifying entry-level and advanced level health education specialists. NCHEC has agreed in principle to only certify students from accredited programs and will move to implement this recommendation when accreditation is widely available and enough time has expired to allow programs to transition to the new accreditation process.)

7. The results of the Task Force should be shared with those professional associations that include public/community health education specialists as members. (Numerous articles have been written in professional journals and presentations made at professional meetings regarding the task force recommendations. In addition, there is a Web site with current news from the Task Force; see Weblinks.)

8. Implementation of the Task Force results will require a profession-wide effort and resources from stakeholders for an extended period of time. (This has occurred as the Task Force continues to function and has successfully lobbied for many of the changes noted above.)

Both the AAHE and SOPHE boards accepted the final Task Force report and then instituted a second committee to transition from the National Task Force recommendations to an implementation phase of the process. Dr. David Birch and Dr. Kathleen Roe cochaired this committee called the National Transition Task Force on Accreditation in Health Education.

The work of this task force culminated in a three-day meeting of health education/promotion professional preparation programs in Dallas, February 23–25, 2006 (Taub, Birch, Auld, Lysoby, & King, 2009). At this Third National Congress on Institutions Preparing Health Educators, accreditation issues were presented, discussed, and debated. Some attendees felt accreditation should move forward as quickly as possible. Others were reluctant to move in the direction of accreditation and wanted more discussion and debate. Several small programs expressed concern that they would not be able to meet accreditation requirements. Some present were concerned that the CEPH was being considered as the accreditation body and that using CEPH would push all health education/promotion programs to become public health programs. Others felt that if the roles and responsibilities utilized by NCHEC were used as the basis of accreditation, CEPH would be a suitable accrediting body. At the end of the conference, most participants supported the initiation of a coordinated accreditation system (Taub et al., 2009). To follow up the work of the National Transition Task Force and the Third National Congress, a third task force was initiated late in 2006. This task force, cochaired by Dr. David Birch and Dr. Randy Cottrell, was named the National Implementation Task Force for Accreditation in Health Education. Its charge was to continue preparing the health education/promotion profession for accreditation (Cottrell et al., 2009, 2012). This Task Force was still active in 2016, but given the substantial progress that has been made on the initial recommendations, discussions about sun setting the National Implementation Task Force for Accreditation in Health Education have begun.

▷ Health Education Program Accreditation

In health education/promotion, accreditation is available through two accrediting bodies. Health education/promotion programs that are affiliated with a college of education and prepared school health education teachers may receive "national recognition" through the Council for Accreditation of Educator Preparation (CAEP). CAEP's mission is to "advance excellent educator preparation through evidence-based accreditation that assures quality and supports continuous improvement to strengthen P-12 student learning" (CAEP, 2016b). As the mission implies, CAEP is dedicated to quality assurance for education in the broad sense. It accredits entire schools of education. Individual program reviews, such as for health education, math education, science education, etc., are a part of the CAEP accreditation process, and successfully reviewed programs receive "National Recognition." School health teacher preparation programs seeking national recognition through CAEP submit a portfolio to CAEP for review based on discipline-specific standards. Specialized Professional Associations (SPAs) recognized by CAEP develop the standards for their respective disciplines and conduct the recognition reviews; thus, professionals with discipline-specific content expertise make recognition decisions for programs such as health education, science, language arts, and math teacher preparation within teacher preparation institutions of higher education. The SPA for health education is currently SHAPE America-Health Education (CAEP, 2016a).

The Council on Education for Public Health (CEPH) accredits public health schools and programs at the graduate and undergraduate levels (CEPH, 2016a). This would include public health programs that have a health education concentration or focus. In the past, only graduate public health programs and undergraduate public health programs in the same unit as a Master of Public Health (MPH) degree program could be accredited. This left many undergraduate health education programs with no accrediting body. Beginning in January 2014, standalone undergraduate programs (those not affiliated with a graduate program) could also be accredited through CEPH. As of March, 2016, 21 Standalone Baccalaureate Programs had applied for accreditation. Four programs had completed their self-studies and undergone a site visit. In June, 2016, CEPH announced the first four standalone undergraduate public health programs to be accredited: East Carolina University, Rutgers University, University of Nebraska at Omaha, and the University of North Carolina Wilmington (CEPH, 2016c).

The accreditation of standalone undergraduate public health programs marks a major milestone for the health education profession. Professional preparation, especially at the undergraduate level, has not been uniform in the profession (Cleary, 1986). Some programs focus more on content, such as drugs, sexuality, stress, and physical fitness, whereas other programs emphasize process courses, such as planning, implementing, and evaluating. Some programs stress only individual behavior change, and others stress only population-based approaches to change. In 1987, the National Task Force on the Preparation and Practice of Health Educators attempted to develop a registry of health education programs. This effort, however, had to be abandoned. There was too much variety in faculty, administrative arrangements, courses, and philosophies of the various professional preparation programs to agree on criteria for inclusion in the registry (Cleary, 1995). There were 273 programs listed in the most recent 2009 edition of the AAHE *Directory of Institutions Offering Undergraduate and Graduate Degree Programs in Health Education* (M. Goldsmith, personal communication, August 3, 2010). Most of these programs were neither approved nor accredited, and there was no professional body monitoring their efforts. This clearly indicates a lack of consistency and quality control in the profession. Hopefully, with the initiation of standalone baccalaureate program accreditation, this situation will be improved and the quality of undergraduate health education professional preparation will be enhanced.

Even with the lack of quality control in the profession, the number of undergraduate public health professional preparation programs has grown significantly over the past 25 years. Many of these programs evolved from community health education programs while others were new. Approximately 50,000 undergraduate students graduated in public health between 1992 and 2012, and half of these graduations occurred after 2008 (Leider et al., 2015).

▷ Responsibilities and Competencies of Health Education Specialists

The skills needed to practice health education/promotion are clearly delineated as responsibilities, competencies, and sub-competencies. **Responsibilities** essentially specify the scope of practice for health education specialists (SOPHE & AAHE, 1997). They provide a general idea of what health education specialists do but do not provide the detail necessary to practice health education/promotion.

Under each responsibility there are four to seven **competencies**. A competency is defined as a "skill or ability necessary for successful performance as a health education specialist" (NCHEC & SOPHE, 2015, p. 89). Each competency is further broken down into multiple **sub-competencies**. A sub-competency is a "cluster of simpler but essential related skills or abilities within a competency" (NCHEC & SOPHE, 2015, p. 90). All students graduating from a health education professional preparation program as well as all practicing health education specialists should be able to demonstrate proficiency in all the health education specialist competencies and sub-competencies.

The most recent set of responsibilities, competencies, and sub-competencies of health education specialists, based on HESPA, is available in the publication, *A Competency-Based Framework for Health Education Specialists 2015* (NCHEC & SOPHE, 2015) and can be found in Appendix A of this text. The number of competencies in the HESPA model is 36 as compared with 34 in HEJA. The total number of sub-competencies in the HESPA 2015 model is now 258 as compared with 223 in HEJA. Of the 258 HESPA sub-competencies, 141 were validated at the entry level, 76 at the advanced 1 level, and 41 at the advanced 2 level (see **Table 6.3**). The additional competencies and sub-competencies reflect the contemporary practice of health education as identified in the HESPA 2015 study (NCHEC & SOPHE, 2015).

The *HESPA 2015* framework should be used by health education specialists and students on a regular basis. This is not a document that should be placed on a shelf to gather dust (see Appendix B). The NCHEC suggests that the competencies be used by students as a personal inventory to assess progress toward becoming a health educator, as a resource when preparing for the CHES/MCHES exam, as a means to assess strengths/weaknesses and direct continuing education efforts, and for professional preparation programs as a guide for curricular development (NCHEC, 2015).

Because the seven major responsibilities identified in the *HESPA 2015 model* are the core of what a health education specialist does, it is important to have a basic understanding of them when entering the profession. The following sections briefly describe each responsibility.

TABLE 6.3 **HESPA 2015 model hierarchical approach**

Level of Practice	Sub-Competencies
Entry-Level (minimum of a baccalaureate degree with professional preparation in the field of health education)	141 entry-level sub-competencies
Advanced 1-Level (minimum of a baccalaureate degree with professional preparation in the field of health education plus various combinations of degree [baccalaureate or master's] and years of experience)	141 entry-level sub-competencies **PLUS** 76 Advanced 1 sub-competencies
Advanced 2-Level (minimum of a doctoral degree in the field of health education, irrespective of years of experience)	141 entry-level sub-competencies **PLUS** 76 Advanced 1 sub-competencies **PLUS** 41 Advanced 2 sub-competencies

Source: National Commission for Health Education Credentialing & Society for Public Health Education. (2015). *A competency-based framework for health education specialists – 2015*. Whitehall, PA: Author. By permission.

Responsibility I: Assess Needs, Resources, and Capacity for Health Education/Promotion

The first major area of responsibility listed for health education specialists involves assessing needs, assets, and the capacity for health education/promotion. This responsibility provides the foundation for program planning (Bensley & Brookins-Fisher, 2009). In fact, "Conducting a needs assessment may be the most critical step in the planning process..." (McKenzie, Neiger, & Thackeray, 2013, p. 72). A **needs assessment** is a process that helps program planners determine what health problems might exist in any given group of people, what assets are available in the community to address the health problems, and the overall capacity of the community to address the health issues. Other terms used to describe this process include *community analysis, community diagnosis*, and *community assessment* (McKenzie et al., 2013).

In a needs assessment, "**Capacity** refers to both individual and collective resources that can be brought to bear for health enhancement" (Gilmore, 2012, p. 9). More specifically, assessing capacity identifies the assets—skills, resources, agencies, groups, and individuals—that can be brought together in a community to solve problems and empower a community. According to the World Health Organization **community empowerment** "refers to the process by which people gain control over the factors and decisions that shape their lives. It is the process by which they increase their assets and attributes and build capacities to gain access, partners, networks and/or a voice, in order to gain control" (World Health Organization, 2016). For that reason, it is critical to include members of the community on any planning team.

All health education specialists, regardless of the setting in which they are employed, must have the skills to assess the needs and capacity of those groups or individuals to whom their programs are directed. For example, a school health education specialist needs to base curriculum on the needs of the students, a health education specialist in the corporate setting needs to plan programs based on the needs of the company's employees, and public health

◄**Figure 6.4** A group of health education specialists meeting to discuss information gathered during the assessment phase that will be used to guide the planning phase

education specialists should base their health education/promotion efforts on the needs of the community they serve (NCHEC, 2015).

Health education/promotion programs should not be based on the whim of the health education specialist or any small group of decision makers. Resources are too valuable to waste on programs that do not address the needs of the population being served. As McKenzie et al. (2013) note, "...failure to perform a needs assessment may lead to a program focus that prevents or delays adequate attention directed to a more important health problem" (p. 72). Conversely, "We know our health education programs are on target when we base them on accurate needs assessment data and a careful interpretation of their meaning" (Doyle & Ward, 2001, p. 124). Ultimately, a well-conceived and well-conducted needs assessment determines if a health education/promotion program is justified. It also defines the nature and scope of a program (Gilmore, 2012).

To conduct a needs assessment, health education specialists should know how to locate and obtain valid sources of information related to their specific population(s) or to populations with similar characteristics. For example, this may entail a literature review or accessing information from local, county, or state health departments. In addition to examining preexisting information, called **secondary data**, it may be necessary for health education specialists to gather data of their own, known as **primary data**. They may have to conduct mail, electronic, and/or telephone surveys; hold focus group meetings (see **Figure 6.4**); and/or use a nominal group process. After all this information is collected, the health education specialist must be able to analyze the data and determine priority areas for health education/promotion programming.

The following example demonstrates the importance of a needs assessment. A health education internship student was placed with the Shriners Hospital for Burned Children in Cincinnati, Ohio. The hospital identified a problem with children being burned around campfires during the summer months and asked the student to develop a fire safety program for young campers. Fortunately, the site supervisor required the student to conduct a needs assessment before planning the program. After conducting focus groups, interviewing camp counselors, and reviewing the literature, it was concluded that campers were the wrong group to target with the program. Instead, a program for the camp leaders and counselors was needed. If the needs assessment had not been done, valuable time and resources would have been spent developing a program for the wrong priority population.

Responsibility II: Plan Health Education/Promotion

Planning involves more than just determining a location and time for a health education/promotion program. Planning begins by reviewing the health needs, problems, concerns, and capacity of the priority population obtained through the needs assessment. Early in the planning process, it is important to recruit interested stakeholders, such as community leaders, representatives from community organizations, resource providers, and representatives of the community population, to support and help develop the program. Without the help of these stakeholders, it may be impossible to develop effective programs. To be effective in the planning process, the health education specialist should have strong written and oral communication skills, leadership ability, and the expertise to help diverse groups of people to reach consensus on issues of interest. Further, as part of the planning process, it may be necessary for the health education specialist to identify and obtain resources to support the program. This often involves the development of grants and/or contracts with outside organizations or funding agencies.

As part of the planning process, health education specialists must be competent to develop goals and objectives specific to the proposed health education/promotion program. These goals and objectives are the foundation on which the program is established. Writing specific and measurable objectives is critical. No health education/promotion program should be initiated without objectives or considered complete until an evaluation of the objectives is conducted. Writing good objectives is a skill you can only obtain through guided practice and experience. After program goals and objectives are written, the next step is to develop appropriate interventions that will meet these goals and objectives.

Many different types of interventions are available to health educators. These interventions can involve educational strategies like brochures, presentations, simulations, health fairs, case studies, role playing, etc. They could also involve changing the social physical environment like removing candy from a vending machine. Sometimes interventions involve community mobilization bringing together like-minded individuals and groups to work on a common problem or issue. Various communication strategies like radio, TV, direct mail, email, and social media can also be utilized as health education strategies. In addition, some strategies involving changing rules, regulations, policies or laws to enhance health, such as instituting nonsmoking policies in a workplace, may be utilized.

Consider the following example of a planning process. A health education specialist, who is working in the university health service wellness center, analyzes the results of a recently conducted needs assessment. Next, the health education specialist recruits a variety of individuals to form a committee that will help develop a plan for the university. This committee includes representatives of the Greek system, student life organization, resident life (dorms), athletics, health education/promotion program, provost's office, campus security, and local chamber of commerce. Together, they review the needs assessment data and agree that alcohol-related incidents are a health problem on campus that needs to be addressed.

First, the planning group uses existing baseline data on alcohol-related incidents to establish written objectives for the overall program. Next, they plan a variety of strategies to increase awareness of alcohol-related problems, modify alcohol-drinking behaviors, and reduce the number of reported alcohol incidents on campus. They organize a campus-wide alcohol awareness day, and they devise strategies with local bar owners to reduce excessive drinking. They also establish an agreement with campus security and the provost to refer any student involved in an alcohol-related incident to a mandatory alcohol education program that they will develop. In addition, they create posters and flyers promoting responsible drinking, train a bevy of peer student leaders to speak to dorm and Greek groups, and plan a variety of nonalcoholic alternative events for the campus community. For each and every strategy, they write specific objectives, establish implementation timelines, assign tasks to committee members, and establish a budget. If the planned strategies are successful, the program objectives will be met.

An important aspect of planning includes observing the **Rule of Sufficiency**. This rule states that any strategies chosen must be sufficiently robust, or effective enough, to ensure the stated objectives have a reasonable chance of being met. For example, in the preceding scenario, do you think the primary objective (e.g., reduce the number of alcohol-related incidents on campus by 20 percent) has a reasonable chance of being reached if all the listed program strategies are implemented? On the other hand, if the only strategy used was to hand out a pamphlet on alcohol abuse to students, the intervention will not be robust enough to achieve the stated objective. In that case, the Rule of Sufficiency would not be met. Either the intervention strategies need to be enhanced, or the program should not be implemented. Time and resources are wasted if interventions are not sufficient to create the desired change. Further, if interventions fail to meet their objectives, then both the reputation of the health education specialist and the health education/promotion profession suffer.

Responsibility III: Implement Health Education/Promotion

After a needs assessment is conducted and analyzed, objectives are written, and intervention strategies are developed, it is time to implement the program. This involves "coordinating the logistics to implement the plan, train volunteers and staff members involved in the implementation, deliver the program, monitor the progress of the program, and evaluate the sustainability of the program" (NCHEC, 2015, p. 80). For many health education specialists, implementation is the most enjoyable of the responsibilities because it involves actually delivering the program.

To successfully implement a program, the health education specialist must have a thorough understanding of the people in the priority population. What is their current level of understanding regarding the issue at hand? What will it take to get the people to participate? Do they need financial assistance or child care? What time of the day should the program be offered? What location(s) would be most convenient? Although some of these questions can be answered from the initial needs assessment, it may also be necessary to obtain additional information about the priority population before proceeding with implementation. As always it is critical to have representation from the priority population on the planning committee as their input is vital to the success of a health education initiative.

When conducting various health promotion and education programs, it is important for the health education specialist to be comfortable using a wide range of educational methods or techniques. In school health, for example, it is not enough to simply lecture to students about "proper" health behaviors. A successful health education specialist uses many teaching strategies such as brainstorming, debate, daily logs, position papers, guest speakers, problem solving, decision making, demonstrations, role playing, drama, music, and current events. In community health, most programs require going beyond developing and distributing a simple pamphlet on a given health topic. Again, a wide variety of strategies should be used, including television, radio, newspapers, billboards, celebrity spokespersons, behavioral contracting, community events, contests, incentives, support groups, social media, and many more. As a general rule, health education specialists should always use multiple intervention activities when planning and implementing programs.

Health education specialists should also include population-based approaches to create health-improvement changes. Instead of focusing on individuals, population-based approaches focus on policies, rules, regulations, and laws to modify behaviors of a priority group or population. For example, instead of working one-on-one with individuals to enhance exercise levels, it might be more effective to work toward funding new walking and biking trails, having bike racks available at bus stations, initiating a city-wide walk/bike-to-work day, advocating for improved pedestrian safety laws, and so forth.

After a program is in place and operating, the responsibility of the health education specialist is not over. The health education specialist should continue to monitor the program to make certain everything is going as planned. If problems are noted, it may be necessary, even while the program is in progress, to revise the objectives or the intervention activities.

When implementing program strategies or interventions, health education specialists may need to apply a variety of sub-competencies such as presentation skills, group facilitation skills, pretest/posttest administration, data collection, and technology utilization, all of which must be demographically and culturally sensitive. During the intervention phase, a health education specialist typically has the most contact with the public. The Code of Ethics for health education specialists (see Appendix A) should be strictly followed, and one should always dress and act in an appropriate professional manner.

Responsibility IV: Conduct Evaluation and Research Related to Health Education/Promotion

Accurate evaluations must be conducted to measure the success of health education/promotion programs. These evaluations help reveal whether or not implemented programs are meeting their specified objectives. Programs not properly evaluated may be wasting valuable time, money, and other resources. Further, an unevaluated program cannot "prove its worth." So, it may risk being reduced or even eliminated when resources are short and downsizing occurs.

To conduct an effective evaluation, the health education specialist must first establish realistic, measurable objectives. As previously mentioned, this is an important part of the planning process. After objectives are in place, the health education specialist must develop a plan that will accurately assess if the program objectives have been met. Depending on the setting, this process may involve developing and administering tests, conducting surveys, observing behavior, tracking epidemiological data, or other methods of data collection. Evaluation plans can be simple or extremely sophisticated, depending on the program being evaluated, the expectations of the program planners, and the requirements of the funding agents.

After data is collected, it must be analyzed and interpreted. Reports are then developed and distributed to the appropriate parties. Ultimately, the evaluation results should be used to modify and improve current or future program efforts. In some cases, evaluation results may indicate that a program needs to be discontinued and funding redirected to other, more productive efforts. Health education specialists must have the fortitude to make these difficult decisions when needed.

In addition to evaluation, research is a vital activity for any profession, including health education/promotion. A profession moves forward and improves in large part as a result of the quality of its research and the new information it generates. **Health education research** can be defined as "a systematic investigation involving the analysis of collected information or data that ultimately is used to enhance health education knowledge or practice, and answers one or more questions about a health-related theory, behavior or phenomenon" (Cottrell & McKenzie, 2011, p. 2). Although more complex research skills are required at advanced levels, entry-level health education specialists should be able to read, synthesize, and use research results to improve their practice.

Responsibility V: Administer and Manage Health Education/Promotion

A great deal of administration, management, and coordination is needed to bring a health education/promotion program to fruition. Even though some administrative tasks may be performed by entry-level health education specialists, administration and management responsibilities are generally handled by professionals at more advanced levels of practice. For example, experienced health education specialists often become program managers or staff supervisors. "Good management and supervisory skills require training in a variety of organizational, psychological and business environments. Good management incorporates effective 'people skills' and knowledge of budgeting, task assignments and performance evaluation" (NCHEC, SOPHE, & AAHE, 2006, p. 33).

Health education specialists must facilitate cooperation among personnel, both within programs and between programs. Some public school systems, for example, have initiated coordinated school health programs. This involves coordinating the activities and services of school nurses, counselors, psychologists, food service personnel, physical educators, health education specialists, teachers, administrators, support staff, parents, and public health agencies. The ultimate goal is to develop both curricular and extracurricular programs to improve the health status of students, faculty, staff, and the community as a whole. Further, health education specialists in school settings may serve as curriculum coordinators or project directors and can be responsible for managing grants and program budgets.

Similar examples can be seen in the community setting. For example, a health department decides to apply for grant funds to reduce the incidence of tobacco use in its community. The health education specialist may form a coalition by bringing together individuals or groups with a vested interest in reducing tobacco use. Coalition members might include representatives from the American Cancer Society, American Lung Association, American Heart Association, local medical society, local dental association, public health department, public school system, and YMCA/YWCA. Coordination and integration of the services offered by these various groups would be critical to the successful development of a grant proposal and ultimately to the success of the funded program. It may even be necessary for the health education specialist to conduct or coordinate in-service training programs to ensure that all coalition members have similar knowledge of tobacco prevention programs. Obviously, administrative and management skills are needed throughout this entire process.

Responsibility VI: Serve as a Health Education/Promotion Resource Person

Health education specialists are often called on to serve as resource persons. It is not unusual for a student to seek out the health teacher for assistance when having a health-related problem. In the corporate setting, health education specialists get questions about a wide range of topics, including nutritional supplements, cancer signs and symptoms, the best type of shoe to wear for jogging, and many more.

Because it is impossible for health education specialists to know all the information that could be needed in a given position, they must have the skills to access resources they need. It may be necessary to visit the library; use computerized health retrieval systems; access health databases; find information on specific diseases; obtain local, regional, state, and national epidemiological data; and so on. It is critical that the health education specialist be able to differentiate valid information from questionable, misleading, false, or fraudulent information. As part of this resourcing process, it may also be necessary for health education specialists to select or develop their own effective educational resources for distribution to their priority populations.

Consider, for example, the entry-level health education specialist who was hired by a large metropolitan hospital. Her duties included developing health education/promotion programs for the community and resource materials for patients. Her first assignment was to develop educational materials on the problem of incontinence in older adults. This subject had not been covered in her professional preparation program. However, because of the skills she had previously learned, she was able to locate a variety of resources on the topic, evaluate their validity, select relevant information, and then develop an educational pamphlet and video on the topic.

Being able to simply retrieve information is not enough. Health education specialists must be able to establish effective consultative relationships with people who seek assistance, whether they are students, clients, employees, or other health education specialists. Health education specialists must instill confidence and communicate effectively in a nonthreatening manner. In some situations, health education specialists may decide to market their skills to individuals or groups as resource consultants. They may even decide to focus their career entirely as a resource person.

Responsibility VII: Communicate and Advocate for Health and Health Education/Promotion, and the Profession

Health education specialists must interact with various groups of people, including other health professionals, consumers, students, employers, employees, and fellow health education specialists. They must be skilled in written communication, oral communication, and mass media use including social media. Health education specialists need to feel comfortable working with individuals, small groups, and large groups, as the situation warrants. In essence, communication is the primary tool of the health education specialist. Without communication skills it is impossible to health educate.

It is often necessary for health education specialists to serve as communication filters between medical doctors/researchers and students or clients. Health education specialists must be able to "translate" difficult scientific concepts so that constituents can understand the information necessary to improve and protect their health. For example, a physician may tell a patient to start an exercise program, reduce fat in the diet, or manage stress better. Although many patients have a general idea of what these recommendations mean, they may not have the knowledge or skills to implement them. Most physicians cannot take the time to teach patients how to incorporate these changes into their lifestyles. Health education specialists can communicate detailed information on exercising safely, teach the client to recognize high-fat foods by reading food labels, and instruct the patient in progressive neuromotor relaxation. This may involve conducting one-on-one instruction, developing a videotape for patients to watch, creating brochures for distribution to patients, teaching classes, or coordinating support groups.

Beyond communicating health information, Responsibility VII requires health education specialists to "advocate" for health and the health education/promotion profession. This means they should initiate and support legislation, rules, policies, and procedures that will enhance the health of the populations with which they work. Health education specialists should be involved in supporting nonsmoking laws, mandatory helmet laws, seat belt laws, antidrug policies, rules to prevent selling "junk foods" in school cafeterias, initiatives to develop walking/biking trails, gun safety laws, and so forth.

Further, health education specialists should "advocate" for their profession. They should educate potential employers about the value of hiring professionally trained and degreed health education specialists with CHES status. When health education specialists hold positions with hiring authority, they should advertise for and hire degreed and certified health education specialists. It is important that health education specialists talk to legislators, policy makers, personnel directors, allied health workers, coworkers, family, and friends about the value of health education/promotion. They should join health education professional associations and support national initiatives designed to move the profession forward. These include the development of National Health Education Standards, updating health education responsibilities, and supporting accreditation efforts. Although advocating for the profession may seem awkward and somewhat akin to "blowing one's own horn," if health education specialists do not promote their profession, who will?

Summary of Responsibilities and Competencies

The responsibilities, competencies, and sub-competencies required for health education specialists do not function independently; they are highly interrelated. All the responsibilities demand excellent communication skills. Conducting an accurate needs assessment requires research skills to identify and gather appropriate resources. Planning should be based on a valid and reliable needs assessment. When implementing programs, be prepared to serve as a resource person. Evaluation relies on goals and objectives established during the planning process. Coordinating people and administering programs are necessary in planning, implementing, and evaluating programs.

It is not enough to be proficient in one, two, or even six of the responsibility areas. All seven responsibilities are critical for effective health education/promotion to take place. It is beyond the scope of this book to teach the reader how to do these tasks. Rather, it is the intent of this text to familiarize readers with the responsibilities, competencies, and skills they will be taught in later classes and ultimately practice in their employment settings.

▷ Multitasking

It is often necessary for health education specialists to use several competency-related skills simultaneously. This requires **multitasking**: the skill of coordinating and completing multiple projects at the same time. In college, health education/promotion students are often given a project at the beginning of a term. There is a specific amount of time to complete the project, and when the term ends the project is completed. In the work world, things do not function this way. Health education specialists work on multiple projects at the same time, and each project is usually in a different stage of completion.

Organization is the key to successful multitasking. For example, one health education/promotion internship student used a visual concept to help her stay organized while working on multiple projects. Using a bulletin board, unfinished projects and tasks were represented by floating balloon images. Once completed, these "balloons" were placed at the bottom of the bulletin board in the hand of a stick figure that represented the health education specialist. Other effective tools for multitasking include spreadsheets, timelines, and "to do" lists. With use of a smartphone, such lists can be readily at one's fingertips for referencing and updating.

▷ Technology

As in most professions, health education specialists must be familiar with and comfortable using computers, smart phones, tablets, and other forms of technology. Because computer software and hardware are constantly changing, it is important to keep up to date on the latest technological aids. Entry-level health education specialists are expected to have required technology skills by the time they enter their internships and certainly by the time they accept their first position. See **Box 6.2** for a list of entry-level computer skills.

In addition to basic computer skills, **social media** skills are becoming a vital component of health education. Social media involves use of the media and other technologies to allow for social interaction. Learning to use such social media as Facebook, Twitter, YouTube, LinkedIn, Myspace, Instagram, Blogger, Skype, and many more is no longer an option. It is a must in many health education settings and positions. Social media can be used for program promotion, social publishing, marketing, personal networks, e-commerce, information sharing, discussion forums, and many other existing and yet to be conceived uses. **Social Networking** is a specific type of social media that has many uses. Social networking involves connecting individuals (or organizations) that are tied (connected) by one or more specific factors, such as friendship, kinship, common interest, financial exchange, occupational or professional interests, or beliefs. More specifically, social networking services can be used by health education specialists to connect people with similar health interests, such as losing weight, exercising, stopping smoking, or reducing stress. They can also be used to link people who have a common cause, such as passing nonsmoking legislation or advocating for gun control. In addition, they are helpful for sending information or updates about programs sponsored by a

---

BOX 6.2

Entry-Level Technology Skills (Not Prioritized)

- Basic word processing/text editing skills including use of writing tools such as spell checkers, electronic thesaurus, etc.
- Basic to advanced electronic-spreadsheet use, beginning with elementary worksheets and progressing to more sophisticated "what-if" analyses
- Introductory statistical analysis software and data entry (assuming that statistics applications are also learned)
- Preparing effective PowerPoint presentations
- Critiquing components of computer-assisted health education software (health assessments to computer-assisted instruction)
- Electronic retrieval of quality health information—search engines, databases, and indexes of health literature

- Electronic health information media literacy, including evaluating the quality of health Web sites
- Using a Web page editor to design and develop effective health-based Web pages. This would include skills needed to upload pages to a server and then marketing the site to specific Internet audiences
- Professional email and discussion list etiquette
- Use of common technological innovations in health education/promotion such as digital video/photography, scanners, personal digital assistants, and computer-assisted interviews and surveys
- Use of various social media formats in communication with clients
- Preparing videos and uploading them to the Internet

Source: Modified from an initial list provided by Dr. Ernesto Randolfi, Montana State University–Billings. Posted to HEDIR Listserve, 2002.

---

given health agency such as the American Lung Association. Social networking has been used to send emails to pregnant women in developing countries to remind them of appointments and to provide educational messages. The possible uses for social networking in health education are limited only by one's imagination and creativity.

▷ Role Modeling

Being a healthy role model is not listed anywhere in the roles and responsibilities of a health education specialist, but it has been discussed and debated within the profession (Bruess, 2003; Davis, 1999) and is worth consideration in an entry level health education course. Some people feel that health education specialists should not be expected to be healthy role models. This expectation may discriminate against professionals who suffer from disease conditions that cause obesity or preclude a regular exercise regimen. Further, they contend that being a healthy role model puts too much pressure on health education specialists, especially because there is no accepted definition for what "healthy" means. On the other hand, many in the profession believe that being a healthy role model is important to effectively carry out the responsibilities of the profession. Some even argue that ethically, health education specialists must be role models.

The authors of this text tend to believe that role modeling is an important aspect of being a health education specialist. The purpose of presenting this issue is to stimulate health education/promotion students to enter the debate. Do you feel health education specialists should be role models? What does it mean to be a role model? Do you think health education specialists who are not role models will be less effective in their work or that those who are role models will be more effective? Are you a role model now for fellow students? Should you be? Do you want to be a role model in the future?

▷ Advanced Study in Health Education

After receiving a bachelor's degree in health education/promotion, students should not stop the educational process. At the very least, health education specialists should continue to learn on their own. One way of doing so is to participate in one or more professional associations (see Chapter 8). Such memberships allow the opportunity to read professional publications and attend state, regional, and national meetings of the associations.

If you are a CHES, an average of 15 continuing education contact hours are *required* each year (75 across five years) to maintain certification. These may be obtained by reading professional journals and submitting responses to questions on selected articles, by attending various professional meetings and workshops, by taking additional coursework, or by participating in other professional development activities.

At some point, health education specialists with a bachelor's degree should consider getting a master's degree. In some areas of the country and in some health education/promotion settings, such as medical care and worksite health education/promotion, the master's degree is often considered the entry-level degree. In other words, to be considered for employment in these settings, the health education specialist must hold an appropriate master's degree (see **Box 6.3**).

In school settings, the master's degree brings additional financial rewards and, in some states, progress toward more permanent teaching certificates or licenses. It is usually advised, however, not to complete a master's degree in teaching prior to obtaining your first teaching position. Hiring a new teacher with a master's degree, versus hiring a new teacher with a bachelor's degree, is more expensive for a school district. This factor may put a person with a master's degree and no teaching experience at a disadvantage in the hiring process.

In community or public health settings, the master's degree may bring additional financial rewards, as well as promotions within the agency. It may also open the door to higher-level positions with other public health agencies or public health departments.

▷ Master's Degree Options

There are multiple types of master's degrees. Typical choices include a Master of Education (**M.Ed.**), Master of Science (**M.S.**), Master of Arts (**M.A.**), Master of Public Health (**M.P.H.**), and Master of Science in Public Health (**M.S.P.H.**) (Bensley & Pope, 1994). Some colleges and universities may offer only one degree option, while others may offer more than one.

The M.Ed. degree is typically found in institutions in which the health education/promotion program is located in a College of Education or Teacher's College. Although many students in these programs focus on school health, this does not mean that everyone who obtains

BOX
6.3

GRADUATE LEVEL STUDY Jovanni V. Reyes

CURRENT POSITION/TITLE: Graduate Research/ Teaching Assistant

EMPLOYER: Texas A&M University

DEGREE/INSTIUTIONS: B.S., Health, Texas A&M University, College Station TX; M.S., Health Education, Texas A&M University, College Station TX

UNDERGRADUATE MAJOR: Health (Emphasis: Allied Health)

GRADUATE MAJOR: Health Education

Background: I was born and raised in a low-socioeconomic status (SES) part of Dallas, Texas, and am the first person in my immediate and extended family to pursue an education after high school. Although my family could never provide funds for my collegiate expenses, I have worked exceptionally hard to acquire awards and resources that will help me further my education. It was in my undergraduate course, "Race, Ethnicity and Health," where I first became interested in the issues of health disparities, health education, and health promotion. I began to realize that I could relate to many of the issues that were discussed. Raised in a low-socioeconomic neighborhood, I have witnessed firsthand the inequalities that minorities experience due to lack of access to quality health care services. These experiences have provided me with a heightened awareness of the actual health issues among minority communities. My research interests include minority health, health disparities, sexual/reproductive health, adolescent risk behaviors, impact of violence on health, and adultification and its impact on health. My current research focuses on the topic of teen pregnancy within minority populations and how the issue in turn affects quality of life. I was raised in a neighborhood where teen pregnancy was the norm. Every year, I saw more and more young pregnant adolescent girls struggling through life, experiencing the consequence of lack of access to information and services. Health issues that are highly prevalent among minorities surround me, and I feel it is my job to educate people about prevention and treatment. I

feel obligated to further my education for the sake of my family and my community. I want to gain as much knowledge as I can so that I can give back to my community. One of the reasons why I chose to further my education is to show both my family and the people of my community that it can be done. With hard work and determination, even children raised in a violence-filled low-socioeconomic neighborhood can defy statistics and be whatever they want to be. I am currently pursuing a terminal research degree in health education with a focus on minority health and health disparities. I am continuing graduate school because I desire to learn more about health education/promotion and health behaviors and how they affect the world around me. This is my inspiration toward becoming a health disparity researcher and educator. My goal is to help fill gaps within the research related to health disparities, and by filling the gaps, I wish to help in eliminating the current inequalities.

Overall impression of graduate school: Being that I was the first in my entire extended family to pursue graduate school, I have to admit that at first the idea was extremely intimidating. I literally had no guidance from family or friends due to the simple fact that I was the only person I knew who had ever chosen to continue school after a bachelor's degree. The first week was tremendously nerve wracking, and it was then that a few professors pulled me aside to talk with me about my transition into graduate school. After talking with them and giving them part of my background, I could see that the professors were truly there to support me in my educational endeavor. I remember one of my professors made us call her by her first name because not only was she our mentor and teacher but from that day on we were her colleagues. The idea that everyone (i.e., faculty, students, and staff) is working together to both promote health

BOX

6.3

continued

and support each other was mind-blowing to me.

What I liked most about graduate school: Graduate school not only opened endless doors of opportunities for me but it also helped me become a better health educator and helped me better understand things around me. Sitting in three-hour classes with my fellow colleagues leads to interesting, and sometimes controversial, conversations. This was my favorite part of graduate school, everyone having an actual conversation and voicing their opinion about various topics. As an undergraduate, some professors limited discussions or avoided certain topics in fear that the conversation would cause some type of riot. The courses I took in my graduate studies were primarily open discussions of different opinions, which often lead to a better understanding of different cultures, races, ethnicities, SES, etc. The more we, as health education specialists, get to know other people, the better we're prepared to educate them.

What I liked least about graduate school: During graduate school, there is definitely going to be an overwhelming number of projects and research opportunities. Initially, I wanted to get as much experience as I could and was really tempted to jump on as many projects as possible. After several talks with a few professors, I began to realize that although numerous opportunities will arise, I only have so many hours in a day. Professors are always going to be working on interesting research projects, but it is important to only "bite off as much as you can chew." The idea of restricting myself from amazing research was devastating to me. In spite of this, when I was finally able to focus on a specific project, I began to see where my passion was. There is always going to be a million really cool research projects, but there are only so many that you can really become passionate about.

Recommendations for health education students considering graduate study: My overall advice to students is to never fear the future. The idea of graduate school can be intimidating and scary, but what students need to know is that the people they meet and network with are there to support them in whatever they choose to do in life. Students usually don't jump for joy when someone recommends that they stay in school a few more years, but graduate school isn't only about sitting in a classroom and gaining new knowledge. It's about applying the knowledge you know to the outside world. It's about making a difference. It's the beginning of a new journey, and along the way you acquire new skills, network with new people, and all of it is beneficial not only to you as an educator but also as a person. Don't be afraid to get out there and push your limits.

this degree must pursue a career in public schools. Some colleges and universities offer M.Ed. degrees which emphasize areas such as community health and corporate health promotion.

The M.S. and M.A. degrees are usually found in universities in which the health education/promotion program is located in colleges other than education. Because there is no accepted accreditation for these programs, schools have much flexibility to develop programs that meet the needs of the local job market. These degrees offer a variety of emphasis areas, including public health, community health education/promotion, and corporate health promotion.

When considering differences between the M.S., M.A., and M.Ed. degrees, remember that the M.S. may be the more scientific or research-oriented degree, whereas the M.A. and M.Ed.

may be more practitioner oriented. This distinction, however, is not always true. Prospective students need to carefully examine the stated mission and degree requirements for any graduate-level health education/promotion program.

As their names imply, the M.P.H. and M.S.P.H. are degree choices for those wishing to work in the broad fields of public health. At one time working in the field of public health meant one would work in a city, county, or state public health department. The definition of public health, however, has been greatly expanded and now includes many other sites including volunteer agencies, public schools, worksites, hospitals, and so forth. The M.S.P.H. degree is typically more research oriented than the M.P.H. degree; otherwise, the degrees are similar. The M.P.H. can be generic or awarded in a variety of specialty areas such as health education, global health, nursing, dietetics, or epidemiology. The M.P.H. with an emphasis in health education/promotion is the degree of most interest to health education specialists. It is similar and often identical to an M.S. or M.A. degree in community health education.

Most M.P.H. degree-granting colleges and universities are accredited by the CEPH. Thus, the requirements to obtain an M.P.H. are more standardized than the requirements to obtain the M.S., M.A., or M.Ed. degrees, which typically are not accredited by any professional body. Resulting in part from accreditation, the M.P.H. degree may enjoy a higher status and more credibility than other health education/promotion degree designations. To obtain M.P.H. accreditation, the curriculum must meet the CEPH standards. To demonstrate that CEPH standards are met, the program develops and writes an extensive and detailed self-study and also hosts a two- to three-day campus visit by a CEPH site visit team.

The M.P.H. in health education/promotion has the reputation of being a more prestigious degree than the M.S., M.A., or M.Ed. There are, however, more health education specialists with M.S., M.A., or M.Ed. degrees than there are with the M.P.H. degree. The 2009 AAHE directory lists 96 institutions that provide master's-level non-M.P.H. health education/promotion degrees (M. Goldsmith, personal communication, August 3, 2010). Many of the institutions that offer non-M.P.H. health education/promotion degrees are now also offering the M.P.H. degree.

As of February 2016 there were 57 accredited schools of public health (up from 48 in 2013) and 110 accredited graduate public health programs (up from 88 in 2013) (CEPH, 2016b). As can be seen, the field of public health is growing. Not all of these public health programs, however, provide a concentration in health education/promotion. From one college to another, there are variations in degree concentration options. Before applying to a graduate program, carefully examine program requirements and master's degree options within the context of your future career goals.

▷ Selecting a Graduate School

Determining which college or university to attend is a decision that goes hand-in-hand with deciding which degree to pursue. In terms of practicality, factors such as cost, financial aid, location, and size must be considered (Cottrell & Hayden, 2007; US News and World Report, 2012). There is no current listing for non-CEPH-accredited community health education programs. AAHE used to maintain a list of all health education professional preparation programs, but with AAHE no longer in existence, that list is not up to date. SOPHE and NCHEC are considering developing a list of all health education professional preparation programs but have yet to do so. The best advice for students at this time is to look on the Web sites of various universities of interest to see what programs they offer. A good, current list of CEPH-accredited schools and programs in public health can be found online at the CEPH's Web site, http://www.ceph.org. Students will still need to look at each CEPH-approved program's Web site to determine which offer a specialization in health education.

College or university reputation is an important factor to consider when selecting a health education/promotion graduate program. There is a definite hierarchy among colleges and universities in the United States. Graduating from one of the more prestigious institutions may lend instant credibility to the graduate degree and enhance job opportunities.

Next, consider the reputation of the health education/promotion program at a given institution. To learn about various programs, bachelor's-level health education specialists can talk to other professionals in the field whom they admire and trust. A visit or call to current or former college professors may also be a good source of information. Contacting recent graduates from a program is also a good way to learn about a particular program and may help in the decision-making process (Cottrell & Hayden, 2007).

After narrowing your list to several programs, carefully review each program's admission requirements and application forms. These can usually be found online and most universities now have electronic applications and electronic references. If you need more information about program curricula or application procedures, contact the program administrator for such information.

▷ Admission Requirements

As an undergraduate health education/promotion student, it is not too early to be concerned about admission requirements to graduate school. Although admission requirements vary greatly from one university to another, the undergraduate grade point average (GPA) has traditionally been an important factor. In general, a student should strive to achieve an overall undergraduate GPA of at least a 3.0 on a 4.0 scale to be considered by most graduate programs. Some institutions do not specify a minimum GPA (Bensley & Pope, 1994). Instead, they tend to use more individual and subjective criteria in their admission process. In either case, it is important for new health education/promotion students to attempt from the first term of their freshman year to achieve the best grades possible. Too often, low grades in the first year or two of college prevent otherwise good students from being accepted into the master's degree program of their choice.

In addition to GPA requirements, most graduate programs require a completed application form, a letter of application, and several letters of reference. To be considered for admission, many programs also require students to submit scores from a standardized performance test such as the Graduate Record Exam or Miller Analogy Test. These scores may be a major component in the decision-making process, or they may simply be used in conjunction with other applicant information to provide a more well-rounded view of the prospective student.

▷ Financing Graduate Study

Funding a graduate degree may not be as burdensome as funding undergraduate education. Many colleges and universities award assistantships or fellowships to graduate students on a competitive basis. Typically, these graduate awards pay all or part of the graduate tuition and provide students with a monthly stipend to cover living expenses during their graduate studies. In return, students agree to work for the health education/promotion program.

If the award is a **graduate teaching assistantship** (or fellowship), the student teaches a specified number of undergraduate courses each term. These are usually introductory health education/promotion courses that meet general university requirements, or they are the first courses for health education/promotion majors. If the award is a **graduate research assistantship** (or fellowship), the student usually works closely with one or more faculty members on a particular research project. Students might be assigned to do literature reviews, assist with data collection, enter data into the computer, or a host of other research-related activities (Cottrell & Hayden, 2007).

Graduate assistantships and fellowships not only provide an excellent alternative for funding graduate education but also provide valuable health education/promotion work experience for the student. Further, a graduate assistantship may provide an advantage in the job market after the degree program is completed.

Summary

Since the late 1970s, many people have dedicated much time and hard work to defining and developing the roles and responsibilities of a health education specialist. The initial stages of this work were known as the Role Delineation Project. Eventually, a set of responsibilities, competencies, and sub-competencies were agreed on for health education specialists, regardless of whether they ultimately wished to work in schools, communities, clinics, or corporate settings. These responsibilities, competencies, and sub-competencies encouraged college and university professional preparation programs to develop their curricula based on a standardized set of skills for all health education/promotion students. These standards were also the basis for establishing individual certification within the profession.

In 1997, three additional responsibilities with accompanying competencies and sub-competencies were identified for graduate preparation in health education/promotion. With the completion of the CUP in 2005, the initial seven responsibilities and the three graduate responsibilities were united into seven revised responsibility areas that are now common to all health education specialists regardless of setting, degree, or experience. In 2015, the results of the HESPA were released, which increased the number of competencies to 36 and sub-competencies to 258. All health education/promotion professional preparation programs should now be training students based on the HESPA 2015 standards.

Accreditation of standalone undergraduate public health education programs is for the first time available through the CEPH. Masters level public health education programs are still accredited via the CEPH. With accreditation now available for all health education programs, it is expected that professional preparation continuity and quality will continue to be enhanced.

Continued study in health education/promotion is necessary to stay current with health information and new techniques for conducting health education/promotion programs. All health education specialists should read professional journals, join one or more professional associations, and take an active role in their functioning. CHESs and MCHESs must obtain continuing education credits to maintain their certification. Most bachelor's-level health education specialists should consider a master's degree at some point in their career. Decisions concerning graduate study should not be taken lightly. Undergraduate health education/promotion students need to be aware of the admission requirements for graduate school and work toward meeting those requirements. Graduate assistantships or fellowships provide an excellent alternative to fund graduate education.

Review Questions

1. Define *credentialing* and explain the differences among certification, licensure, and accreditation.

2. Outline the major events of the Role Delineation Project. What is the significance of the CUP HEJA 2010 and HESPA 2015? As a health education specialist, why should you be proud of these efforts?

3. Review the "Responsibilities and Competencies for Entry-Level Health Educators" (Appendix B). Do you think they are more focused on health content or the process skills needed to be a health education specialist? Defend your position and explain why you believe the health education/promotion profession has moved in this direction.

4. Identify two ways health education specialists can stay up to date in the field.

5. Explain the importance of accreditation for standalone undergraduate public health education programs.

6. What are the differences among the following academic degrees: M.A., M.Ed., M.S., M.P.H., and M.S.P.H.?

7. What technology skills are important for current and future health education specialists?

8. Briefly describe the process for applying to graduate school and discuss the potential benefits of serving as a graduate assistant.

Case Study

Reba is a junior level undergraduate student majoring in public health with a concentration in community health education. She has been asked by one of her faculty members to attend a recruiting event for high school seniors. The purpose of the event is to allow high school seniors the opportunity to interact with college students who are in a major the high school seniors are considering. After a brief presentation, Reba is answering questions from the seniors. One of the high school students asks, "You mention that your public health studies program is accredited by CEPH. Why is that important to me in considering which college program to attend?" The next question she gets is, "You mentioned that students graduating from your program are eligible to take an exam to be a Certified Health Education Specialist. What are the advantages of obtaining this certification?" How would you respond to these two questions?

Critical Thinking Questions

1. If Helen Cleary and her contemporaries had not begun the Role Delineation Project, and if there were no certification (CHES) available to health education specialists, how

do you think the profession would be different today? Think in terms of professional preparation, recognition, employment opportunities, and so on.

2. An accreditation system is now available for all graduate and undergraduate public health education/promotion professional preparation programs. How do you think enhanced opportunities for accreditation will impact the profession? What do you see as the potential positive outcomes and the potential negative outcomes of accreditation? Do you feel that only students graduating from accredited programs should be allowed to sit for the CHES exam?

3. Review the National Health Education Competencies that resulted from the HESPA 2015 model (see Appendix B). Do you feel they accurately represent professional practice? Why or why not? What changes do you think should be made in terms of eliminating competencies, adding competencies, or moving sub-competencies from one level to the other?

 ## Activities

1. Read each competency and entry-level sub-competency of a health education specialist (see Appendix B). Score each competency and sub-competency using the following scale:

    a. I currently have the skill to meet this competency/sub-competency.

    b. I am uncertain if I have the skill to meet this competency/sub-competency.

    c. I do not have the skill to meet this competency/sub-competency.

    After rating each competency and sub-competency, make a list of things you can do to enhance your skills. Keep this table and periodically reevaluate your skills throughout your program of study.

2. Identify one or more universities you may wish to attend for graduate school. Go online and read about the program, its curriculum, degrees offered, financial aid and graduate assistant opportunities, and application procedures.

3. Make an appointment with a professor at your school to talk about graduate school. Ask about schools the professor attended and the degrees earned. Finally, ask for advice on what degree to earn and what school to attend.

Weblinks

1. http://www.nchec.org/

    National Commission for Health Education Credentialing (NCHEC)

    Use this Web site to learn more about becoming a CHES. The site provides helpful information about health education certification including application procedures.

2. http://www.ceph.org/

    Council on Education for Public Health

    The Council is responsible for accrediting programs in public health. A complete list of accredited schools and programs of public health can be found at this site. This site can help identify accredited public health education graduate programs to which one may want to apply.

The four Web sites below all contain good information on selecting a graduate program to attend.

3. http://www.usnews.com/education/best-graduate-schools/articles/us-news-ranks-best-graduate-schools

4. http://www.princetonreview.com/grad-school-advice/choosing-a-school

5. http://www.nextscientist.com/choose-graduate-school-program/

6. http://www.gradschools.com/get-informed/before-you-apply/choosing-graduate-program

References

Allegrante, J. P., Airhihenbuwa, C. O., Auld, M. E., Birch, D. A., Roe, K. M., & Smith, B. J. (2004). Toward a unified system of accreditation for professional preparation in health education: Final report of the National Task force on Accreditation in Health Education. *Health Education & Behavior, 31* (6), 668–683.

Allegrante, J. P., Barry, M. M., Airhihenbuwa, C. O., Auld, M. E., Collins, J. L., et al. (2009). Domains of core competency, standards, and quality assurance for building global capacity in health promotion: The Galway Consensus Conference Statement. *Health Education & Behavior, 36* (3), 476–482.

Allegrante, J. P., Barry, M. M., Auld, M. E., & Lamarre, M. (2012). Galway revisited: Tracking global progress in core competencies and quality assurance for health education and health promotion. *Health Education & Behavior. 39* (6), 643–647.

Allegrante, J. P., Barry, M. M., Auld, M. E., Lamarre, M., & Taub, A. (2009). Toward international collaboration on credentialing in health promotion and health education: The Galway Consensus Conference. *Health Education & Behavior, 36* (3), 427–438.

American Association for Health Education (AAHE), National Commission for Health Education Credentialing (NCHEC), & Society for Public Health Education (SOPHE). (2010). Health Educator Job Analysis—2010: Executive summary and recommendations. Retrieved February 20, 2016, from http://www.sophe.org/HEJA2010.cfm.

Bensley, L. B., Jr., & Pope, A. J. (1994). A study of graduate bulletins to determine general information and graduation requirements for master's degree programs in health education. *Journal of Health Education, 25* (3), 165–171.

Bensley, R. J., & Brookins-Fisher, J. (2009). *Community health education methods: A practical guide* (2nd ed.). Boston: Jones and Bartlett Publishers.

Bruess, C. (2003). The importance of health educators as role models. *American Journal of Health Education, 34* (4), 237–239.

Cleary, H. P. (1986). Issues in the credentialing of health education specialists: A review of the state of the art. In William B. Ward (Ed.), *Advances in health education and promotion,* (pp. 129–154). Greenwich, CT: Jai Press, Inc.

Cleary, H. P. (1995). *The credentialing of health educators: An historical account 1970–1990.* New York: The National Commission for Health Education Credentialing, Inc.

Cottrell, R. R., Auld, M. E., Birch, D. A., Taub, A., King, L. R., et al. (2012). Progress and directions in professional credentialing for health education in the United States. *Health Education and Behavior, 39* (6), 681–694.

Cottrell, R. R., & Hayden, J. (2007). The why, when, what, where and how of graduate school. *Health Promotion Practice, 8* (1), 16–21.

Cottrell, R. R., Lysoby, L., Rasar King, L., Airhihenbuwa, C. O., Roe, K. M., et al. (2009). Current developments in accreditation and certification for health promotion and education: A perspective on systems of quality assurance in the United States. *Health Education & Behavior, 36* (3), 451–463.

Cottrell, R. R., & McKenzie, J. F. (2011). *Health promotion and education research methods.* Boston: Jones and Bartlett Publishers.

Council on Education for Public Health. (2016a). *Accreditation Criteria and Procedures.* Retrieved February 20, 2016, http://ceph.org/criteria-procedures/

Council on Education for Public Health. (2016b). *Accredited Schools & Programs.* Retrieved February 27, 2016, from http://ceph.org/accredited/.

Council on Education for Public Health. (2016c). *Standalone Baccalaureate Programs.* Retrieved July 24, 2016 from: http://ceph.org/accredited/#baccalaureate.

Council for Accreditation of Educator Preparation. (2016a). *SHAPE America health education.* Retrieved July 27, 2016 from http://caepnet.org/accreditation/caep-accreditation/spa-standards-and-report-forms/shape-health-ed.

Council for Accreditation of Educator Preparation. (2016b). *Vision, mission, & goals.* Retrieved July 27, 2016 from http://caepnet.org/about/vision-mission-goals.

Davis, T. M. (1999). Health educators as positive health role models. *Journal of Health Education, 30* (1), 60–61.

Doyle, E., & Ward, S. (2001). *The process of community health education and promotion.* Mountain View, CA: Mayfield Publishing.

Gilmore, G. D. (2012). *Needs and capacity assessment strategies for health education and health promotion.* Boston: Jones and Bartlett.

Gilmore, G. D., Olsen, L. T., Taub, A., & Connell, D. (2005). Overview of the National Health Educator Competencies Update Project, 1998–2004. *American Journal of Health Education, 36* (6), 363–370.

International Union for Health Promotion and Education. (2016). The IUHPE European Health Promotion Accreditation System Overview. Retrieved February 20, 2016, from http://www.iuhpe.org/index.php/en/the-accreditation-system.

Joint Committee for Graduate Standards. (1996). *National Congress for Institutions Preparing Graduate Health Educators.* Program Booklet, 1.

Leider, J. P., Castrucci, B. C., Plepys, C. M., Blakely, C., Burke, E., & Sprague, J. B. (2015). Characterizing the growth of the undergraduate public health major: U.S., 1992–2012. *Public Health Reports.* 130, 104–113.

McKenzie, J. F., Neiger, B. L., & Thackeray, R. (2013). *Planning, implementing & evaluating health promotion programs* (6th ed.). Boston: Pearson Education, Inc.

National Commission for Health Education Credentialing. (1996). *A competency-based framework for professional development of certified health education specialists.* New York: National Commission for Health Education Credentialing.

National Commission for Health Education Credentialing. (2015). *The health education specialist: A companion guide for professional excellence* (7th ed.). Whitehall, PA: Author.

National Commission for Health Education Credentialing. (2016a). *Areas of responsibility for health education specialists. 2015.* Retrieved February 20, 2016, from http://www.nchec.org/responsibilities-and-competencies.

National Commission for Health Education Credentialing. (2016b). *Eligibility for the CHES exam.* Retrieved March 3, 2016, from http://www.nchec.org/exam/eligible/ches/.

National Commission for Health Education Credentialing. (2016c). *Mission and purpose.* Retrieved August 19, 2013, from http://www.nchec.org/aboutnchec/mission/.

National Commission for Health Education Credentialing. (2016d). *NCHEC receives distinguished recognition.* Retrieved February 20, 2016, from http://www.nchec.org/news/posts/nchec-receives-distinguished-recognition

National Commission for Health Education Credentialing. (2016e). *Why certify? Credentialing and benefits of certification.* Retrieved February 20, 2016, from http://www.nchec.org/credentialing/credential/.

National Commission for Health Education Credentialing & Society for Public Health Education. (2015). *A competency-based framework for health education specialists—2015.* Whitehall, PA: Author.

National Commission for Health Education Credentialing, Society for Public Health Education, & American Association for Health Education. (2006). *A competency-based framework for health educators—2006.* NCHEC: Whitehall, PA.

National Task Force on the Preparation and Practice of Health Educators. (1985). *Framework for the development of competency-based curricula for entry level health educators.* New York: National Commission for Health Education Credentialing, Inc.

National Transition Task Force on Accreditation in Health Education. (2016). *What is accreditation?* Retrieved February 20, 2016, from http://www.healthedaccred.org/docs/home/Benefits%20of%20accred.pdf.

Quality Assurance Solutions. (2016). *Quality assurance definition.* Retrieved February 20, 2016, from http://www.quality-assurance-solutions.com/Quality-Assurance-Definition.html.

Society for Public Health Education. (2000). Future directions for quality assurance of professional preparation in health education. *News & Views, 27* (3), 5.

Society for Public Health Education & American Association for Health Education (1997). *Standards for the preparation of graduate-level health educators*. Washington, DC: Author

Speller, V., Parish, R., Davison, H., & Zilnyk, A. (2012). Developing consensus on the CompHP professional standards for health promotion in Europe. *Health Education & Behavior, 39* (6), 663–671.

Taub, A., Birch, D. A., Auld, M. E., Lysoby, L., & King, L. R. (2009). Strengthening quality assurance in health education: Recent milestones and future directions. *Health Promotion Practice, 10* (2), 192–200.

US News and World Report. (2012). 7 critical steps to find the right grad school. Retrieved February 27, 2016, from http://www.usnews.com/education/best-graduate-schools/articles/2012/04/06/7-critical-steps-to-find-the-right-grad-school.

World Health Organization. (2016). Track 1: Community empowerment. Retrieved February 27, 2016, from http://www.who.int/healthpromotion/conferences/7gchp/track1/en/.

The Settings for Health Education/ Promotion

Chapter Objectives

After reading this chapter and answering the questions at the end, you should be able to:

- Identify the four major settings in which health education specialists are employed.

- Describe the major responsibilities for health education specialists in the four major settings.

- Discuss the advantages and disadvantages of the four major settings.

- Explain the qualifications and major responsibilities of health education specialists working in colleges and universities.

- Identify a variety of "nontraditional" settings in which health education specialists may be employed.

- State several action steps that can be taken to help procure one's first job in health education/promotion.

Today, most Americans live a healthier and longer life than ever before. Despite this fact, it is clear that many, if not most, Americans are not living at their optimal level of health. Hereditary, environmental, societal, and behavioral factors predispose too many U.S. citizens to disease, suffering, disability, and premature death. Health education specialists are professionally trained to help individuals and communities reduce their health risks. According to the U.S. Department of Labor Bureau of Labor Statistics (2016), there were 115,700 health education specialists employed in the United States in 2014 earning a median annual wage of $42,450 or a median hourly wage of $20.41. The job outlook for 2014–2024 is for health education positions to grow at a rate of 13 percent, which is considered faster growth than for the average profession. The challenge for health education specialists is to help people reduce their risk for disease and death and increase the probability of a long, happy, and productive life.

To meet this challenge, health education specialists conduct programs in a variety of settings (Society for Public Health Education [SOPHE], 2014). The use of multiple settings is important because it allows health education specialists to reach the greatest number of people in the most convenient, efficient, and effective ways possible. Although settings differ, "The concept of a 'generic role' common to all health educators, regardless of work setting, emerged and formed the basis for the credentialing process for health education specialists" (National Commission for Health Education Credentialing, 2016). While the goals of health education/promotion and the competencies needed to carry out the responsibilities are nearly the same in all settings, the actual duties of a specific job may differ greatly from setting to setting. For example, some positions may involve more assessing and planning while others may involve more research and evaluation, and still others may involve direct education of individuals and groups.

Professional preparation programs in health education/promotion should prepare students to meet the various competencies and sub-competencies of a health education specialist and thus prepare students for employment in one or more of four major settings. These settings are schools, hospitals/clinics, public/community health agencies, and business/industry. On obtaining a terminal degree, students from any of these settings may seek employment as college or university health education faculty. In addition, health education specialists can work in a variety of nontraditional employment areas.

This chapter discusses each of the four major settings for health education/promotion. After a short introduction to the setting, a description of one day in the career of a health education specialist from that particular setting is presented. This is designed to give the reader a general idea of what a workday is like. Because of the great diversity in duties from one health education specialist to another, even within the same setting, it is impossible to say that this is a typical day. For most health education specialists, there is no such thing as a typical day. Following the description is a section that describes additional responsibilities that might be assigned to health education specialists in the setting. Again, this is not intended to be an exhaustive list but rather to further the reader's understanding of job responsibilities in that setting. Finally, each section ends with a listing of some advantages and disadvantages for that setting. As students become interested in one or more settings, they are encouraged to contact, interview, and job shadow health education specialists working in those settings.

▷ School Health Education/Promotion

School health is more than just the health educator teaching in the classroom, although that is certainly a very important component. School health also involves a physically and socially healthy environment, health services such as nursing and athletic training, a good nutrition program that provides healthy and appetizing meals, physical education and athletics, programs to promote the health of faculty/staff, counseling and psychological services, and community buy in and involvement (American School Health Association, 2016). **School health education/promotion instruction**, as the name implies, primarily involves instructing school-age children about health and health-related behaviors. The initial impetus for school health stemmed from the terrible epidemics of the 1800s and the efforts of the Women's Christian Temperance Movement to promote abstinence from alcohol in the early 1900s. Many states mandated school health education/promotion to inform students about these health hazards. Unfortunately, these mandates have seldom been strictly enforced. Further, teachers often have been underqualified, with only an academic minor or a few elective courses to prepare them for the health classroom. Frequently they hold a dual certification in health education/promotion and physical education with the majority of their professional preparation being in physical education. As a result, the quality of school health programs often has been compromised (Breckon, Harvey, & Lancaster, 1998; Naidoo & Wills, 2000).

Despite these limitations, the potential for school districts and health instruction programs in particular to impact students is tremendous. Jalloh (2007) noted that "school-based health education is an opportunity waiting to be taken advantage of; an opportunity for you to discover the best way to influence positive health-related change in the lives of youth and to maximize the use of some education dollars to achieve synergistic health and education goals" (p. 18). It is easier and more effective to establish healthy behaviors in childhood than it is to change unhealthy behaviors in adulthood. The goal of health education/promotion in schools is to help students adopt and maintain healthy behaviors (Joint Committee on National Health Education Standards, 2007). Each school day provides the opportunity to reach 50.1 million public school students and 4.9 million private school students. The 98,500 schools in the United States (National Center for Educational Statistics, 2016) should provide a laboratory where students can eat healthy foods, participate in physical activity, and learn how to take care of their health and well-being. The results of a recent comprehensive literature review found, "Schools can improve the health and learning of students by supporting opportunities to learn about and practice healthy behaviors, providing school health services, creating safe and positive school environments, and engaging families and community" (Michael, Merlo, Basch, Wentzel, & Weschler, 2015, p. 740).

The sophistication of school health education/promotion instruction has increased dramatically over the years. Today's school health education specialist needs to be well trained and prepared to deliver a comprehensive and demanding curriculum. Comparing the 1922 "Rules of Good Health" with the 2007 National Health Education Standards (Joint Committee on National Health Education Standards, 2007) clearly illustrates this point (see **Tables 7.1** and **7.2**).

When the school health education/promotion component is made part of a broader, district-wide approach known as the **Whole School, Whole Community, Whole Child Model (WSCC)**, the potential to impact students in a positive way is even greater as is the alignment between student health and educational outcomes (Lewallen, Hunt, Potts-Datema, Zaza, & Giles, 2015). The WSCC Model is based on the original work of Allensworth and Kolbe (1987), who were the first to envision a comprehensive and coordinated school health program. They called this a **coordinated school health**. They defined it as

> an integrated set of planned, sequential, school-affiliated strategies, activities, and services designed to promote the optimal physical, emotional, social, and educational development of students. The program involves and is supportive of families and is determined by the local community based on community needs, resources, standards and requirements. It is coordinated by a multidisciplinary team and accountable to the community for program quality and effectiveness. (p. 60)

The new WSCC Model focuses on student health and learning, addresses critical education and health outcomes, encourages collaborations, and engages community resources (Lewallen et al., 2015).

A health education specialist choosing to work in the school setting will find a challenging and rewarding career. Given the number of school districts in the United States, it is obvious that a large number of people teach health education/promotion in the schools. Unfortunately, many of these people are not health education specialists. Some school districts

TABLE 7.1 **Rules of Good Health—1922**

1. Take a full bath more than once a week.
2. Brush teeth at least once a day.
3. Sleep long hours with window open.
4. Drink as much milk as possible, but no coffee or tea.
5. Eat some vegetables or fruit every day.
6. Drink at least four glasses of water a day.
7. Play part of everyday outdoors.
8. Have a bowel movement every morning.

Source: "Rules of the health game" in Milk and Our School Children, U.S. Dept. of the Interior, Bureau of Education, Health Education, No. 11 (1922).

have used biology, physical education, home economics or family life, and consumer science teachers to teach health. Even when certified health education teachers are employed, they may have only a minor in health education/promotion and are not fully prepared. A further problem confounding the employment situation in the schools is that the requirement for health education/promotion is usually less than the requirements for other academic subjects. Students typically need only one or two semesters of health education instruction to graduate from high school, whereas they probably are required to complete four years of English. With such a minimal requirement for health education, the number of health teachers needed and the resulting demand for health teachers are lower than in other teaching fields. The bottom line is that, in many parts of the country, it is difficult to obtain a job in school health.

Those students who are really committed to being outstanding school health teachers, however, should not be deterred from this career path. With time, dedication, networking, and perseverance, those who really want to teach health in the schools can usually find employment. Substitute teaching, coaching, and volunteering are good ways to make oneself known in a school district and increase the likelihood of eventual employment. Students are

TABLE 7.2 **National Health Education Standards—2007**

1. Students will comprehend concepts related to health promotion and disease prevention to enhance health.
2. Students will analyze the influence of family, peers, culture, media, technology, and other factors on health behaviors.
3. Students will demonstrate the ability to access valid information and products and services to enhance health.
4. Students will demonstrate the ability to use interpersonal communication skills to enhance health and avoid or reduce health risks.
5. Students will demonstrate the ability to use decision-making skills to enhance health.
6. Students will demonstrate the ability to use goal-setting skills to enhance health.
7. Students will demonstrate the ability to practice health-enhancing behaviors and avoid or reduce health risks.
8. Students will demonstrate the ability to advocate for personal, family, and community health.

Source: Reprinted with permission from the American Cancer Society. *National health education standards: Achieving excellence,* 2nd ed. Atlanta, GA: American Cancer Society, 2007. http://www.cancer.org/bookstore.

▶ **Figure 7.1** Food service is one component of a coordinated school health program.

encouraged to talk to their own professors to determine the job market for school health education/promotion in their area.

Beyond teaching in the classroom, the school health education specialist should also take a leadership role in advocating for and the development of school health policy. Policies are written statements that guide the school district related to many health issues (McKenzie & Pinger, 2015). For example, a school district may have policies related to tobacco use on school property, the food and snack items available in the cafeteria (see **Figure 7.1**), safety measures, violence, suicide, staff wellness programs, community advisory committees, and many more issues. Further, once policy is developed, it needs to be carefully implemented and then monitored. Policy work is not easy, but it is extremely important for a school district. It is often the policy work that provides the most visibility to a coordinated school health education program and individual school health education specialists. When school boards, administrators, and the community know about and are proud of the health education program, that program is a success.

A Day in the Career of a School Health Education Specialist

At 5:45 A.M. the alarm goes off, and Ms. Bell's day starts. Ms. Bell teaches seventh- and eighth-grade health at a junior high school in a suburban school district. After going through the normal morning routine, she arrives at the school building around 7:00 A.M. There is a half-hour before homeroom, so she picks up her mail and duplicates a test that she prepared the night before for her eighth-grade health class. She then heads for her homeroom to meet the students. Essentially, homeroom involves administrative responsibilities and a considerable amount of paperwork.

In homeroom she takes attendance, gets a lunch count, listens to announcements over the loudspeaker, and collects money from a fruit sale fund-raiser. The fruit sale is being conducted by the PTA to raise money for new computers in the school. The PTA used to sell candy, but because of a new district policy that Ms. Bell and the Coordinated School Health team advocated for, candy sales are no longer allowed as fund raisers. Selling candy to raise money is counterproductive to the health message the school is trying to promote.

At 7:45 A.M. the first period starts. This school has eight 50-minute periods, with only four minutes between periods. In the first three periods, Ms. Bell teaches seventh-grade health. Today's lesson is on refusal skills related to alcohol and drug use. Ms. Bell has written three scenarios that students could find themselves in. The scenarios are open ended, so after each one Ms. Bell leads a discussion on how to use refusal skills to get out of a bad situation. She then asks students to role-play the situations to gain further practice in using refusal skills. Unfortunately, only two of her three classes will get this lesson today. The second-period class is one day behind because of an assembly that was held a week ago. Ms. Bell has to find a way to catch this group up with the rest of the classes.

Ms. Bell's fourth period is divided in half. The first half, she has lunch room duty. It is her responsibility to monitor the lunch room while students are eating. This is a noisy and somewhat stressful duty. In today's lunch room, two boys become unruly and nearly get into a fight. She sends them to the office for discipline, but the situation is still upsetting.

The second half of fourth period is Ms. Bell's lunch time. She usually has 25 minutes to eat lunch and relax before fifth period begins. Today, however, she must use part of that time to drop by the office for a follow-up discussion with the assistant principal concerning the incident with the two boys in the lunch room.

In fifth period, Ms. Bell teaches eighth-grade health. Today is a test day. While the students are taking their test, Ms. Bell works at her computer to update the online Web page that lists student assignments for the week. She must keep her online Web page up-to-date so that parents can be constantly informed of what is happening in the class and what assignments their children have due.

Sixth period is Ms. Bell's planning period. Today she tries to make a phone call to the parents of one of her students who is having problems in health class, but no one is home. She then grades the test papers from her previous class and records the grades. She averages the grades and starts to develop interim reports for the fifth-period class, but she runs out of time. Seventh and eighth periods are also eighth-grade health classes. While students take their tests, Ms. Bell grades papers from the previous classes and works on developing her interim reports. She must develop an interim report for each student that is then distributed to the parents.

School ends for the students at 2:57 P.M. After monitoring the hall while students leave the building, Ms. Bell hurries to the cafeteria for the monthly teachers' meeting. General information and announcements are presented by the principal. The meeting ends at 4:00 P.M.

In addition to her teaching responsibilities, Ms. Bell coaches the junior high girls' volleyball team. Practice usually goes from 3:15 P.M. to 5:00 P.M. Today's practice will go from 4:00 P.M. to 5:30 P.M. because of the teachers' meeting. After practice, Ms. Bell waits until the last girl leaves the locker room, then returns to her classroom to prepare for the next day's classes. She leaves the school at around 6:00 P.M.

After dinner and her family responsibilities, Ms. Bell spends 20 minutes on the phone with the student's parents who were not at home when she tried to call earlier in the day. She then finishes grading the tests she gave in class and continues working on interim reports. It will take her at least one more evening to finish the interims. At 11:00 P.M. she turns off the light and goes to bed. Tomorrow will start again at 5:45 A.M.

Additional Responsibilities

In addition to the lesson planning, grading, parent meetings, disciplining, coaching, and the various administrative duties, teachers may have still more responsibilities. They may be involved in curriculum development, the review of materials for classroom use, the chaperoning of dances or other after-school activities, fund-raising, and the advising of student groups such as yearbook, debate, or student council. Many teachers now keep active Web pages that can be accessed by students and parents. These Web pages may contain announcements, assignments, and grades or progress reports. Teachers need to be responsive to their email accounts because parent, student, and school district communication is often conducted in this manner. School health education specialists should also be active members of their professional organizations such as the American School Health Association and/or the Society for Public Health Education. This allows them to network with other health education specialists and to stay up to date in the field. Finally, school health education specialists should be strong advocates for health and health education/promotion (see **Box 7.1**). They must make certain that fellow faculty, administrators, school boards, and the community as a whole are aware of the unique contributions of a school health program. (See **Table 7.3**.)

TABLE 7.3 **Advantages and disadvantages of working in school health education/promotion**

Advantages

- Health education specialists have the ability to work with young people during their developmental years.
- Health education specialists have the potential to prevent harmful health behaviors from forming instead of working with older people after such behaviors have been formed.
- Health education specialists have the opportunity to impact all students because health education/promotion is usually a required course.
- A graduate degree is not needed for entry-level employment.
- There is good job security.
- Summer months are free and there are nice vacation periods in December and in spring.
- Benefits are good.
- There is a multifaceted career ladder.
- There are typically good health and retirement benefit programs.

Disadvantages

- Good health education specialists usually spend many long hours at their job, including weekends and evenings.
- Health education specialists may have relatively low status in a school district when compared with teachers of more traditional subjects such as math, science, and English.
- Pay is low when compared with professionals in other fields but comparable with that of other health education specialists.
- Student discipline problems are often seen as a major disadvantage.
- Summer "free time" may be consumed with summer employment that is needed to compensate for the low salary or returning to college for additional required coursework.
- It is difficult dealing with conservative school boards, parents, and community groups when teaching controversial issues such as sex education and drug education.
- Resources may be limited to support the program.

Practitioner's Perspective

SCHOOL HEALTH EDUCATION/PROMOTION Carolyn Conley

CURRENT POSITION: Teacher, Health and Physical Education

EMPLOYER: South Carolina Public Schools

DEGREE/INSTITUTION: B.S., University of Toledo, 2010, Health Education and Physical Education

Describe your past and current professional positions and how you came to hold the job you now hold (How did you obtain the position?): After graduating from the Health Education Program at the University of Toledo in the winter of 2010, I decided to take a little vacation and lived with my sister for a few months in California as I searched and applied for Health and Physical Education jobs through the Internet. I had never been a fan of Ohio winters so besides looking through a few Ohio teacher job search sites, I was also looking in North and South Carolina, Florida, Georgia, and California. I spent no less than three hours each day searching and applying for positions without much luck. I moved back to Ohio in April after being contacted by a public charter school that immediately needed a part-time PE teacher. When I arrived home, I also was accepted to three local school districts to substitute teach. For the remainder of the 2011 school year, I worked as many hours as I could in all four positions.

After many disappointing leads and a few job offers in places I was not interested in working, I was contacted by the administrators from a Title I high school in rural South Carolina. It was the first week of August and they needed to quickly fill a health and physical education position. After receiving an employment offer, I took a quick drive down to South Carolina to make sure that the school was a fit for me. The town was very small without much to offer a girl in her 20s, but the weather was great, the people seemed friendly, and the teaching position was full-time. At this point in the search it was hard to pass up a job. I have now finished my second year in this position.

Describe the duties of your current position: In my current position, I have a lot of different and eclectic duties. In addition to teaching two health education classes, three Freshmen Focus classes, and one physical education class, I have normal responsibilities like every teacher has, such as parent/teacher conferences, lunch duty, faculty meetings, graduation assignments, etc. I also coach two varsity sports: volleyball and softball; am a site coordinator for implementation of a sexual health curriculum; run a "Safer Choices" peer group as part of the sexual health program; and am the high school liaison for the American Cancer Society's Relay for Life program.

Describe what you like most about this position: The thing I like most about this position is that I have a lot of freedom to do what I want with the classes I teach and the groups I lead. I have to stick to basic standards but can mold my lessons around them in creative ways and have fun with my students. I also like the relationships I have been able to make with the students. Since I was the outsider in their community, it was initially difficult to gain the students' trust. Now after two years the students and community know me better. When my students see me in the grocery store and see me running through their neighborhoods, they know I am a real person just like everyone else. It is also really good for them and the community to see that I follow a healthy lifestyle, exercise regularly, and in general, practice what I teach in class.

Describe what you like least about this position: The thing I like least about this position is the lack of organization, collaboration, and standards within the school building. The expectations for teachers and students are low and that is the level at which everyone performs. While I enjoy the freedom to mold my curriculum, at the same time there needs to be oversight and evaluation to be sure standards are met. It

BOX 7.1 *continued*

is hard to stay passionate and motivated when no one cares what you're doing. There needs to be more accountability and higher expectations. Teachers and administrators also need to work together more and to be on the same page to do the best they can to better the students.

What health education responsibilities (assessing, planning, implementing, evaluating, resourcing, communicating, advocating) do you use in your position? As a health educator, it is my responsibility to plan my overall curriculum and outline for the school year. I assess what concepts need specific focus in the community where the school is located and plan health education units to meet those needs throughout the year. I do research before implementing each unit to make sure I have the most up-to-date information possible and carry out the lessons I have planned in the most creative and effective ways possible. I evaluate each student in relation to the objectives that I establish. To be the most effective teacher I can be, I communicate with other teachers, administrators, and parents through phone calls, emails, letters, and personal conversations.

What recommendations/ advice do you have for current health education students who would like to eventually be school health educators? My advice to health education students would be to find one or more passionate health education faculty/ professional mentors, learn all you can from them, and maintain contact with them after graduation. You will need these people to keep you motivated, write letters of recommendation, and give you advice. I initially found teaching to be very challenging, especially in a position that is not fully supported and where there are no other health educators. I constantly have to advocate for health and health education to make sure it remains a priority for the school and community. I feel like my job is the most important one in the school, and the field of health education is crucial for human happiness and success. You have to keep your passion even when you have terrible days at school. Force yourself to be positive, relax, and look at the big picture. Remember that you are making a huge difference. Challenge yourself every day to be better than you were yesterday.

▷ Public or Community Health Education/Promotion

Within the health education/promotion profession, there has been much discussion concerning the terms community health education/promotion and public health education/promotion. Some believe these two terms are synonymous whereas others feel there are unique differences between them. It is the opinion of the authors that the terms are more alike than different and that the field is gradually evolving to accept the term public health education/promotion. Both community health education/promotion and public health education/promotion students have similar skill sets, meet the competencies of the National Commission for Health Education Credentialing, and compete for similar jobs in departments of public health and community health agencies. A survey of professional preparation programs (Miller, Birch, & Cottrell, 2010) found that 72.3 percent of respondents reported making modifications to their existing undergraduate health education/promotion program or concentration within the past three years to take on a more public health focus. Sixty-three percent of the programs surveyed indicated they would seek accreditation as a public health education/promotion program when available whereas only 19 percent indicated they would not seek accreditation as a public health education/promotion program. For that reason the authors use the term *public health education/promotion* to include both community health education/promotion and public health education/promotion programs.

Public health programs target individuals, local communities, states, and the nation. There is a reciprocal relationship between these various targets. Over the years, it has become clear that the health of a community is closely linked to the individual health of community members. Likewise, the collective behaviors, attitudes, and beliefs of everyone who lives in the community profoundly affect the community's health. Indeed, the underlying premise of *Healthy People 2020* was that the health of the individual is almost inseparable from the health of the larger community, and that the health of every community in every state and territory determines the overall health status of the nation. This explains why the vision for *Healthy People 2020* is "A society in which all people live long, healthy lives" (U.S. Department of Health and Human Services, 2016).

The most likely sources of employment for public/community health education specialists are voluntary health agencies and public health agencies. **Voluntary health agencies** are created by concerned citizens to deal with health needs not met by governmental agencies (McKenzie & Pinger, 2015). "Their missions can be public education, professional education, patient education, research, direct services and support to or for people directly affected by a specific health or medical problem. They may also serve families, friends, or loved ones of those affected" (Daitz, 2007, p. 4). As their name implies, they rely heavily on volunteer help and donations. There are usually paid staff members who are responsible for administration, volunteer recruitment and coordination, program development, and fund-raising. Health education specialists are hired to plan, implement, and evaluate the education component of the agency's programs. They often, however, are involved in other aspects of the agency as well. Voluntary health agencies are usually nonprofits and are funded by such means as private donations, grants, fund-raisers, and possibly United Way contributions. Examples of voluntary health agencies include the American Cancer Society (see **Figure 7.2**), American Heart Association, and American Lung Association. Most of these large, well-known voluntary agencies have national, state, and local divisions.

In addition to the large national voluntary associations, there are many other nonprofit health-related organizations that provide a variety of services to the public. One such organization is Smile North Carolina, which is a part of the Smiles Program mobile dentists. See **Box 7.2** for more information about working in such a program.

▶ **Figure 7.2** The American Cancer Society is a nationwide voluntary health organization dedicated to eliminating cancer as a major health problem by preventing cancer, saving lives from cancer, and diminishing suffering from cancer through research, education, advocacy, and service. Health education specialists often work for voluntary agencies such as the American Cancer Society.

COMMUNITY AGENCY Jennifer C. O'Donnell

CURRENT POSITION: Oral Health Educator
EMPLOYER: Smile NC
DEGREE/INSTITUTION/MAJOR: B.S., University of
North Carolina Wilmington, 2012, Community
Health Education

**Describe your past and current profes-
sional positions and how you came to hold
the job you now hold (How did you obtain
the position?):** Working as an Oral Health
Educator has been my first health-related
job since graduation. During college, I
worked on two internships, both dealing
with different aspects of community health.
Each internship provided me with important experience that helped prepare me
for my current role. I worked with Project
Tobacco Free UNC, which was trying to
change the state constitution to allow state
universities to create their own tobacco
use policies, including the decision to be a
tobacco-free campus. While with this project, I worked on many initiatives, including
letter writing campaigns to the Board of
Governors, speaking with state legislators,
creating and implementing a smoking prevention workshop for middle schoolers, and
joining advocacy initiatives to help turn a
local beach into a smoke-free beach. For my
second internship, I worked as a campus
representative for NARAL Pro-choice North
Carolina, the state subsidiary of a national
reproductive rights organization. I was a
founding member of NARAL Pro-Choice NC
at the University of North Carolina Wilmington and drafted the constitution to become
a school-sponsored organization.

After graduation, I took a month off to
help transition from the role of full-time
student back into the role of mother to
two elementary-school-aged children.
While searching for health-related jobs
on Indeed.com, I found this job listed and
realized that it would be a perfect fit with
my desire to help people and be involved in
raising my children. This position was the
first and only position I applied for post-
graduation. I was contacted for an initial
telephone interview and was hired during
a follow-up Skype interview a few days
after I applied for the job.

**Job responsibilities in
your current position:** As
an Oral Health Educator for
Smile NC, my main priority
is to increase the number
of children who are able to
receive preventative and re-
storative dental services. I do this in three
ways. Firstly, I encourage administrators,
directors, and other key people to allow us
to offer our services to the children in their
communities. I also work to remain in communities by strengthening relationships
between my organization and the stakeholders to be able to continue to educate
and provide care to the children already in
our care. Lastly, I spend time with these
children educating them about how to have
a healthy mouth, and getting them excited
about healthy teeth to open conversations
with their parents. I spend a lot of time on
the road, traveling to various communities, day cares, schools, and administrative
offices across the eastern part of North
Carolina.

**Describe what you like most about
this position:** I feel so fortunate to have
the ability to work for an organization
that provides direct and indirect help to
children across the state, especially those
from disadvantaged backgrounds. North
Carolina has a large number of children
with limited access or have no access to
dental services. There are many communities with a large part of their population that live in extreme poverty. Poor
oral health can lead to reduced academic
achievement, as 58 hours per 100 elementary students and 80 hours per 100 high
school students are missed due to dental
problems each year. (Seirawan, Faust, &
Mulligan, 2012). I feel that I am helping
these children have a chance at a better
future. I love that we find a way to help
every child who has parental consent. No
child is turned away because they can't
afford to pay.

I love talking with the children about
their teeth. To me, so many things about
dental health are obvious, but they are not

BOX

7.2

continued

obvious to many of the students I work with. I now understand better than ever how misinformation, fear, and a lack of resources contribute to poor health outcomes. In a short period of time, I can teach proper brushing techniques, help alleviate fears about going to the dentist, improve the self-esteem of those with dental restorations, and give hope to those who've never been to the dentist. I love seeing the pride in the faces of students when they answer tricky anatomy questions correctly. I love feeling the joy and gratitude of the students when they receive a new toothbrush. It breaks my heart to hear that some of these kids didn't even have a toothbrush of their own. I also love talking with the parents and teachers of the students. They play such an influential role in the health of students

Describe what you like least about this position: In all honesty, I love every aspect of my job. Every workday is different, every school I visit has a different way for me to get the information to the students, and the long car rides provide me the opportunity to listen to audiobooks! The hardest part of my job is that the main office is in Michigan, while I operate out of my home office in North Carolina. Even though there are regular email, telephone, and teleconferencing communications with the main office and Oral Health Educators across the country, I don't always feel as if I am part of a larger team.

What health education responsibilities (assessing, planning, implementing, evaluating, resourcing, communicating, advocating) do you use in your position? There are many health education responsibilities that I use in my job. I have had to plan and implement school assemblies, create and teach lesson plans for various age groups, and constantly update and improve ways to disperse as much age-appropriate, retainable information as possible in a short amount of time. Currently, I do not assess the needs of each community, but other employees use data collected from

the census to target schools with a large percentage of students living in poverty or have students receiving free or reduced school lunches. At the end of the school year, the State Manager compiles a report for each specific community. These reports detail the schools serviced, the number of students seen, the number of cleanings, sealants, and cavities corrected, and the estimated number of classroom hours saved by having these services performed. I present this information to community stakeholders, including school system administrators and nurses. During these meetings, I also try to strengthen the relationship between the communities and my program by addressing any concerns and offering suggestions on how to increase student participation.

Communication is the most important part of my job. I have to speak to people of all ages in ways that enable them to learn and retain information. While it is easy to speak with a classroom filled with eager kindergarteners while entertaining them with a puppet with gigantic teeth, it becomes challenging to find ways to engage apathetic middle schoolers (showing and explaining real x-rays works wonders!).

My job includes the opportunity for a lot of advocacy. I need to develop ways to explain to community officials why our mobile dental unit will help their community, and I teach children how to advocate for themselves while talking with their parents about the possibility of receiving dental care at their school.

What recommendations/advice do you have for current health education students who would like to eventually be working in a community agency? I actually have two things I'd recommend to a current health education student who would like to work in a community agency. The first and most important would be to discover your passion and find a way to incorporate it into your career. Participate

BOX 7.2 *continued*

in relevant experiences, internships, and volunteer opportunities that will help expand your résumé. A résumé filled with pertinent experiences will help you land an interview. Demonstrate your passion when you speak to interviewers so they will want to bring that passion into their team. There is no greater feeling than having the ability to get paid while working on something you love. This will increase your life satisfaction and make you a more effective health educator.

The second thing I would recommend would be to become extremely proficient in health communications. This is such a diverse field, with diverse situations in which we need to convey information.

Whether it is helping a senior citizen take their prescriptions correctly and consistently, encouraging local politicians to help provide funding for a safe driving program, or organizing a community to help prevent a cement plant from moving into town, we will need to find a way to convince people of the importance of our information. The ability to find a way to help any demographic in a manner that helps them understand, learn, and retain information is what health education is all about. Effective written and oral communication is the key to improving the health of an individual, community, state, or nation.

Public health agencies, or official governmental health agencies, are usually financed through public tax monies. Government has long been responsible for doing for the people as a whole what individuals cannot do for themselves. Thus, governments provide police protection, educational systems, clean air and water, and many other important services. Departments of public health, thus, are formed to coordinate and provide health services to a community. Health departments may be organized by the city, county, state, or federal government. They operate primarily with paid staff and typically provide health education/promotion services as part of their total program. They may also seek grants and hire health education specialists on grant funds. Public health agencies are known for their bureaucracies, protocols, policies, and procedures. It often takes considerable time to accomplish tasks, and work often needs to be reviewed and approved by higher-level administrators. On the positive side, public health agencies often work with the groups of people most in need of health services and offer good benefit packages for employees (Hall, 2007). **Table 7.4** contains a partial list of agencies that have programs for which public health education specialists may be employed.

More diversity in terms of job responsibilities exists in the public/community health education/promotion settings than in the other major settings in which health education specialists are employed. This is as a result of the large number of community and public health agencies that exist and the vast differences in their missions, goals, and objectives. In some agencies, health education specialists serve administrative functions such as coordinating volunteers, budgeting, fund-raising, program planning, and serving as liaisons to other agencies and groups. They often use population-based strategies such as advocating for laws, policies, rules, and regulations that impact health. In other public/community agencies, the health education specialist may be more involved in direct program delivery to the clientele of that agency and/or the community at large. Most frequently, however, health education specialists are involved in a little bit of everything.

TABLE 7.4 **Possible sources of employment in public/community health education/promotion**

State, local, city health departments
U.S. Public Health Service
U.S. Food and Drug Administration
U.S. or state departments of agriculture
U.S. or state departments of transportation
County extension services
U.S. Department of Health and Human Services (USDHHS)
U.S. Centers for Disease Control and Prevention (CDC)
National Institutes of Health (NIH)
Environmental Protection Agency (EPA)
Health Resources and Services Administration (HRSA)
Substance Abuse and Mental Health Services Administration (SAMHSA)
Indian Health Service
U.S. or state penal institutions
Voluntary health agencies
Private health agencies/foundations

A Day in the Career of a Community Health Education Specialist

Mr. Hernandez is a certified health education specialist (CHES) working for the county health department. He arrives at the health department around 8:30 A.M.. He spends a half hour looking through his email, listening to his voice mail and going through his paper mail. Today at 9:00 A.M. is the weekly staff meeting that he must attend. This is run by the Health Commissioner and includes all staff working at the health department. At each staff meeting Mr. Hernandez is expected to give a brief five minute report on what is happening in the health education division. At this meeting he also learns what is happening in the other divisions of the health department. It is not unusual for staff in one division to assist staff in another division with projects or initiatives they may have.

After the staff meeting, Mr. Hernandez has a couple hours before lunch to respond to his email and voice messages and work on a new grant proposal to fund a health education program for seasonal migrant workers. At 12:00 P.M., Mr. Hernandez breaks for lunch. He usually eats lunch at his desk while reading journal articles from *Health Promotion Practice*. This is one of the journals published by SOPHE, of which Mr. Hernandez is a member. He finds many of the articles in this journal relate directly to his work and often provide ideas for new initiatives or for how he can better do his job.

At 1:00 P.M., Mr. Hernandez has a meeting scheduled with a group of bicycling enthusiasts and bicycle shop owners regarding the development of a biking safety program for the county. Data have shown that the number of bicycle accidents in this county is higher than for other counties in the state. This group will consider measures that may be taken to modify this problem.

At 2:00 P.M., Mr. Hernandez has a meeting with a local newspaper reporter. The reporter is doing a story on food poisoning during the summer months and how to prevent it. Mr. Hernandez only had one nutrition course in college, and this is not his area of expertise.

He spent considerable time yesterday afternoon researching food poisoning and calling a dietician friend at the local hospital to confirm the information he will give the reporter. At 2:30 P.M., Mr. Hernandez heads over to the high school for a 3:00 P.M. meeting. He is part of the "Health Team" in the school district, and they are in the process of trying to develop and have approved a policy that soft drinks and candy cannot be sold in the lunchroom when school lunches are being served. This is controversial as some students oppose the policy and the vending machine company is lobbying against it. Today's meeting is to develop the actual wording for the policy that will be presented to the school board and to brainstorm other community organizations and groups that might provide additional support for the proposed policy.

At 4:00 P.M., when the school meeting ends, Mr. Hernandez heads back to the health department to load his car with various health department pamphlets and displays. The local mall is having a health fair from 5:00 P.M. to 9:00 P.M. this evening. He, along with many other community organizations, will be there to display their materials and answer questions the public may have about health issues or health department services. Mr. Hernandez frequently has to work evenings and weekends as part of his job. He does receive comp time for the hours he works beyond the normal work week, which allows him to take some additional days off during the year.

Additional Responsibilities

Mr. Hernandez is actually one of three health education specialists working at the health department. The other two health education specialists are working on grants. One is working on a grant to improve safety issues for elderly residents. This involves educating these residents on how to prevent falls and the importance of smoke and carbon monoxide detectors in their homes. The grant also provides financial resources to install safety features in bathrooms and to purchase smoke and carbon monoxide detectors for those who cannot afford these improvements. The other health educator is working on a grant to help the county and its residents prepare for a potential natural disaster such as an earthquake, hurricane, or tornado. This grant will last for just one year, and then the health education specialist will have to find another funding source or will need to seek other employment.

Mr. Hernandez is an actual employee of the county health department, and his job is not dependent on grants. In addition to his previously described work, Mr. Hernandez is the information/public relations officer for the health department. He is responsible for responding to questions called into the health department by county residents. Whenever a health-related news story breaks, local residents will often call the health department with questions. Recently he has been addressing many questions about the Zika virus and whether local mosquitoes carry the virus. Further, Mr. Hernandez is also the person who interfaces with the media when they have questions. As a result he is often on the TV or radio talking about health issues.

As can be seen from the example above, public/community health education specialists are involved in numerous and varied activities (see **Box 7.3**). Planning, implementing, and evaluating programs and events are major tasks, but, in conducting these tasks, health education specialists get involved in grant writing, fund-raising, coalition building, committee work, budgeting, general administration, public speaking, volunteer recruitment, grant writing, policy development, media relations, and advocacy (see **Table 7.5**).

PUBLIC HEALTH EDUCATOR Ashton Putnam

CURRENT POSITION/TITLE: Public Health Educator II

EMPLOYER: Forsyth County, North Carolina Department of Public Health
799 Highland Avenue
Winston-Salem, NC 27101

DEGREE/INSTITUTION/YEAR: B.S., University of North Carolina Wilmington, 2011

MAJOR/MINOR: Major: Community Health Education Minor: None

How I obtained my job: After completing my degree at the University of North Carolina Wilmington, I began working as a project manager for a marketing research organization in Charlotte, NC. Although this opportunity contributed to my professional growth and development, it was not in my chosen field of health education. I continued to pursue a career in the field of health education, and in the spring of 2012, I accepted a Public Health Educator position at the Forsyth County Department of Public Health in Winston-Salem, NC. This role made it possible for me to work in a variety of capacities within the Maternal and Child Health unit including program planning, curriculum implementation, group facilitation, advocacy, quality improvement, and evaluation. I also gained experience in conducting home visits with high-risk families to reduce infant mortality rates by addressing health education priority areas. Additionally, I coordinated an advisory board and organized community outreach activities to promote and improve health outcomes.

The following year, I was promoted to a Public Health Educator II, and this is the position I currently occupy. The function of my position includes supervisory responsibilities and management of staff, administrative duties and budgets, adherence to proper and effective program operations, grant writing, and policy compliance. I participate in the community health assessment and action plan development as well as collaborate with neighboring partners for community initiatives and

projects. Working in local, county government has provided me with exposure to the fundamental factors associated with advancing the health and well-being of others and successfully contributing to the practice of health education.

How I utilize the health education competencies in my job: In my position at the local health department, I use the health education competencies continuously and work with my colleagues to support them in their designated roles as well. For example, one evidence-based toddler parenting program that we implemented required assessing the need of our priority population, reviewing planning models, establishing goals and objectives within the curriculum, implementing a 14-week program with an identified cohort, collecting and analyzing data post-series, properly managing fiscal resources and using positive outcomes for program sustainability. This is just one of numerous instances where I regularly use the health education competencies. I also use the competency areas in advancing policy changes, influencing decision makers, leading advocacy initiatives, growing prevention projects, and identifying areas of program expansion. Applying these standards and principles throughout your work in the health education field will guide your practices to encourage effective change.

What I like most about my job: My position provides a unique opportunity to interact with diverse populations, improve the health and well-being of individuals, promote change in the workplace and the community, work with dynamic partnering agencies, enhance my leadership skills, and gain personal satisfaction. I have had the chance to explore various aspects of Maternal and Child Health in the Public Health sector, and an ongoing project

BOX 7.3

continued

that brings me fulfillment is the work and efforts I do with the local coalition of Safe Kids Worldwide, an organization dedicated to preventing injuries in children and ensuring their safety. I have worked with this coalition since my first role at the health department and continue to do so, as this network has had a profound impact on keeping children safe through raising awareness and educating families. I also enjoy helping staff build and develop their talents in health education and strive for quality and effective program implementation and outcomes.

What I like least about my job: Working in a supervisory role has decreased my direct contact with program participants, which is why I initially entered the field of Public Health. While working in the field has great rewards, it can also present difficulties such as trying to reach high risk, transient populations. Funding from the state that supports local health department programs is highly competitive and has limitations, so the need to continuously seek resources and work with partners is an ongoing challenge. On the positive side, state funding limitations have allowed me to further develop my health education skills in grant writing, collaborative impact planning, and utilizing data to demonstrate evidence of change.

Recommendations for those preparing to be health education specialists: Individuals preparing to be health education specialists who seek career longevity in the field must remain committed to hard work and retain a passion for the profession. To be effective, you should strive to be a life-long learner with a commitment to explore professional development opportunities. Join professional organizations prior to leaving your undergraduate program and stay connected through attending and presenting at conferences and networking whenever possible. Arrange adequate preparation time for the Certified Health Education Specialist (CHES) exam prior to graduation. Obtaining CHES credentials demonstrates your competencies and readiness for working as a health educator. Seek leadership and internship opportunities to gain experience and build relationships with schools, public health agencies, hospitals, and community partners, as this may open doors that will lead to future career opportunities.

The Role of health education specialists in the future: Health Educators will have an ever-increasing role in communities, hospitals, schools, and public health agencies as a part of the comprehensive healthcare system. As health care is evolving in societal, demographic, cultural, and institutional realms, health education specialists will be a vital contributor to primary prevention. We must strive to be more proactive rather than reactive to chronic health issues and healthcare costs in this country. Health education specialists, using theories and evidence-based practices, can work together with healthcare providers to plan, implement, and evaluate programs to decrease health risk behaviors. Reducing risk behaviors and significantly improving healthy behaviors will assist in the efforts of lowering morbidity and mortality rates in the United States. Health education specialists possess knowledge of current practices, facilitation skills, and, in partnership with clinicians, can offer well-versed and holistic care in the systematic reform of health care. I believe the future for health education specialists is bright, exciting, and transformative. They will not only have a positive influence on improving health behaviors and reducing health care costs, but will leave a lasting impression on the lives they touch in a profound way.

TABLE 7.5 **Advantages and disadvantages of working in public/community health education/promotion**

Advantages

- Job responsibilities are highly varied and changing.
- There is a strong emphasis on prevention.
- There is usually a high community profile.
- Health education specialists work with multiple groups of people.
- There is a high degree of self-satisfaction.
- These positions typically offer good benefit packages.
- These positions typically allow flex time when working evenings or weekends.

Disadvantages

- Pay may be low, particularly in voluntary agencies.
- When hired directly by a community or public health agency, job security tends to be good. In such situations, the health education specialist is said to be employed on **hard money**. Sometimes, however, these agencies hire health education specialists on money secured through grants, which is known as **soft money**. In these situations, positions are terminated when grant funding is discontinued, so job security can be a concern.
- Relying heavily on volunteers can be frustrating. Although most volunteers are great, some do not demonstrate the same level of commitment as might a paid employee.
- There never seems to be enough money to run all the programs that need to be offered in the way they should be offered.
- These positions often require irregular hours that may include evenings and weekends.
- There is a lot of bureaucracy in public health agencies.

▷ Work-Site Health Education/Promotion

In describing Work-Site Health Promotion programs, the Centers for Disease Control and Prevention (CDC) refers to them as "a coordinated and comprehensive set of strategies which include programs, policies, benefits, environmental supports, and links to the surrounding community designed to meet the health and safety needs of all employees" (CDC, 2016b). Certainly, the workplace and the health of workers are closely related. Worksites should not only protect the safety of employees, but provide employees with opportunities to enhance their overall health and well-being. Since the mid-1970s, business and industry in the United States have been offering work-site health promotion programs for their employees. Why are health education specialists interested in working in these settings, why are worksites interested in offering these programs, and why are employees interested in participating in such programs? For health education specialists, work-site wellness programs offer an additional setting for them to reach segments of the population that are not easily accessed through traditional community health programs. For worksites and employees, the CDC (2016c) notes numerous potential benefits that can be seen in **Table 7.6**.

In the United States, annual healthcare expenditures reached 3 trillion dollars in 2014 or an average of $9,523 for every man, woman, and child living in the United States. Overall,

TABLE 7.6 **Overview of potential benefits of workplace health programs to employers and employees**

For Employers:

- Lower healthcare and disability costs
- Enhanced employee productivity
- Reduced employee absenteeism
- Decreased rates of illness and injuries
- Enhanced corporate image
- Improved employee morale
- Improved employee recruitment and retention
- Increased organizational commitment and creation of a culture of health

For Employees:

- Increased well-being, self-image, and self-esteem
- Improved coping skills with stress or other factors affecting health
- Improved health status
- Lower costs for acute health issues
- Lower out-of-pocket costs for healthcare services (e.g., reduced premiums, deductibles, co-payments)
- Increased access to health promotion resources and social support
- Improved job satisfaction
- Safer and more supportive work environment

Centers for Disease Control and Prevention. (2016). Workplace health promotion: How employers can benefit. Downloaded April 12, 2016, from http://www.cdc.gov/workplacehealthpromotion/businesscase/benefits/index.html

healthcare expenditures accounted for 17.5 percent of the gross domestic product in the USA (Centers for Medicare & Medicaid Services, 2016). Just as points of reference, $253 billion was spent on health care in 1980, $714 billion was spent in 1990, $1.6 trillion in 2002, and in 2010, the amount spent was $2.6 trillion. Healthcare costs are projected to be nearly 20 percent or one fifth of the GDP in 2020 (California Health Care Foundation, 2013). Approximately one fourth of these healthcare costs are picked up by business and industry (Fronstin & Roebuck, 2015a). Starbucks, for example, pays more for its U.S. employees' health insurance each year than it does for coffee (Rubleski, 2007). Can work-site health promotion programs reduce these costs? According to the Wellness Councils of America (2006), the advantages of work-site health promotion are no longer a matter of speculation. In 2006, there were more than 600 articles that provided both circumstantial and direct evidence of the value of work-site health promotion programs. The tangible benefits include reduced sick leave absenteeism, reduced use of health benefits, reduced workers' compensation costs, reduced injuries, and reduced presenteeism losses (losses resulting from poor productivity in those employees who are present). Beyond the tangible benefits there are also intangible benefits including improved employee morale, increased employee loyalty, less organizational conflict, a more productive workforce, and improved employee decision-making ability.

Goetzel and Pronk (2010) conducted a systematic review of 51 work-site health promotion studies. They found that certain health behaviors, biometric measures, and financial outcomes could be influenced through work-site health promotion programs although the effect sizes for these improvements were modest when compared to clinical trials. The impact, however, of modest changes when applied to large groups of people combined with the relatively low cost of work-site programs when compared with clinical interventions confirmed their value. They went on to say that

> Many of the programs considered in the worksite review fall under the broad umbrella of primary prevention (e.g., encouraging workers to be more physically active; providing them with education about and access to a healthy diet; teaching techniques for managing stress; helping employees stop smoking; and mandating seat belt use) and thus may achieve long-lasting population based health improvements at a low cost. Further, it was observed that health promotion interventions delivered at the worksite can be efficiently and cost-effectively provided, especially when company leadership, norms, culture, and policies are aligned to support adoption of healthy habits and prevention practices. (p. S224)

Health promotion programs at worksites differ greatly from site to site (Chenoweth, 2011; Fronstin & Roebuck, 2015b). Some are extensive, include elaborate facilities, and are conducted by full-time staff members hired by the company; others are minimal programs that may include only a brown bag lunch speaker's program or a discount at the local YMCA or health club (Chenoweth, 2011). **Figure 7.3** shows the percentage of companies offering different programs by company size. There is also a wide variety of health promotion activities that can be offered at any site. For a list of work-site health promotion activities, see **Table 7.7**.

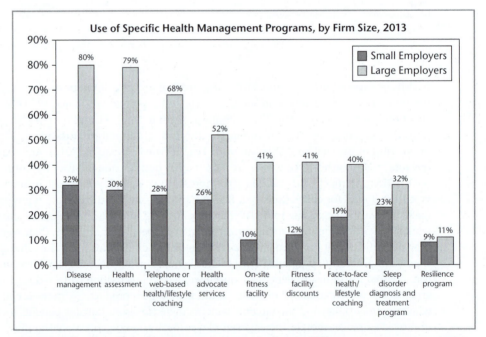

▲ **Figure 7.3** Use of specific health management programs by firm size 2013 Source: Adapted from Fronstin, P., and Roebuck, M.C., "Financial Incentives, Workplace Wellness Program Participation, and Utilization of Health Care Services and Spending", EBRI Issue Brief, no. 417, (Employee benefit Research Institute, Aug. 2015).

TABLE 7.7 **Work-site health promotion activities**

Smoking cessation	Mammography screenings	Newsletters
Smoke-free policies	Cancer risk awareness	Lending libraries
Stress management	Cardiovascular risk	Physical examinations
Weight loss	awareness	Counseling hot lines
Exercise/physical fitness	Skin cancer screenings	Hypertension screenings
Nutrition	Flu shots	HIV/AIDS prevention
Safety	Health fairs	Paycheck stuffers
First aid & CPR	Bulletin boards	Web site development

The proportion of employers who provide work-site health promotion programs has increased over the years, especially among larger employers. Despite these increased numbers for large employers, more needs to be done. Many of these large employers have only minimal health promotion offerings. The majority of U.S. employees work in small and medium-sized companies that are much less likely to offer any health promotion opportunities. Certain types of employers, such as retailers, seldom offer health promotion programs, and any employer with a high rate of workforce turnover has no motivation to offer health promotion programs.

Work-site health promotion received a significant boost from the passage of the Patient Protection and Affordable Care Act. As a result of the wellness and prevention provisions in this act, a national work-site health policies and programs survey was done to more thoroughly assess what employers were doing in relation to work-site health promotion. In 2011, five-year grants to small employers (less than 100 employees) were made available to provide technical assistance and other resources to establish wellness programs for employees. In 2014, employers were permitted to provide employee rewards in the form of insurance premium discounts, waivers of cost-sharing requirements, and so forth for employees participating in wellness programs and meeting certain health-related standards (Society for Public Health Education [SOPHE], 2013).

Even with incentives, questions exist regarding the ability of work-site programs to attract employees who are less well and at higher risk. In other words, do only the motivated and healthy employees participate? One recent study specifically designed to determine the impact of financial incentives concluded, ". . . financial incentives—on the order of $240 per employee per year—were successful at encouraging widespread participation in this employer's workplace wellness program . . . these incentives brought in less-healthy individuals—those arguably in most need of the program" (Fronstin & Roebuck, 2015a, p. 19).

Though positions exist in the work-site health promotion setting that are strictly health education/promotion, more frequently expertise in exercise testing and prescription is also required. This is because many work-site health promotion programs are centered around a fitness center. It is often the fitness center that is the most visible aspect of a work-site health promotion program and attracts many employees to health promotion activities. Therefore, skills related to exercise are important, and these skills are not part of the competencies required by a health education specialist. As a result, health education specialists preparing for employment in work-site health promotion should strongly consider a minor or second major in exercise science (see **Box 7.4**). Peabody and Linnan (2007) recommend that those wanting

BOX

7.4

Practitioner's Perspective

WORKSITE HEALTH PROMOTION Nicole Gaudette

CURRENT POSITION: Manager, Health Education & Wellness

EMPLOYER: Geneia

DEGREES/INSTITUTION: M.P.H., Boston University

MAJOR: Social and Behavioral Science Concentration

Job history: After graduating from Boston University with my Master of Public Health degree and participating in multiple innovating internships in Boston, I moved back to my hometown in Pennsylvania. I was offered employment at Global Secure Systems in a grant-funded, one-year position as a Public Health Training and Outreach Specialist. In this role I independently designed and delivered interactive presentations catered to the individual needs of Pennsylvania participants within an alert network system. I managed and administered the logistical components of this alert network, coupled with the creation of novel documents and protocols. While directing this system, I communicated and disseminated pertinent information regarding the significance of this network at the same time establishing effective working relationships with city, government, and community agencies.

After completion of this one-year role, I moved to Capital BlueCross as a Health Education Consultant. In this role I delivered professional consultation and high-level wellness implementation to employer groups, individual members, and the community for health management programming and employee lifestyle enhancement in the workplace. I also evaluated health prevention and promotion strategies, specific to diverse work environments, for application and execution of programs and synthesis of program validity and cost-benefit to group customers. Another job responsibility was the generation of specific recommendations for customer-specific reference through research of employee population needs based on disease prevalence, utilization, associated costs, and trends designed to impact positive health outcomes. After five years in the health education and wellness unit, I have advanced from

Consultant to Team Lead to Manager of the unit.

My current job responsibilities: I am the Manager for a team of health education specialists. Within my scope of job duties I supervise seven individuals whose main function is to support employer groups for health management programming. As a team we have staff meetings once every two weeks, case reviews every quarter, intrinsic motivation skill building sessions once a month, and individual one-on-one meetings every two weeks, all which I develop, coordinate, and lead. Having a healthy work culture is vital in my view so I focus on staff members in various ways, such as creating consistent awards and recognition processes, clearly communicating new program development, assessing motivation of staff for change, and development of novel implementation strategies for staff-led programming. Being a compelling role model for change as the team leader is crucial with exemplification of a positive attitude and stance on changes. With changes and as part of a sound communication strategy, I conduct feedback loops to evaluate specific procedures within health and wellness to assess job duties and functions and analyze individual performance. As the manager, I also attend finalist presentations and answer request proposal summaries both for prospective and current group customers.

What I like most about my position: The best part of my position is working within a team of fun, passionate, energetic, knowledgeable, and inspiring individuals. We genuinely have a healthy and happy work environment that makes every day enjoyable and something I look forward to each day. We function in a high-energy, fast-paced environment that generates different and exciting days. As a unit we steadfastly support one another and are true team members, just like a professional sports team, who have concern, care, and perpetual encouragement for everyone.

BOX 7.4 *continued*

What I like least about my position: One of the biggest challenges in my position is the variety of tasks and pace of schedule that I face. In many cases, we support a large and wide-ranging set of customers and maintain a large customer base with assorted sets of needs and objectives. As our product offerings and success relies on tailoring of our products and services to meet the unique needs of a customer, it is not uncommon that, week-to-week, there is a different set of tasks with fluctuating schedules to perform. To meet this challenge, I find that dedicating time each week to organizing and planning is essential. This strategy includes detailed preparation of near-term activities and high-level scoping of longer-term activities. Implementing this planning cycle allows me to be proactive in identifying and scheduling specific tasks to ensure that the output of my and my unit's work exceeds customer's expectations and is completed and conducted on schedule.

Recommendations for future students: There are so many opportunities within the realm of health education and wellness. I would encourage students to follow their passion that will enhance their intrinsic motivation for traveling down their chosen path. It is important to inherently motivate yourself in ways that can lead to heightened success in the area you have chosen. Doing something you like keeps you motivated because it is enjoyable. Through choosing to do something you have satisfaction in doing, it is important to seek out and master optimal challenges. The reward for choosing a path such as this is that it will foster your sense of what you enjoy doing, and it will allow for accomplishment of and provide an enhanced view of what you want to do thereby making you a positive contributor to society.

A day in the career of a health education and wellness manager: Every day is a bit different depending on the immediate needs of staff members and/or employer groups with whom we work. Being connected to staff members is essential as decisions and feedback are at times needed promptly. Meetings typically infiltrate into the day very quickly, making being adaptable essential and a strong skill set for this position. At times, employer group requests arise that need to be addressed in a time-sensitive manner. These get boosted to the top of the list of the day for priority completion. There is always an open door guiding principle for staff members to discuss challenging group situations or anything that needs senior level support. There is also a lot of interaction within the Clinical Management department as a whole within a day. Many of the scheduled meetings involve various projects and/or initiatives in the department, and interacting and dialoguing with these individuals is important to move forward in a productive, streamlined manner.

careers in the work-site setting consider getting two degrees: one a more generalist degree (e.g., health education, public health, or health promotion) and the second a specialist degree (e.g., exercise physiology, nutrition science, nursing, or athletic training). They indicate that it does not matter which degree is the undergraduate and which is the graduate but that an individual with both a generalist and a specialist degree "will have many more options than someone with two degrees in either field" (Peabody & Linnan, 2007, p. 31). Beyond specialty expertise, a master's degree is also required for many entry-level health education/promotion positions in business and industry. In addition to the Certified Health Education Specialist (CHES) or Master Certified Health Education Specialist (MCHES) credential, certifications more specific to exercise are available from the American College of Sports Medicine and may be required at some work-site settings. Certifications for specific aspects of work-site health promotion, such as aerobic dance, first aid, and cardiopulmonary resuscitation (CPR), and for smoking cessation instructors are also available and encouraged. In general, the more degrees, certifications, and credentials one has, the better one will compete for work-site health promotion positions.

A Day in the Career of a Work-Site Health Education Specialist

The day begins early for Alisa. The fitness center opens promptly at 5:00 A.M. so that employees who start work at 6:00 A.M. have time to work out before beginning their shift. Alisa has to be there at 4:45 A.M. to open the doors, turn on the lights, and greet the first members. The first two hours of her day are spent "working the floor." This means she greets members as they enter the facility; walks around the machines, providing instruction where needed; chats with the members; answers health-related questions; and basically makes everyone feel important and welcome. By 7:00 A.M., all the shift workers have left the fitness facility and, by 9:00 A.M., the managerial employees have cleared out.

From 9:00 A.M. to 11:00 A.M. is a slow time in the center. A few retired employees and spouses use the machines, but this is basically the time for Alisa to get other tasks done. She begins by laundering the dirty towels and folding those that come out of the dryer. Next she provides the routine maintenance to the machines. This involves cleaning them with disinfectant and applying a lubricant to the moving parts. Once this is completed, Alisa has about an hour to work at her desk. Today she is writing an article on the different types of dietary fats, to be included in the Wellness Center newsletter she publishes each month. The newsletter is distributed to all active employees and retirees of the company. Alisa is always amazed at how important writing skills are to her position in work-site health promotion.

Between 11:00 A.M. and 12:15 P.M., Alisa teaches two aerobics classes for the employees. The first is a beginners' class for new members. The second is supposed to be a more advanced class. Unfortunately, many of the shift employees have no choice in their lunch time, so Alisa ends up with some very advanced members in the beginners' class and some beginners in the advanced class. This is frustrating and could be avoided if there were another fitness center employee. There are, however, only two employees in the center, and Rob, the other health education specialist, must work the floor with the lunch crowd while Alisa teaches. Alisa is going to pursue the possibility of hiring a part-time aerobics instructor just for the lunch hours. This would allow her to offer a beginning and an advanced class at each time slot.

From 12:15 P.M. to 1:00 P.M., Alisa runs an ongoing weigh loss support group for employees. All participants bring a brown bag lunch that is supposed to contain food appropriate for a weight-loss diet. They weigh in weekly, and Alisa provides each participant with a voluntary body composition (fat vs. lean) analysis every three months. At least twice a week, Alisa prepares a 20-minute lecture on a weight-loss topic or invites a guest speaker from the community. The same issue concerning lunch breaks also impacts the weight loss support class. Some employees who take lunch break from 11:00–12:00 are not able to participate.

At 1:00 P.M., the employees are back at their work stations, and there is again a quiet time in the health promotion center. Alisa spends the next hour eating lunch at her desk and working on a new incentive program for employees to join the health promotion center that will be offered next month. She has to develop all the brochures, promotional material, and registration forms and arrange for the purchase of incentive items.

At 2:00 P.M., she has a meeting with upper management of the company. She has been advocating for the company to establish a no-smoking policy for the past five years. Two years ago, the company did restrict smoking to specified smoking areas, which was a major accomplishment. Today she will present a proposal to phase out all smoking over a one-year period. Alisa would be responsible for offering several smoking cessation classes over the 12-month period before the no-smoking policy takes effect. She has already decided that her next advocacy effort will be to have more healthy alternatives available in the vending machines, snack rooms, and cafeteria. She has begun a literature review to learn what other companies have done to improve the nutrition of their employees.

By 2:30 P.M., she is back in the health promotion center. The second-shift employees are in the center now ahead of their shifts, so Alisa is again working the floor. Today she has to do initial fitness assessments on three new employees. This involves running the employees through a standardized series of tests. Based on the results of these tests and each employee's fitness objectives, she prescribes an individualized exercise program for each employee. She then takes the employees through the fitness center and teaches them how to use the equipment and maintain a record of their progress.

By 3:30 P.M., Alisa is finished with the assessments. Because she had the early shift, opening the facility, she is finished for the day. Rob, who came in later, will stay and close the facility at 8:00 P.M.

Additional Responsibilities

The responsibilities involved in working in a corporate health promotion center are many and varied. In some facilities, maintaining records such as who is using the center, which programs are most popular, fitness assessment results, and health profiles are major tasks. Fortunately, there are software programs available to assist with this. There are always many little things that need to be done, such as the creation and updating of bulletin boards, equipment maintenance, and towel distribution and laundering. Many times, annual health fairs, company-wide health screenings, and flu shot programs are the responsibility of the health promotion staff. In addition, advocating for population-based, corporate-wide policies, rules, and regulations to enhance the health of employees is important. These policies, rules, or regulations may relate to tobacco use, food service, safety, violence, stress, and so forth.

Being a health education specialist in a work-site setting is not easy. It is imperative that work-site health education professionals stay up to date with health information and the operational processes of running a work-site program. As noted by the American College of Sports Medicine (2003), "the worksite health promotion professional needs to have a good handle on where to find the information, knowledge, resources and expertise that are needed to access the underlying foundations on which programs are built, the operational processes that allow programs to flourish, and the motivation to continually keep a heads-up attitude toward new and innovative strategies that allow well-established programs to maintain their cutting edge" (p. xi). See **Table 7.8** for a listing of the advantages and disadvantages of employment in work-site health education/promotion.

Those who combine health education/promotion with a fitness background may find employment in settings beyond the business world. See **Table 7.9** for a partial listing of employment opportunities for those with both health education/promotion and exercise training.

TABLE 7.8 **Advantages and disadvantages of working in work-site health promotion**

Advantages

- It affords excellent opportunities for prevention.
- It provides access to individuals who may not participate in community programs.
- Health education specialists work with multiple and diverse groups of people, including everyone from upper management to shift workers.
- Most health education specialists in the corporate setting enjoy their positions and report a high degree of job satisfaction.
- Pay is usually higher than in other health education settings. Benefits are usually good, but they vary considerably from employer to employer.
- Health education specialists have access to fitness facilities for personal use.

Disadvantages

- Hours are long and irregular. To cover employees on all shifts in a company may necessitate health education specialists' working hours early in the morning or late in the evening. It is not unusual to work more than eight hours a day.
- Upward mobility may be a problem. Typically, there are only one or two managerial positions in health promotion at any given worksite. This makes it difficult for health education specialists to move up. In addition, those holding managerial positions as directors of health and fitness have nowhere to move up in a company unless they are willing to get out of the health promotion field.
- Health promotion programs and fitness centers often seem to be low on a company's priority list. Such programs are often the first to receive budget cuts in difficult times and often seem to be short of the staff necessary to run optimal programs.
- Some companies subcontract their health promotion and fitness programs to outside vendors. Some of these outside vendors hire part-time health education specialists, pay lower wages, and provide few or no benefits.
- Health education specialists have strong pressure to be extremely fit and be healthy role models for other employees.

TABLE 7.9 **Employment opportunities in health education/promotion with an emphasis in exercise and fitness**

Corporations, business, and industry	Outside commercial vendors that provide programs to worksites
Corporate/industrial parks	
YMCAs/YWCAs	Entrepreneurial enterprises (aerobics studios, consulting, club owner, personal training)
Private health and fitness clubs	
Special-population clubs (women, elderly, etc.)	Fitness product/service companies (sales and marketing)
Community parks & recreation programs	Condos and apartment complexes
Colleges/universities	Hotels
Hospitals	Spas
Sports medicine centers	Resorts and cruise lines
Insurance companies that offer health education/promotion programs to their corporate clients	

▷ Health Education/Promotion in Healthcare Settings

Positions are available for health education specialists in a variety of **healthcare settings**, including clinics, hospitals, and managed care organizations (McKenzie, Neiger, & Thackeray, 2013). "Typically in the medical care field, health education specialists serve as administrators, directors, managers, and coordinators, supporting and consulting on health education programs and services" (Totzkay-Sitar & Cornett, 2007, p. 8). Health education specialists have also been used in healthcare settings to provide patient education (Byrd, Hoke, & Gottlieb, 2007). For example, a patient is diagnosed with heart disease or an increased risk for heart disease. That patient is then referred to the health education specialist for information about exercise, nutrition, weight control, stress management, smoking cessation, and so on. This could involve one-on-one education or counseling sessions with the patient, or it might involve group programs in which multiple patients receive the same program at the same time.

In hospitals and other healthcare settings, health education specialists have also been hired to direct health and fitness programs for company employees, much the same as in other work-site settings (Breckon et al., 1998) (see **Figure 7.4**). Sometimes these programs are also open as an outreach service to community members. Other times, health education specialists are responsible for developing and conducting health and fitness programs specifically designed for community members through fitness facilities that are affiliated with the hospital (see **Box 7.5**).

Unfortunately, patient education has not emerged as a major source of employment for health education specialists. Although it seems like an ideal activity for health education specialists, third-party reimbursement is not provided by health insurance companies to cover a health education specialist. Third-party reimbursement refers to the system whereby healthcare providers can submit their bills to the patient's insurance company for reimbursement (McKenzie & Pinger, 2015). Thus, patient education does not happen or it may be done by nurses who can also serve other functions in the healthcare setting

▶ **Figure 7.4** Hospitals employ health education specialists to provide programs for employees, patients, or the community at large.

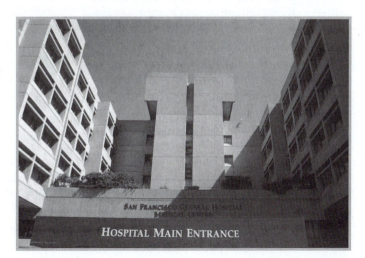

HOSPITAL MAIN ENTRANCE

PATIENT EDUCATOR Heather Rhodes

CURRENT POSITION/TITLE: Health Educator

EMPLOYER: IU Health Ball Memorial Family Medicine Residency Center

DEGREE/INSTITUTION/YEAR: B.S. Ball State University, 2007

MAJOR: Health Science

Job responsibilities: My job as the Health Educator for the Family Medicine Residency Center includes a wide range of responsibilities. I receive referrals from our resident physicians to educate clinic patients about a number of health topics, such as diabetes management, healthy nutrition, smoking cessation, and weight loss. All of our family medicine residents are responsible for completing a set number of community service hours throughout their residency, and I serve as the coordinator for all community outreach activities. I also serve as the coordinator for our Reach Out and Read program, a program that offers free books to children ages six months to five years during their well-child visits. I am very involved in the community and serve on a number of local boards and councils that all promote health and wellness as well as provide education to the commu-nity. I am responsible for displaying timely and appropriate health information on 26 bulletin boards throughout the clinic. I offer group smoking cessation classes in the com-munity and also serve as a resource for the IU Health Ball Memorial Cancer Center by providing one-on-one cessation counseling to their patients. I serve as the supervisor for a number of interns, both health education and administrative, who spend time at our facility. In addition, I have recently started conducting intake and education sessions with our newly pregnant patients in which I gather all pertinent information for their doc-tor and educate them about what to expect throughout pregnancy.

How I obtained my job: I stayed in touch with my internship supervisor after gradu-ation, and she shared that the job was available. I was familiar with the position as I had shadowed the previous Health Ed-ucator as a part of curriculum requirements

for one of my health science classes, and she had offered me an internship there as well. The job required a four-year degree as well as a CHES certification, and I possessed both. I felt that it was the perfect fit because my favorite part of my internship was the one-on-one education that I was able to give during health screenings. My previous job was telephone-based health coaching, which made me realize that I really desired to work with patients face to face. I had the valuable health coaching experience, which I feel made me a great candidate for the position.

What I like most about my job: I love the fact that I get to try and help people and make a difference in their lives on a daily basis. I also really enjoy the variety that my job provides. I am given a great deal of freedom to be creative and expand my position in new ways. Another thing I appreciate about my job is the positive and family-oriented work environment. Ev-eryone is passionate about helping others, and we all work as a team to provide our patients with the best care possible.

What I like least about my job: The big-gest challenge of my job and what I some-times like least is the fact that I am the only educator in the facility. There are no other health education specialists to bounce ideas off of and collaborate with. As a re-sult, I have to wear many hats and try to be available in all areas as much as possible. I love having the variety, but because my job provides a little more flexibility, I am given a wide variety of extra tasks that others may not have the ability to complete due to more rigid schedules.

How my work relates to the responsi-bilities and competencies of a health education specialist: As part of my job, I am constantly assessing the needs of my patients on an individual basis. I am assessing their learning levels as well as readiness to change so that I can really

BOX 7.5 *continued*

tailor information to the patient in a way that will make it most valuable for them. On a larger scale, I have had several opportunities to partner with outside agencies to provide health education/promotion programs for the community. In each instance, we work together to assess needs, plan, implement, and evaluate our programs. I serve as a resource person within our clinic and help residents find appropriate services, information, organizations, etc. that can meet the needs of their patients. I also serve as a resource for the community by participating in health fairs as well as local boards and councils.

Recommendations for those preparing to be health education specialists: For those who are preparing to be health education specialists, I would encourage you to make the most of your health science classes and learn all you can. Your classes will help prepare you for the CHES exam and will provide you with the necessary framework to start your career successfully. I also think it is always beneficial to take every opportunity to gain practical experience with program planning and health education through volunteering, research, and part-time work. Work on building your knowledge base about chronic disease management, nutrition, and other important health and wellness topics. Choose

wisely when picking your internship site as this will really help you determine your desired career path after graduation. It will give you valuable hands-on experience and will either confirm that you are on the right path or can help you find a new direction.

The role of health education specialist in the future: I think that the sky is the limit when it comes to the role of the health education specialist in the future. Over the last eight years, my career has continued to evolve and grow. I think that opportunities will expand beyond the typical clinical and program-planning settings, and there will be more of a need for educators to work with specific groups of the population in behavioral modification/educational programs. For example, over the next year there will be a shift in my job responsibilities, including how and where I educate patients. I will still be educating patients in our clinic, but I will also be part of a diabetes home visit education program focusing on the whole family unit as well as a Centering Pregnancy group in which women receive more extensive education and support throughout pregnancy with a small group of women with similar due dates.

that are reimbursable. Although health insurance companies are certainly concerned about reducing healthcare costs, their strategies to date have been more short term. The impact of health promotion and education programs may not be seen for years, and cause-and-effect relationships are difficult to establish. Therefore, without the availability of third-party payment, there is a major disincentive for hospitals, clinics, and private practice physicians to offer health promotion and education services to their patients. In response to this problem, SOPHE has made third-party reimbursement one of its major advocacy issues.

Of all healthcare settings, health maintenance organizations (HMOs) have been most receptive to hiring health education specialists. The first HMOs were established in the 1970s as a result of federal money that was made available to help with start-up costs and to study the effectiveness of this healthcare delivery mechanism. In essence, patients belonging to an HMO pay one set fee for all their medical services in a given year. It therefore benefits the HMO to provide preventive health services and health education/promotion programs to keep their patients healthy. The fewer services a patient uses, the greater the cost benefit to the HMO. In the initial HMO legislation, one of the criteria for establishing an HMO was providing health education/promotion. Unfortunately, there were no stipulations on the professional preparation of the health education/promotion provider. Often, nurses or other individuals with little or no health education/promotion preparation or experience were given the responsibility of providing health education/promotion programs. As a result, some HMOs have developed outstanding health education/promotion programs with health education specialists, whereas others do very little.

There is, however, reason to be optimistic about future employment opportunities in healthcare settings for health education specialists. The Health Promoting Hospitals Network (HPH), initiated by the World Health Organization (WHO), functions to incorporate more health promotion and education programs in hospitals worldwide (The International Network of Health Promoting Hospitals and Health Services, 2016). With changes in the U.S. medical care system rapidly occurring, the increased emphasis on cost-cutting measures, and movement toward more managed care, it is likely that prevention will take a higher profile in the future. As these changes occur, health education specialists will be the best prepared professionals to assume responsibility for helping individuals adopt healthy lifestyles.

A Day in the Career of a Healthcare Setting Health Education Specialist

Mary's day begins at 8:30 A.M., when she arrives at the hospital, picks up her mail, and proceeds to her office where she reviews her email and phone messages. She is the only health education specialist employed by this large metropolitan hospital, but she does have a secretary/assistant who works closely with her to carry out the duties of the position.

At 9:00 A.M., Mary has to attend the weekly staff meeting. This is a meeting with all department heads at the hospital. Much of the agenda does not concern Mary directly, but it is important for her to know what is going on in all departments. At today's meeting, it was decided to have an open house for the public to see the newly renovated obstetrics wing of the hospital. Mary is given the responsibility of planning and advertising this event.

At 10:00 A.M., Mary has an appointment with the administrative head of the Cardiac Rehabilitation Program at the hospital. The purpose of the meeting is to begin planning the development of two brochures that will eventually be distributed to all cardiac rehabilitation patients and will be posted on the hospital education Web site that Mary maintains. One brochure will be on stress-management strategies and the other on different types of dietary fat. They brainstorm ideas, and Mary agrees to develop a rough draft of the content of the brochures for the administrative head to review prior to their next meeting. They will also discuss graphics, layout, and production at the next meeting.

At 11:00 A.M., Mary leaves the hospital to drive to one of the local malls. The mall has decided to conduct a three-day health fair, and the hospital has agreed to be a co-sponsor of the event. Today is a planning meeting for all of the agencies and businesses that will participate. In addition to serving on the planning committee, Mary is responsible for setting up the hospital's display and coordinating nurses and physicians to work in several screening stations.

During the health fair, Mary will be at the hospital's booth all day, handing out materials, answering questions, and promoting the hospital's community outreach health promotion programs.

After lunch, Mary returns to the hospital around 1:00 P.M. and spends the next two hours working on the hospital's health and wellness newsletter. As a public service and to promote the hospital, Mary is responsible for developing a newsletter every other month that is mailed to all households in the hospital's immediate service area. Each edition of the newsletter features one department in the hospital and contains several additional articles about health and wellness. Mary writes much of each newsletter, using information she obtains from the Internet and from a variety of health journals and newsletters to which she subscribes. She designs and formats the newsletter with a desktop publishing program she has on her computer. She marvels at how important good writing skills are to her position.

At 3:00 P.M., Mary leads a weight-loss support group for hospital employees. Most of the participants are nurses and housekeeping staff from either the first or second shift. At each session, participants weigh in, share their experiences over the previous week, and listen to a 20-minute presentation designed to enhance their weight-loss program. Mary is responsible for each week's presentation. In addition, she provides participants with healthy recipes, exercise tips, motivational incentives, and recognition awards. The weight loss support group also has a Web site that Mary maintains where additional recipes and information on weight loss are posted. In the future Mary plans to expand the Web site and develop an online hospital-based weight-loss program that will be made available to the entire community.

After class, Mary returns phone calls, answers emails, and ties up loose ends until it is time for her to go home at 5:00 P.M. It is not unusual for Mary to take some work home in the evenings or on weekends. Tonight, however, Mary must return to the hospital at 7:30 P.M. to teach a stress-management class for the community. The stress class is part of the hospital's on-going community outreach program. Each month a different health topic is taught, and Mary is responsible for either teaching the class or lining up the instructor/speaker for the class.

Additional Responsibilities

Health education specialists working in healthcare settings are involved in numerous and varied activities. The actual responsibilities can differ greatly from one healthcare setting to another. Planning, implementing, and evaluating programs and events are certainly major tasks. Health education specialists may also be involved in grant writing, one-on-one or group patient education services, publicity, public relations, employee wellness activities, and various collaborative efforts with other hospital staff, community agencies, or departments of public health.

Administration is a major responsibility of many health education specialists working in hospitals. They are often hired as managers, directors, or coordinators of programs. Hospitals often adopt a "team" approach to health education/promotion, in which doctors, nurses, physical therapists, and other health specialists are all part of the team. Health education specialists plan and coordinate the programs and serve as resources for the other team members, who actually present the programs. In this type of position, the health education specialist provides little direct client service (Breckon et al., 1998). (See **Table 7.10**.)

TABLE 7.10 **Advantages and disadvantages of working in a healthcare setting**

Advantages

- Job responsibilities are highly varied and changing.
- There is increased credibility due to the healthcare connection.
- There is usually a high community profile.
- Health education specialists work with multiple groups of people.
- Wages and benefits are good.
- There is a high degree of self-satisfaction.

Disadvantages

- Health education/promotion may have low status and low priority within healthcare settings.
- Health education specialists must continually justify the program's value.
- Jobs are difficult to obtain.
- Turf issues over educational responsibilities can develop.
- Hours may be long and irregular.
- Some medical doctors may be difficult to work with.

▷ Health Education/Promotion in Colleges and Universities

Colleges and universities are another source of employment for health education specialists. Within the college setting, there are typically two types of positions that health education specialists hold. The first is an academic, or faculty, position, and the second is as a health education specialist in a student health service or wellness center.

As a faculty member, the health education specialist typically has three major responsibilities: teaching, community and professional service, and scholarly research (Preparing Future Faculty, 2016). The amount of emphasis on each of these major responsibilities is dependent on the institution. In large research institutions, faculty may spend most of their time writing grants and conducting research. In smaller four-year colleges, teaching may be the major responsibility. In addition to the major responsibilities, faculty may be asked to advise students, serve on committees, coordinate or lead student groups, attend professional conferences, and accept administrative duties.

The minimum qualification for working as a faculty member in the college/university setting is usually a doctoral degree in health education/promotion. Though some junior colleges and small four-year schools may hire faculty with only a master's degree, most tenure-track positions require a doctorate. In addition, depending on the position for which one is applying, it may be necessary to have had prior experience or academic training in school health, public/community health, or work-site health promotion. Holding or being eligible for a CHES or MCHES credential is often listed as a preference or requirement for faculty positions.

For a health education specialist in a university health service or wellness center, the major responsibility is to plan, implement, and evaluate health education/promotion programs for program participants (see **Box 7.6**). In some universities, the program participants are students, whereas in others it is the faculty and staff. Often both groups are included as program participants. In addition to program planning, the health education specialist may be responsible for maintaining a resource library; maintaining a Web site; one-on-one advising with students; developing and coordinating a peer education program; speaking to residence hall, fraternity, and sorority groups; conducting incentive programs; and planning special events.

BOX 7.6

UNIVERSITY WELLNESS CENTER Elizabeth D. Peeler

CURRENT POSITION: Health Educator, Office of Health, Alcohol, and Drug Education

EMPLOYER: Ball State University

DEGREE INFORMATION:

UNDERGRADUATE: Appalachian State University (Bachelor of Science)

MAJOR: Cell/Molecular Biology

MINOR(S): Art History and Chemistry

GRADUATE: University of South Carolina (Master in Science of Public Health)

CONCENTRATION: Health Promotion, Education, and Behavior

How I got into health education: I stumbled my way into health education as a pre-med freshman at Appalachian State University. I applied to be a Wellness Peer Educator to show medical schools that I had the skills to communicate to patients on how to change their health behaviors to become healthier. Little did I know that by joining this organization I would change my career path from medicine to public health.

My current job responsibilities: As the Office of Health, Alcohol, and Drug Education health educator at Ball State University, I present to student groups on a number of different health topics, and plan, implement, and evaluate campus-wide events to promote better health while managing two grants. Both grants focus on alcohol consumption and harm reduction among college students. I oversee the Peer Health Educators and a graduate assistant at Ball State University who are responsible for providing peer-to-peer health education. I am responsible for administering the American College Health Association – National College Health Assessment and other surveys to determine student health needs. Based on needs assessments and climate surveys, I am responsible for strategic planning within my office.

I collaborate with a number of offices and departments on campus to better serve the needs of our students. As such, I serve on a number of campus and community committees. I also engage with the outside community to build rapport and relationships to address any issues that may arise

off-campus. As well, I participate in national professional organizations through conferences, coalitions, and committees to further health education and health promotion in higher education.

How I obtained my job: After I graduated with my master's, I decided to focus my attention on obtaining a health education position at an academic institution. I came across the announcement of a health educator position at Ball State University and submitted my cover letter along with my CV, list of references, and transcripts to the search committee for review. I was contacted for a 30-minute phone interview followed by an in-person interview at Ball State. I received the job offer two weeks after the in-person interview and happily accepted the position.

How I utilize health education/promotion in my job: I utilize a number of different theories and models in my programs. Most commonly, I use the Socio-Ecological Model, Transtheoretical Model, and Health Belief Model to inform my programming. I use process, impact, and outcome evaluations to measure behavior and culture change. Needs assessments and climate surveys are administered to help inform my programming on the current needs of students. I also use community and stakeholder engagement to organize and disseminate health promotion programming. I collect, analyze, and report data on my programs' reach and effectiveness to university administrators and community leaders.

What I like most about my job: There are so many things I love about my job, I cannot possibly mention them all. While there are definitely challenges working with college-aged students, their energy, enthusiasm, and creativity more than makes up for the challenges they present. Without students' input into programs, events, and initiatives, I would not be able to do my job. Students are the key stakeholders, and

BOX

7.6

continued

they must be fully engaged to change the climate and culture in a university.

I also enjoy working with different disciplines across campus to bring better programs and initiatives to students. By working collaboratively with different departments, I am able to ensure that I am approaching all needs of the students. Some departments I have worked with include student life, residence life, campus police, dining services, and recreation services.

What I like least about my job: With any position in public health, there seems to be never enough resources to go around. This leads to stress in trying to figure out how to implement programs, but it also encourages creativity. Further, it can be incredibly frustrating to work on improving students' health but not see immediate changes in their behaviors. Behavior change is not instantaneous, and health educators must learn patience.

Recommendations for those preparing to be health education specialists: For future health education specialists, I suggest finding a mentor in their field of choice. I have been very lucky in finding a number of mentors in my field that have helped me immensely whether that has been professionally, academically, or even personally.

I also recommend completing observations, practicums, and internships in different settings. You may find that you prefer a clinical setting over an office setting or vice-versa. Interning is also a great networking opportunity to help better prepare you for the field.

Another important recommendation that often gets overlooked for health education specialists is the importance of research. The fundamentals of research help immensely when reading the literature to help in developing cutting edge, evidence-based programs. Research is also vital when trying to justify the importance of a needed resource or program.

The role of health education specialists in the future: Based on my experience as a health educator, future health education specialists are going to be utilized more in clinical settings to change health behavior than they currently are. Health coaching will become a part of the clinical experience for patients who need to change health behaviors for a healthier and more productive life. Health education specialists are also going to be utilized more in administrator roles to better address the needs of the community.

▷ International Opportunities

Health education/promotion specialists may wish to consider working in global health for all or a portion of their careers. There is great need for professionals with health education/promotion skills in many low- and middle-income countries. These positions often require special dedication because the living and working conditions may be more challenging than those experienced in the United States. For health education specialists so inclined, however, the rewards in terms of personal satisfaction and accomplishment can be tremendous. Further, the experience gained by planning, implementing, and evaluating health promotion and education programs in foreign countries can be invaluable to one's professional development (see **Box 7.7**).

Working in developing countries often requires the health education specialist to examine different health problems and to try different approaches. For example, instead of helping

GLOBAL HEALTH Emily Miller

CURRENT POSITION/TITLE: International Medical Programs Coordinator; Tena, Ecuador

EMPLOYER: Timmy Global Health

DEGREE/INSTITUTION/YEAR: Bachelor of Science, Ball State University, 2013

MAJOR/MINOR: Health Science/Spanish

My global health experience: Global health is an all-encompassing term that refers to health equity and prosperity both locally and globally. During my freshman year of college, I became actively involved in global health. In 2009, I participated in an international medical brigade hosted by the Ball State University Timmy Global Health chapter (BSU Timmy). Our team of students and doctors visited five rural communities surrounding Quito, Ecuador, and treated over 500 patients in the span of one week. Throughout the week, I was given the opportunity to collect patient history, record patient vitals, shadow medical professionals of various specialties, administer fluoride for all the children, and manage a mobile pharmacy.

Along with this clinical experience, I was also given the opportunity to further expand on several health education initiatives. Water sanitation, dental hygiene, malnutrition, and prenatal care are the four main health disparities within these communities. Waterborne parasites are extremely common within these communities, so it is important to teach community members how to properly boil and treat their water source in order to lessen and/ or eliminate this illness. Dental hygiene is another major health concern, particularly among the children. Many children will arrive to the clinic with a mouthful of cavities, so teaching proper brushing and flossing techniques is very important in promoting good oral hygiene. All pregnant mothers are also given prenatal vitamins for which I explained the importance of prenatal care and encouraged the mothers to receive periodic check-ups prior to their delivery. Although medical treatment is important, primary and secondary prevention are imperative. Health education plays a major role in the prevention of communicable diseases and the overall offset of chronic diseases.

To say it was an enriching experience is an understatement—this first trip to Ecuador revolutionized my view of health. The various determinants of health (i.e., social, political, environmental, biological, etc.) play a significant role in the health outcomes of poor, rural communities. For example, the majority of patients we treat during brigades do not have regular access to a health clinic. Furthermore, several patients must walk over five hours to reach a mobile clinic, while others must wait several months before the next mobile clinic is in their area. The field of global health attempts to minimize these determinants through various interventions and programs. This initial experience granted me the opportunity to intern with the organization and eventually obtain my current position.

How I obtained this experience: I obtained this experience through the Timmy Global Health chapter at Ball State University (BSU Timmy). The organization has nearly 30 university chapters across the United States, and I was fortunate enough to have a chapter at my school. Being originally from Texas, I had never heard of the organization, so this was a great opportunity to learn more about the organization and get involved in global health. Stemming from my experience with the BSU Timmy chapter, I was able to work my way up and intern at the organization headquarters in Indianapolis. Consequently, I worked closely with the organization staff and was fortunate enough to receive my current position as an international medical programs coordinator. In this position, my responsibilities include organizing medical brigades, coordinating meetings among the community health workers, developing and implementing health education programs, and conducting research, all of which tie in nicely with the seven areas of health education responsibilities.

BOX

7.7

continued

Why I have chosen to work in global health: Health is a fundamental human right, and everyone deserves the opportunity to a happy and fruitful life. Unlike the majority of the world's population, I was born into a privileged, healthy life. I believe it is my responsibility to give back to those less fortunate to ensure that the communities with whom I work are given the same opportunities and health resources that I received throughout my numerous stages in life.

What I like most about working in global health: Working in global health allows me to combine my three passions in life: health, servitude, and travel. After my first medical brigade in Quito, Ecuador, I was immediately hooked. The demand for health education in poor, rural communities is undeniable, and the broad scope of this field allows me to address an endless list of health disparities. My particular position as a medical programs coordinator gives me the ability to provide health services and resources to individuals who otherwise lack such amenities. Simply teaching an individual how to properly wash their hands or treat their water drastically impacts their health. These seemingly small accomplishments play a much larger role in these communities, which make this occupation all the more enjoyable and rewarding.

What I like least about working in global health: Working in global health is a never-ending endeavor. Unfortunately, there are millions of individuals and families living in abject poverty with little opportunity to improve their circumstances. As a health education specialist, I am limited in the amount of work I can do in these communities, and unfortunately, several circumstances (e.g., social, environmental, biological, etc.) are out of my control. For example, the poverty level and isolated location of these communities limits the amount of health resources and services they are able to receive. Additionally, the patriarchal or 'machismo' culture within these communities greatly hinders the health status of

women and children. Furthermore, shifting community health behaviors is not a short-term process. After investing a lot of time and energy and waiting patiently for my work's impact to unfold, I am continually learning the full impact of my job.

Health education responsibilities I use in my global health work: My work in global health allows me to encompass all seven areas of health education responsibilities. Alongside my responsibilities as a medical programs coordinator, I also received a grant through Timmy Global Health to design and implement a women's health program in Tena, Ecuador. Through these combined duties, I am able to address each area of health education responsibilities. Specifically, in order to understand my international communities, it is imperative that I assess the needs, assets, and capacity for health education within my adopted community (Area I). Once I determine the level of health intervention needed, I am able to plan, implement, and evaluate my health education program(s) (Areas II–IV). Research is another important component of the health education process, which allows one to understand, evaluate, and improve existing and future health programs within their community (Area IV). Within my occupation, I am also able to administer and manage health education within my community health programs (Area V), serving as a health education resource person and advocate for health and health education (Area VI–VII). Needless to say, my work in global health has given me the opportunity to exercise all seven areas of health education responsibilities.

Recommendations for other health education specialists who would like to work in global health: One advantage of working in global health is the ability to work anywhere in the world. Begin your exploration in the classroom and enroll in global health courses. If your school does

BOX 7.7 *continued*

not offer courses in global health, MIT offers free international health courses (https://www.edx.org/ and http://ocw.mit.edu/index.htm). For those interested in tackling modern global health issues, consider volunteering for both local and international health organizations (e.g., health clinics that serve impoverished communities, homeless shelters, health education facilities, etc.). It is important to note that it is not absolutely necessary to travel to another country to experience poverty and disease; there are countless communities here in the United States that desperately need help, as well. However, to fully understand the complexities of health disparities around the globe, consider studying abroad in an impoverished country and make sure to study the language beforehand. Last, but not least, remain curious; make a point to explore and cultivate your interests.

people reduce high-fat, high-cholesterol diets, as in the United States, the health education specialist may be helping people deal with problems of starvation, malnutrition, and parasitic and bacterial infections. Instead of dealing with heart disease and lung cancer, the health education specialist in a developing country may be facing schistosomiasis, diarrhea, and ascariasis and tapeworm infections.

Consider the case of Sofia. Sofia was working as a community health education specialist for the health department in a rural community of about two thousand people in a developing country. The water source for this community consisted of several large ponds. These ponds were the only source of drinking water and were also used for bathing, clothes washing, and care of animals. Many people were getting sick with severe diarrhea, and there had been several deaths among the elderly and very young. To alleviate this problem, it was decided to develop an educational campaign to get people to boil their water before consumption. Sofia was given the responsibility for developing this campaign. There were no local newspapers or radio stations and no billboards, and many of the people could not read. After consulting with local leaders, it was decided that the best way to spread the information would be through word of mouth using a "mobile communication system." This was accomplished by hooking up an old stereo system to a car battery and driving around the community, broadcasting information about the importance of boiling water. In addition, Sofia set up several demonstrations around the community about how to boil water effectively. These sessions were also advertised via the "mobile communication system."

As can be seen from Sofia's experience, health education specialists working in foreign countries must be able to develop creative, innovative programs to solve identified health problems. Most often, these programs must be low-cost, easily developed and implemented, acceptable to the social and cultural norms of the community, and available to all aspects of the public. It is imperative that these programs be developed in conjunction with the local people being served. It is also helpful when programs are sponsored by organizations seen as credible by the priority population.

One of the best ways to begin a career in international health is to volunteer with the Peace Corps. Health education/promotion professionals are in demand by the Peace Corps, and students should begin the application process early in their senior year. Many colleges and

TABLE 7.11 **International health organizations**

National Council for International Health
American Association for World Health
World Health Organization (WHO)
Joint United Nations Program on HIV and AIDS (UNAIDS)
Pan American Health Organization
U.S. Agency for International Development (USAID)
Foundations such as the Bill and Melinda Gates Foundation
Nongovernmental organizations such as Save the Children
CDC Coordinating Office for Global Health

universities are visited by Peace Corps recruiters every year, and talking to one of these Peace Corps volunteers is a good place to start. Faculty members on your campus may have been former Peace Corps volunteers and talking to these individuals can provide valuable insight into the Peace Corps experience. Some colleges and universities have developed Peace Corps Prep Programs, which provide students with a certificate upon completion of a specific set of classes and an approved internship experience. Students completing the Peace Corps Prep Program are not guaranteed entry into the Peace Corps, but they are given strong consideration.

There are many advantages to volunteering with the Peace Corps. The Peace Corps provides volunteers with some of the best language and technical training in the world. Each Peace Corps volunteer is granted a monthly allowance for housing, food, clothing, and miscellaneous expenses. Free dental and medical care are provided, as well as free transportation to the placement setting and 24 vacation days per year. Deferment of federal student loans is also possible while serving in the Peace Corps. After completing the two-year experience, volunteers are given a post-service readjustment allowance of $8,000. They are also given preference for federal jobs and have enhanced scholarship and assistantship opportunities at many major colleges and universities (Peace Corps, 2016). In addition, a successful Peace Corps experience may serve as a stepping stone to paid positions in other international health organizations (see **Table 7.11**).

The CDC is expanding its presence overseas. This may create future opportunities for health education specialists. "CDC is committed to ensuring that people around the world will live safer, healthier, and longer lives through the achievement of its Global Health Goals: Global Health Promotion, Global Health Protection, and Global Health Diplomacy" (CDC, 2016a).

▷ Nontraditional Health Education/Promotion Positions

In addition to the traditional settings for health education/promotion that have been described in this chapter, there are a variety of nontraditional jobs that health education specialists may wish to consider. These positions may or may not carry the title of health education specialist. In some cases, they require the health education specialist to use their skills and competencies in different or unique ways. Further, it is often necessary for health education specialists to sell themselves to get these positions because the person(s) doing the hiring may be unfamiliar with the skills and training of a health education specialist.

Given health education specialists' knowledge of health and fitness, sales positions related to health and fitness products are a real possibility. Pharmacy sales, fitness equipment sales, and the sales of health-related textbooks are all areas in which health education specialists have found employment. Life and health insurance are two additional options to consider in the area of sales.

By emphasizing the communication competencies that are part of the professional training in health education/promotion, the health education specialist may seek employment in journalism, TV, or radio. Television stations often have a regular health or medical reporter who does feature stories on health-related issues. Newspapers may have a health column that could and should be written by a health education specialist. Writing articles for health-related Web sites or actually developing Web sites for health-related organizations are other possibilities (see **Box 7.8**). Again, it is necessary for health education specialists to sell themselves to obtain these positions. Taking elective classes or minors in media, communications, and journalism and doing one's internship in these settings also may assist those interested in this career field.

BOX

7.8

Practitioner's Perspective

NONTRADITIONAL HEALTH EDUCATION/PROMOTION POSITIONS Patricia Stewart

CURRENT POSITION: Education Program Consultant

EMPLOYER: The Children's Health Market, publishers of The Great Body Shop, Comprehensive Health Education Curriculum Program

DEGREE: B.S.ED, Dakota State University, Madison, South Dakota; Major – Physical Education; Minor – Health Education

Current job responsibilities: My responsibilities as a Program Consultant for The Children's Health Market are to communicate with public and private schools through sales calls and marketing to promote The Great Body Shop Health Education Curriculum. I serve as a health education curriculum resource for school districts in the Northwest and Upper Midwest regions of the United States. I network with State Department of Education Directors and Coordinators working in Pre-K through Secondary Education who focus on Health and Physical Education. As school districts adopt the curriculum, I provide a variety of training designs to meet the needs of school districts. I represent the company at a variety of education conferences representing Pre-K through Grade 9 focusing on a wide range of health issues from social-emotional learning (SEL), drug and alcohol prevention, comprehensive health education, and character education. I also network with university professors in the field of health education and with hospital administration and insurance companies who may be interested in supporting public/community health aspects of our primary prevention program serving children and their families.

It is also my responsibility to maintain a current knowledge of state and national initiatives that will serve as opportunities or barriers for adoption of health curriculum in schools. I know the National and State(s) Health Education Standards and how health education aligns to Common Core for English Language Arts. I utilize CDC's Health Education Curriculum Assessment Tool and School Health Index in my curriculum work with schools. On an annual basis, our company reviews and updates the health curriculum, and I am asked to review and provide editorial suggestions to assist in that process.

Health Education/promotion responsibilities I use most in my job: Although my job is nontraditional, I use many of the core responsibilities of a health education specialist.

BOX 7.8 *continued*

1. **Assess Needs:** This often involves an initial conversation with a school administrator, curriculum director, or health specialist who I may contact through a cold call or at a professional development conference. I need to be an attentive listener to understand what their goals and needs are for health education for their student population at their school or center. When individuals feel that you are in tune with their needs, they may be more open to further exploring the "fit" of our curriculum. For example, The Great Body Shop is a comprehensive health education curriculum covering multiple health topics that are integrated throughout the variety of lessons and units. Although a curriculum director may only want to purchase materials focused on one or two topics, we believe a comprehensive health approach is most effective. It is important to demonstrate how these topics of his/her focused interest are covered in different ways using a variety of strategies across the curriculum to reinforce the knowledge and skills of students. Sometimes we are able to persuade them to consider this integrated approach as a more effective way to build knowledge and skills. Acknowledging possible funding and classroom time challenges is important as well.

2. **Plan and Implement the Program:** I work closely with school district personnel to plan and design training that meets the needs of the teachers implementing the curriculum. It may be a training for all of the staff or a train the trainer model. Training may be face-to-face or via conference call or webinar. It is important to encourage and support training needs to create an environment that will sustain a quality health education program. The initial training and on-going follow-up and technical assistance are vital to the successful implementation and sustainability of any curriculum. During training

and presentations, my knowledge and enthusiasm have to be evident to help motivate others to want to teach health.

3. **Evaluate:** Following conference presentations and school training provided to customers, I gather feedback through formal evaluations, phone calls, and emails to determine the success of meeting the training goals and objectives. When schools pilot the curriculum, we evaluate the implementation process to measure progress and ease of use. I am continually communicating with school staff on the ease of implementation seeking their ideas and suggestions for improvement.

4. **Act as a Resource:** I serve as the main contact for school districts in approximately 10 states implementing the health curriculum. Effective verbal and written communication skills are important in providing technical assistance. I answer initial questions from schools regarding their consideration of our program versus other health curricula. It is important to help guide their curriculum adoption process professionally and honestly. There may be instances where our product does not meet the goal or need of the school district, and it is important to be honest about that fact.

How I got my job: I taught health and physical education at the secondary level in two school districts in South Dakota for thirteen years. Part of my teaching experience was in the Sisseton School District, which had a high percentage of Native American students giving me insight into cultural differences related to health risks and the challenges that poverty adds in accessing quality health services. My professional experience led me to a position in the South Dakota Department of Education (SDDOE) as the Title IX and Equal Education

BOX 7.8

continued

Opportunities Director where I began to promote and train students and adults on the importance of equity based on gender, race, and national origin. I learned to write grants and have spent much of my career writing and directing grants from the U.S. Department of Education or the Department of Health and Human Services (DHHS). I have worked in both South Dakota and Idaho as the Director of the Coordinated School Health Program (CSHP) guiding schools toward a coordinated approach to school health. In my position in state departments of education, I began to provide more presentations and training to adults focusing my teaching skills around meeting the needs of adult learners. I experienced first-hand the importance of communication skills and networking. I believe my knowledge of school health, my training skills with a variety of age groups and diverse populations, and my passion for health education and curriculum design have led me to my current job.

What I like about my job: I appreciate the flexibility and the diversity of my work. As an independent consultant, I am able to work from home on my own schedule and determine my work load and travel schedule to meet the needs of my family. Every day provides the opportunity to talk about health education with school staff and others from across the country. I do not manage or supervise others but am in control of my own schedule and workload. I enjoy working and am highly self-motivated, which is key to being a successful independent consultant. My favorite activity is conducting a training for a school district implementing The Great Body Shop! It is

my love of teaching that led me into education in the first place. What I didn't consider, then, is just how important "selling" what you are teaching is to engaging people at any age!

What I like least about my job: Since I am an independent consultant and not an employee of the company, I do not receive benefits. Being an independent consultant requires attention to business details that one may not have considered when employed full-time by a company covering all benefits. I also miss face-to-face interactions that one would have in the workplace although I do maintain regular contact through emails or phone calls.

Recommendations for those preparing to be health educators: To be successful, you must remain committed to the hard work and be passionate about what you do and why you do it. Be dedicated to the profession and strive to be a lifelong learner with a commitment to seeking professional development. Join your professional organization(s) even before leaving your undergraduate program and stay connected by attending, presenting, and seeking leadership opportunities. Seek opportunities for internships to get experience and begin that professional networking process. Network and develop relationships with school, community, and state partners—one never knows how these partnerships may open doors of opportunity to benefit the people and programs one is currently working with or provide a new, challenging career opportunity.

Health education specialists should always be alert to unique job opportunities, many of which may not even carry the title of health education specialist. One health education specialist, for example, was hired by a state mental hospital as a "Teacher II." His job was to provide drug education to patients who had a history of drug problems and sex education to patients who had a history of sex problems. The remainder of his work schedule involved tutoring patients in math and science who were studying to obtain their high school general equivalency diploma.

▷ Landing That First Job

At first, it may seem unusual to discuss landing one's first job in an introductory text, but it is never too early to consider the issue of future employment. There are several actions students can take during their college years to enhance their chances of obtaining employment. By following the suggestions made in this section, a student will be far ahead of those who wait until the end of their degree program to address these issues.

No matter what the setting in which a health education specialist hopes to eventually work, landing the first job can be a frustrating experience. Students often find themselves in a dilemma. Employers want their new employees to have had "experience," but where are students supposed to get experience if they can't get hired? There are several possible answers to this question. One way to gain experience is to obtain part-time or summer employment in one's preferred health education/promotion setting. Typically, there are many more students looking for this type of employment than there are employment situations. Should such an opportunity be available, however, it is an excellent way to gain experience before graduation. Another way to obtain experience is to volunteer time in the chosen health education/promotion setting. Most professional health education specialists working in the field are more than willing to accept and use the volunteer time of health education/promotion students. In addition to experience, volunteering also begins the important process of **networking**. Networking involves establishing and maintaining a wide range of contacts in the field that may be of help when looking for a job and in carrying out one's job responsibilities once hired.

Many health education/promotion programs now offer **service learning** opportunities to their students (Cleary, Kaiser-Drobney, Ubbes, Stuhldreher, & Birch, 1998). Organized service learning opportunities provide course credit for students to work with a community agency to meet an identified community need. For example university students helped elderly residents of a low socioeconomic area of the city to develop community vegetable gardens. Not only did they help with cultivation, planting, and harvesting, but they also provided education messages about healthy diet.

This service learning experience provided hands-on, practical, real-world experience that students could not obtain from the classroom. Service learning can also be beneficial in broadening one's professional network, which is so important in the health education/promotion field. Take advantage of as many service learning opportunities as possible. The experience and networking gained through service learning can give new health education/promotion professionals a tremendous advantage in the job market.

Carefully planning internships and practicums can help students obtain their first professional position (see **Box 7.9**). Required field experiences are often the best way to obtain practical experience in one's chosen setting. Students should consider what they would like to be doing five years after graduation and select an experience that closely matches that goal. Frequently students are hired by the agency after completing their practicum or internship experience.

In addition to obtaining experience, students should strive to obtain an excellent academic record. When there is heavy competition for an open position, one of the first strategies in making hiring decisions is to examine grade point average. This is not to say that the person with the highest grade point average is always the best person or will always get the

STUDENT INTERN Jeremy Herzberg

BOX 7.9

Practitioner's Perspective

MAJOR/INSTITUTION: *Community Health; Central Michigan University, Graduation May 2016*

INTERNSHIP ORGANIZATION: *Gratiot Family Practice; Alma, Michigan*

Internship placement: My career goal is to become a physician assistant in an urban setting where I can easily use my health education skills to augment my medical practice. In this career path, I hope to utilize my skills I have obtained from public health to help educate my patients as well as changing the mentality of our health system as a whole. My hopes are to contribute to the change of our healthcare system from a strictly disease care system to a disease prevention system.

I have worked during my college career as an EMT in Saginaw, Michigan. Naturally, I wanted my internship to be as close to a clinical setting as I could. My professor, knowing this, suggested Gratiot Family Practice, a private practice just south of where I attended school for my internship site.

Internship description: Interning at a private practice gave me many opportunities that would not have been available had I done my internship in a nonclinical setting. Not only was I able to shadow the doctors and PAs to learn about the practice of medicine, but I was able learn how medicine and public health education have the potential to interact at the primary care level. My internship location was extremely primary prevention oriented. Instead of waiting for an illness to develop and then treating the patient, we strived to educate and empower patients to be conscious and take action with their own health. In other words, we wanted to give patients the tools to get healthy and stay healthy in all aspects of their lives. Being able to observe and work with providers who shared this view on medicine was a truly humbling and exceptionally valuable experience.

I was given a lot of autonomy when it came to projects I worked on for the practice. One of my main goals was to get patients more involved or aware of the opportunities in their local community. So, with the help of local nonprofits in the area, I was able to introduce a community bulletin board in the waiting room for patients to access. This board had flyers from all around the community with event schedules, services offered, and volunteer opportunities that patients could partake in. This was well received by patients in the practice. Overall, I feel the contributions I made during my internship had a positive impact on the practice and its patients.

Pros and cons of my internship: I loved the autonomy of my internship and the opportunity I had to learn about how medicine and public health education should interact. Everyone was very supportive of me and always interested in ideas that I brought to the table. I learned a lot about the true needs of the patients we strive to help in our local communities as well as their expectations when it comes to medical care. However, I did experience the frustration that we as public health educators witness when we interact with patients who do not care for their health. Try as we might, sometimes people are just too set in their old habits to change. Overall, my internship experience was truly humbling and rewarding.

Internship importance: As an aspiring physician assistant with an astute interest in public health education, this internship really served as the bridge between my two passions. Prior to internship, I hadn't really the slightest clue on how I would utilize my public health background in my future career in medicine. However, after observing and working with providers who share these same passions as myself, I was able to learn how medicine and public health education can and should work together to benefit the patient. This experience was really the epitome of my undergraduate career. All of the class work I had conducted up to this point was finally put

continued

BOX 7.9

into practice. I learned a lot about program planning as well as educating patients, hands on, in a variety of areas.

Recommendations for those preparing to be health education specialists: When thinking about your future in the health education field, try to really understand where your passion lies. For example, ask yourself, "Do I like the clinical side?" or "Do I like policies, writing grants, or developing programs?" Maybe even, "Do I want to work with a specific population such as children, HIV, or underserved areas?" Whatever your passion is, find it and run

with it! Don't let anyone tell you or suggest otherwise. Working in an area that you are not passionate about can lead to personal disappointment and frustration as well as have a negative impact on those you work with. Your internship is your opportunity to find that setting you love, so choose wisely. Don't take the easy way out. If you can find that area where you wake up every day and say, "I have the best job in the world!"—then everything else will fall into place, I guarantee it.

job. But, when there are 50 applications for one job, grade point average is an easy way to begin limiting the field.

Develop a well-organized, professional-looking portfolio. A **portfolio** is a collection of evidence that enables students to demonstrate mastery of desired course or program outcomes/competencies. In health education/promotion, the responsibilities, competencies, and subcompetencies should be emphasized. Many health education/promotion programs now require portfolios as part of their professional preparation programs. Even if the portfolio is not required, students should develop a portfolio on their own. Thompson and Bybee (2004) note that a portfolio is a "living document that is ever-changing with the increasing depth of knowledge and experience of the individual" (p. 52). They go on to identify five basic elements that should be included in any portfolio: (1) table of contents, (2) résumé, (3) education and credentials, (4) samples of work, and (5) references. The samples of work could include such exhibits as student papers or course projects, audio- or videotapes of students giving a presentation, analyses of student work by professors or outside reviewers, student goal statements, reflections, and summaries (Cleary & Birch, 1996, 1997). Another way to design the portfolio is to structure it around the NCHEC health education specialist competencies. Essentially, exhibits are included in the portfolio for each competency. Students may also want to consider developing the portfolio in an electronic format instead of the more traditional notebook or binder. In addition to providing more flexibility in the way exhibits are presented and displayed, an electronic format also provides the opportunity to showcase one's creativity and to demonstrate technology skills to potential employers (McKenzie, Cleary, McKenzie, & Stephen, 2002). Imagine the impact on a prospective employer when a new health education specialist provides a well-developed, attractive portfolio that clearly demonstrates health education responsibilities and competencies.

Your résumé is extremely important in obtaining your first job. The résumé is your advertisement for yourself. It is the first item of yours that most prospective employers will see. It will create a first and lasting impression of you. What you include in the résumé and how you present the information may make a difference in whether or not you are hired. You

TABLE 7.12 **Résumé—Words of wisdom**

Out-of-Date Résumé (Overused Clichés)	More Effective Résumé (Be Specific—Provide Examples)
Results Oriented	Describe a problem that you solved
Team Player	Describe a team project you were part of and the results
Excellent Communication Skills	Demonstrate how your communication skills produced meaningful results
Strong Work Ethic	Provide an example of how you went "above and beyond" to produce results
Meets or Exceeds Expectations	Explain how you were recognized for your effort/work

Source: Jeff Brizzolara, Ph.D., MPH, MBA. Chief Clinical Officer, Viverae Health Care, Inc. Used by permission.

should start now to involve yourself in experiences that will look good on your résumé. As you develop your résumé, make sure that there are no spelling or grammar errors. One former student actually lost a job opportunity because of three spelling errors on her résumé. The more specific you can be in describing your accomplishments on the résumé, the better. Jeff Brizzolara, a health education specialist and Chief Clinical Officer for Viverae Health Care, has some suggestions on how to be more specific; these can be seen in **Table 7.12** .

Beyond the portfolio and résumé, consider what certifications are going to be important in landing your first job and carefully plan to make sure they are awarded either before graduation or as soon after graduation as possible. All professional health education specialists should pursue the CHES and MCHES credential. In the future, this may be a prerequisite for many health promotion and education positions. Other certifications should be obtained depending on work setting and need.

Get to know your faculty. They are a great source of information about jobs and how to compete for them successfully. Often employers contact faculty directly, asking for the names of students who might be interested in a particular position. But unless a faculty member knows a student by name and knows that the student is in the job market, there is little the faculty member can do.

Most colleges and universities have placement centers that provide a variety of services to students, including help in developing an effective resume. They may also assist by maintaining a list of job openings, providing workshops or handouts on interviewing skills, and establishing reference files for students. The placement center at the University of North Carolina Wilmington provides in-depth trainings for students on how to use LinkedIn to help land a job. It would be a good idea to contact the placement center well before graduation to determine when and how to access its services.

A final suggestion is to join one or more of the health education professional associations (see Chapter 8). Employers are typically impressed when they see that a young professional has been a member of a professional association and perhaps has attended one or more professional meetings. "Professional meetings and conferences are filled with opportunities . . . . Where else can you find hundreds, even thousands, of education professionals from all over the world coming together to share cutting-edge knowledge through presentations, sessions, workshops, socials, and other events, than at professional meetings and conferences?" (Dixon-Terry, 2004,

p. 16). If your campus has a student health association or a chapter of Eta Sigma Gamma, the professional health education/promotion honorary, try to get involved. Eta Sigma Gamma recognizes high academic achievement, provides opportunities to obtain valuable leadership experience, and allows students to plan, implement, and evaluate various service projects and social activities.

In addition to the aforementioned suggestions, one caution is in order. Be careful what you place on social networking Web sites such as Facebook and Twitter. Prospective employers are savvy and often will look online to see what additional information they can find about you. "Susan Masterson, a recruiter with TeamHealth in Knoxville, TN, said, using social networking sites is a strategy that anyone in recruiting, whether it be physicians or otherwise, needs to incorporate in their plan. It's here. It's here to stay" (Dolan 2009). Health education/promotion internship site supervisors have even looked online before accepting a student for internship. One author of this text actually received a letter from a prospective employer indicating that he had not hired the author's student because of offensive content he found online. Further, he admonished the program to caution students about what they include online. Students posting questionable information online seems to be a somewhat common practice. According to an *AMNews* article, in one study 60 percent of U.S. medical schools surveyed reported incidents of students posting unprofessional content online (Dolan, 2009). What is questionable content is difficult to define. Certainly pictures involving sex, alcohol, or drugs are not appropriate, but anything that causes doubt should be removed. Students should also restrict who can be friends and can access their information as much as possible.

Students who follow the aforementioned suggestions will be better positioned to obtain initial employment in the health promotion and education profession. This is a good time to be a health education specialist, and the future looks even brighter than the present. According to the U.S. Department of Labor Bureau of Labor Statistics (2016), the number of health education jobs in 2014 was 115,700. The growth rate for health education jobs between 2014 and 2024 is expected to be 13 percent, which places health education in the "faster than average" growth rate category.

▷ Excelling in Your Health Education/Promotion Career

Landing a job is merely the first step in becoming a successful health education specialist. Once you have the job, it is critical that you excel in the job. This is important for two reasons. First you must excel to demonstrate that you are an important and contributing member of the organization that hired you and to enhance your career potential. Second, you need to excel to help further the health education/promotion profession. Your work reflects on all health education specialists and may determine whether your organization or other organizations will hire more health education specialists in the future.

What does it take to excel in health education/promotion? Obviously, one must demonstrate the ability to meet the competencies and sub-competencies of a health education specialist, but one must also meet the standards of a good employee. Numerous authors writing about careers in health education/promotion have elaborated on what is needed to excel as an employee in a health education/promotion position. In talking about how to excel in a voluntary health agency position, one author wrote, "Completing your tasks and projects on time, under budget, and with minimum problems is your most obvious goal, but do not underestimate the value of attitude, spirit, and the ability to work under pressure and with difficult people. A positive, can-do attitude, a willingness to learn new and different skills on the job, and the ability to work in an environment that values teamwork is a 'must'" (Daitz, 2007, pp. 5–6). Other authors writing about working in health and medical care note, "Being successful means meeting and exceeding the expectations of the job and showing initiative in achieving organizational goals" (Totzkay-Sitar & Cornett, 2007, pp. 9–10). In discussing federal health education/promotion positions, Howze (2007) said, "With any job, success requires continually showing how you add value to the organization. For example, many federal agencies are struggling to find workers with language skills, so consider becoming fluent in a second language" (p. 13). And finally, if you are trying to excel in a public health department position (see **Box 7.10**), "Become known as a high achiever/performer and a good team player. Make a positive and lasting impression on your supervisor as well as upper level managers with whom you may have contact through your assignments. Anticipate what needs to be done" (Hall, 2007, p. 17).

BOX

7.10

Practitioner's Perspective

EMPLOYER OF HEALTH EDUCATION SPECIALISTS Louise Villejo

CURRENT POSITION: Executive Director, Patient Education Office

EMPLOYER: University of Texas MD Anderson Cancer Center

DEGREE/INSTITUTION: University of Houston, B.S.; University of Texas School of Public Health, MPH

MAJOR: Health Administration

My employment history: I have been privileged to serve MD Anderson Cancer Center patients and their family members for the last 31 years. I began as a health education coordinator in the Patient Education Office and was promoted to director in 1984. Before I came to MD Anderson I did an internship at the National Cancer Institute as a health communications intern and felt that this opportunity had a major impact on my career. I was able to experience health education/promotion program planning from a national public health perspective. After college, I worked for an organization that provided administrative support to migrant healthcare centers across the southwest and saw how important these organizations were in addressing the disparities of access to basic health care.

My current job responsibilities: In my current position I am responsible for developing and directing a system-wide infrastructure so that patients/family members and clinical staff have access to the wide array of health education programs and resources developed by our team and interdisciplinary healthcare providers.

I work with staff to ensure our strategic initiatives to develop or improve cancer patient education programs are in line with the institutional goals and assist the organization to meet regulatory compliance standards. We engage patients/family members using patient- and family-centered methodologies to inform our efforts. I believe that it is my responsibility to make sure we are developing cutting-edge educational resources while also ensuring that we address health literacy and the educational needs of diverse populations.

An essential skill when working in a health care environment is collaborating with the healthcare team. I work with every multidisciplinary disease-site center in the institution, and our patient education programs address cancer across the continuum of care from prevention, screening, treatment, recovery, surveillance, relapse, and survivorship or hospice.

My goal is to continually educate leadership and staff of the importance of using best and evidence-based practice and engaging patients/family members in

BOX
7.10

continued

their care. The bottom line is helping the patients/family members participate in their care, develop the skills they need, and improve their health outcomes.

To do this work it is critical to recruit, train, and retain a cadre of highly trained health educators. I have eight health educators on staff, and they must confidently lead the clinical team in patient education program and resource development.

People management and planning, directing, and monitoring a program budget are also my key responsibilities.

How I develop a job description: The organization has a framework for developing job descriptions that I follow, which includes overall function and scope, essential job functions, supervision given and received, physical requirements, certifications, education, and experience. I use the seven areas of responsibilities of a health education specialist as the framework for the essential job functions. I start by outlining what we need done and list the specific responsibilities, competencies, skills, and abilities that are needed. It is always helpful to have other managers, staff, and someone from Human Resources review the draft to make sure it is clear and is in the appropriate format.

What I look for in reviewing applications: When I am reviewing applications for a position, I develop a spreadsheet and include column headings of the most important aspects of the position, for example, education and experience in management, health education program development, budget, strategic planning, personnel management, etc. This helps me prioritize at a glance characteristics of preferred candidates to interview.

What I look for in an interview: As when reviewing applications, I develop an interview guide and interviewee spreadsheet. The guide makes sure that I am asking each applicant similar questions. I use it strictly as a guide and not a rigid interview script. The interviewee spreadsheet does provide at a glance an accurate comparison of applicants. Beyond the interview guide, however, I delve deeper into their work experience and try to understand why they are interested in the position. I try to determine their leadership style and experience working with diverse groups.

I am thrilled if they are able to frame their experiences in the health education specialist's seven areas of responsibility. Even a newly graduated student with little work experience can use their class projects and volunteer activities. Bringing a well-prepared portfolio of work products is a plus.

Recommendations for health education specialists looking for employment: Health educators looking for employment should work their networks, join one or more professional organizations, attend meetings, and contact leadership. Sites liked LinkedIn and a growing number of mobile job search apps can assist in networking and provide job opportunities. The networking is not only critical for your job search but is key for a public health professional. Public health work relies strongly on collaborations to leverage limited assets and build capacity.

Volunteering with nonprofits is another way to build your portfolio. If you want to develop or sharpen your skills, volunteer to participate or co-lead a project.

Network with everyone you know and discuss what type of position you are looking for and your experience and background. Even if they are not in the field they might know someone you can contact. Call all of your professional contacts and don't forget your professors. Ask each person you talk to if they would recommend someone else that you can contact. Don't just ask them if they have a job opening, ask broader questions to assist you to understand all the field has to offer. Ask them about what they do and how they got into the field. Most people are very willing to help and connect you with others if they do not have a job opening. Don't stop looking even if you get an interview, keep reaching out and applying for positions. You don't want to lose momentum if you don't get that job.

Read everything you can regarding advice on job-hunting and interviewing.

BOX

7.10

continued

Looking for employment is a full-time job. Organize and keep track of your efforts. If you get an interview, be prepared, follow-up with a thank you letter, and ask when they expect to fill the position. Have your elevator speech prepared regarding why it is important to hire an academically trained health education specialist. Let them know how interested you are and what a great fit you would be and why. Don't hesitate to follow-up several times if necessary. Be upbeat and ask specific questions.

From my perspective as someone who hires health educators, I recommend that health education specialists looking for employment submit high-quality, well-written letters of application and résumés, focus on the responsibilities and competencies required in a position, and tie those to your training as a certified health education specialist. Be well-prepared for any interview opportunities, be well-versed on the organization to which one is applying, have questions ready for interviewers about the job duties and responsibilities, dress professionally, and demonstrate a sense of self-assurance and confidence.

The aforementioned quotes clearly indicate that, regardless of the setting, you must go beyond simply meeting the minimum expectations of the job to be a good employee and a good health education specialist. To excel you must go the extra mile and do the unexpected as well as the expected. You need to be a good "people person," demonstrate a positive attitude, and be willing to learn and take on new tasks. These are the things that will separate you from other employees and establish you as a truly outstanding health education specialist.

Summary

There are many settings in which a health education specialist can seek employment. In this chapter, we have discussed in detail health education/promotion positions in schools, public/ community health agencies, worksites, healthcare facilities, colleges and universities, and international settings. In addition, we have examined the potential for employment in nontraditional settings and have considered what introductory-level undergraduate students can do to help themselves obtain their first job. Finally, we discussed what it takes to be successful in a health education/promotion position.

Review Questions

1. Identify four major settings and two nontraditional settings in which health education specialists are employed.

2. Compare and contrast the roles and responsibilities of health education specialists working in schools, public and community health agencies, worksites, and healthcare facilities. How are all of these settings similar? How are they different?

3. What is the difference between a position funded with hard money and a position funded with soft money? Which position is preferable and why?

4. Explain why it might be said that health education/promotion has never reached its real potential in the healthcare setting. What factors have kept health education/promotion positions at a minimal level in this setting?

5. What is networking and why is it important in health education/promotion?

6. What can introductory-level health education/promotion students do now that might help them land their first job after graduation?

▷ Case Study

Marla has a B.S. degree in health education/promotion and is CHES certified. For the past five years, since graduating from college, she has been working as a health education specialist for a private vendor who then contracts with companies to offer health education/promotion and fitness services to their employees. During this time the vendor has placed her at three different corporations. All three corporations have been extremely satisfied with her services and the vendor/employer has also given her positive evaluations.

Marla has started to question her long-term potential with this company. She feels that her $30,000 annual salary is too low, and she gets no retirement, dental, vision, or pharmacy benefits. With her current employer, there is no opportunity for promotion, and raises are small and infrequent. She has two specific goals for the future. One, she wants to continue working in health education/promotion, but she is open to working in any setting. Two, she wants to earn a higher salary and have better benefits. If you were advising Marla, identify options you could suggest. What things could she do to make herself more marketable? What additional education or professional development does she need? What does she need to do in terms of networking? What types of positions and settings should she be considering? Outline a plan for Marla in the next 12 months that will help her to realize the two goals she has established.

▷ Critical Thinking Questions

1. Select any health education/promotion setting and give specific examples of how a health education specialist working in that setting would need to use all seven responsibilities of a health education specialist (i.e., when thinking about assessment at the work-site setting, a health education specialist might have to assess the health needs of employees, assess the current health behaviors of employees, assess how responsive employees would be to a given health promotion program, assess upper management support for a given program, etc.).

2. If you were in a position to hire a new health education specialist, what qualities, traits, and experiences would you look for in making your hiring decision? Compare this with the qualities, traits, and experiences you currently possess. Make a list of things you could do to enhance your marketability prior to graduation.

▷ Activities

1. Select the one setting you think you would most like to work in. Develop a short essay describing why you prefer this setting to other health education/promotion settings and what you think you will need to do to land a job in that setting.

2. Visit a health education/promotion professional who works in the setting in which you would most like to be employed. Develop a job description for this person's position that explains the qualifications and responsibilities needed for the job.

3. Examine the online classified ads of a major-city Sunday newspaper as well as any online employment sites you can find. Identify jobs that specifically ask for a health education specialist. Next, look through the same classified ads/job listings and identify jobs that do not specify a health education specialist but require competencies and skills similar to those of a health education specialist. Compare your results with others in the class.

4. Interview someone who is responsible for hiring health education specialists. Find out what that person looks for in a letter of application, a vita, and a personal interview.

5. Contact the placement office at your institution. Determine what services it offers and when these services should be accessed.

 # Weblinks

1. http://www.bls.gov
   U.S. Bureau of Labor Statistics

   Go to this Web site and run a search for "health education specialists." Review the various documents you find to determine workforce size, average salaries, states with most health education specialists employed, states with highest average salaries, metropolitan areas with highest average salaries, and other important information about health education specialists.

2. http://www.peacecorps.gov
   Peace Corps

   This Web site provides information about the Peace Corps, what volunteers do, where the Peace Corps is active, benefits of Peace Corps service, how to become a Peace Corps volunteer, and much more.

3. http://www.welcoa.org
   Wellness Council of America

   The Free Resources section of this site indexes a number of free work-site health promotion resources that can be easily downloaded in PDF format.

4. http://www.cdc.gov/nccdphp/dnpao/hwi
   Centers for Disease Control and Prevention's Healthier Worksite Initiative

   This Web site contains strategies and resources related to nutrition, physical activity, and obesity as well as media tools and policy resources to help one plan, implement, and evaluate work-site wellness programs.

5. http://www.cjhp.org
   Californian Journal of Health Promotion

   Use the Past Issues section to access Volume 5, Issue 2 of the *Californian Journal of Health Promotion* and specifically an article written by Byrd, Hoke, and Gottlieb titled "Integrating Health Education into Clinical Settings." This is an excellent article that describes a successful use of health education specialists in a clinical setting.

6. http://www.cjhp.org

Californian Journal of Health Promotion

Use the Past Issues section to access Volume 2, Issue 1 of the *Californian Journal of Health Promotion* and specifically an article by Eleanor Dixon Terry titled "Attending Professional Health Education Meetings: What's In It for the Student and New Professional." This is an excellent article with good advice for students or new professionals attending their first professional health education/promotion meeting.

7. http://www.acha.org

American College Health Association

In the Publications section of the Web site, go to the Guidelines, Recommendations, and White Papers area. There you can download a document titled "Guidelines for Hiring Health Promotion Professionals in Higher Education." Compare yourself against the guidelines and recommendations presented in this document. While this document was designed specifically for health education specialists working in college or university wellness programs, many of these guidelines and recommendations would be appropriate for employers in other settings.

References

Allensworth, D., & Kolbe, L. (1987). The comprehensive school health program: Exploring an expanded concept. *Journal of School Health, 57,* 409–412.

American College of Sports Medicine (ACSM). (2003). *ACSM's worksite health promotion manual.* Champaign, IL: Human Kinetics.

American School Health Association (ASHA). (2016). *What is school health?* Retrieved April 16, 2016, from http://www.ashaweb.org/about/what-is-school-health/.

Breckon, J., Harvey, J. R., & Lancaster, R. B. (1998). *Community health education: Settings, roles, and skills for the 21st century.* Gaithersburg, MD: Aspen Publishers, Inc.

Byrd, T. L., Hoke, M. M., & Gottlieb, N. H. (2007). Integrating health education into clinical settings. *Californian Journal of Health Promotion, 5* (2): 18–28.

California Health Care Foundation. (2013). *California health care almanac.* Retrieved June 3, 2013, from http://www.chcf.org/~/media/MEDIA%20LIBRARY%20Files/PDF/H/PDF%20HealthCareCosts12.pdf.

Centers for Disease Control and Prevention (CDC). (2016a). Jobs and opportunities around the world. Retrieved April 16, 2016, from http://www.cdc.gov/globalhealth/employment/.

Centers for Disease Control and Prevention (CDC). (2016b). *Workplace health promotion: Glossary terms.* Retrieved April 12, 2016, from http://www.cdc.gov/workplacehealthpromotion/glossary/index.html.

Centers for Disease Control and Prevention (CDC). (2016c). *Workplace health promotion: How employers can benefit.* Retrieved April 12, 2016, from http://www.cdc.gov/workplacehealthpromotion/businesscase/benefits/index.html.

Centers for Medicare & Medicaid Services. (2016). *National health expenditure data: Historical.* Retrieved April 16, 2016, from https://www.cms.gov/research-statistics-data-and-systems/statistics-trends-and-reports/nationalhealthexpenddata/nationalhealthaccountshistorical.html.

Chenoweth, D. H. (2011). *Worksite health promotion* (3rd ed.). Champaign, IL: Human Kinetics.

Cleary, M. J., & Birch, D. A. (1996). Using portfolios for assessment in the college personal health course. *Journal of Health Education, 27* (2), 92–96.

Cleary, M. J., & Birch, D. A. (1997). How prospective school health education specialists can build a portfolio to communicate professional expertise. *Journal of School Health, 67* (6), 228–231.

Cleary, M. J., Kaiser-Drobney, A. E., Ubbes, V. E., Stuhldreher, W. L., & Birch, D. A. (1998). Service learning in the "third sector": Implications for professional preparation. *Journal of Health Education, 29* (5), 304–311.

Daitz, S. J. (2007). Health education careers at nonprofit voluntary health agencies. *Health Education Monograph, 24* (1), 4–6.

Dixon-Terry, E. (2004). Attending professional health education meetings: What's in it for the student and new professional? *Californian Journal of Health Promotion, 2* (1), 16–21.

Dolan, P. L. (2009). Social media behavior could threaten your reputation, job prospects. AMNews. Retrieved October 13, 2009, from http://www.ama-assn.org/amednews/2009/10/12/bil21012.htm.

Fronstin, P., & Roebuck, M. C. (2015a). Financial incentives and workplace wellness-program participation. *Employee Benefit Research Institute, Issue Brief #412.*

Fronstin, P., & Roebuck, M. C. (2015b). Financial incentives, workplace wellness program participating, and utilization of health care services and spending. *Employee Benefit Research Institute, Issue Brief #417.*

Goetzel, R. Z., & Pronk, N. P. (2010). Worksite health promotion: How much do we really know about what works. *American Journal of Preventive Medicine, 38* (2) Supplement 2, S223–S225.

Hall, J. Y. (2007). Entering and navigating a health education career in the local public sector. *The Health Education Monograph, 24* (1), 15–17.

Howze, E. H. (2007). Health education jobs in the federal government. *The Health Education Monograph, 24* (1), 11–14.

International Network of Health Promoting Hospitals and Health Services. (2016). Development. Retrieved April 16, 2016, from http://www.hphnet.org/index.php?option=com_content&view=article&id=22&Item id=4.

Jalloh, M. G. (2007). Health education careers in schools. *The Health Education Monograph, 24* (1), 18–22.

Joint Committee on National Health Education Standards (JCNHES). (2007). *National Health Education Standards: Achieving excellence* (2nd ed.). Atlanta: American Cancer Society.

Lewallen, T. C., Hunt, H., Potts-Datema, W., Zaza, S., & Giles, W. (2015). The Whole School, Whole Commuity, Whole Child Model: A new approach for improving educational attainment and healthy development for students. *Journal of School Health, 85* (11), 729–739.

McKenzie, J. F., Cleary, M. J., McKenzie, B. L., & Stephen, C. E. (2002). E-portfolios: Their creation and use by pre-service health education specialists. *International Electronic Journal of Health Education, 55,* 79–83.

McKenzie, J. F., Neiger, B. L., & Thackeray, R. (2013). *Planning, implementing, & evaluating health promotion programs* (6th ed.). Boston, MA: Pearson Education, Inc.

McKenzie, J. F., & Pinger, R. R. (2015). *An introduction to community and public health* (8th ed.). Burlington, MA: Jones & Bartlett Learning.

Michael, S. L., Merlo, C. L., Basch, C. E., Wentzel, K. R., & Wechsler, H. (2015). Critical connections: Health and academics. *Journal of School Health, 85,* 740–758.

Miller, B., Birch, D., & Cottrell, R. R. (2010). Current status and future plans for undergraduate public/community health education program accreditation. *American Journal of Health Education, 41* (5), 301–307.

Naidoo, J., & Wills, J. (2000). *Health promotion: Foundations for practice* (2nd ed.). Edinburgh, Scotland: Bailliere Tindall.

National Center for Educational Statistics (NCES). (2016). *Back to school statistics.* Retrieved April 16, 2016, from http://nces.ed.gov/fastfacts/display.asp?id=372.

National Commission for Health Education Credentialing (NCHEC). (2016). *Role Delineation Project.* Retrieved April 12, 2016, from http://www.nchec.org/health-educator-job-analysis-projects.

Peabody, K. L., & Linnan, L. A. (2007). Careers in worksite health promotion. *The Health Education Monograph, 24* (1), 29–32.

Peace Corps. (2016). *Peace Corps: What are the benefits?* Retrieved April 16, 2016, from http://www.peacecorps.gov/volunteer/learn/whyvol/.

Preparing Future Faculty. (2016). Faculty roles and responsibilities. Retrieved April 16, 2016, from http://www.preparing-faculty.org/PFFWeb.Roles.htm.

Rubleski, J. (2007). Embracing workplace wellness. *Absolute Advantage, 6* (5), 30–33.

Seirawan, H., Faust, S., & Mulligan, R. (2012). The impact of oral health on the academic performance of disadvantaged children. *American Journal of Public Health, 102* (9), 1729–1734.

Society for Public Health Education (SOPHE). (2013). *Wellness & prevention provisions in the Patient Protection and Affordable Care Act (H.R. 3590).* Retrieved June 3, 2013, from http://www.sophe.org/Sophe/PDF/Health%20 Care%20Reform.pdf.

Society for Public Health Education (SOPHE). (2014). *What is a health education specialist?* Retrieved March 27, 2016, from: http://sophe.org/healthedspecialist.cfm.

Thompson, S. E., & Bybee, R. F. (2004). Professional portfolios for health education specialists and other allied health professionals. *Californian Journal of Health Promotion, 2* (1), 52–55.

Totzkay-Sitar, C., & Cornett, S. (2007). Health education options in health and medical care. *The Health Education Monograph, 24* (1), 7–10.

U.S. Department of Health and Human Services. (2016). *About Healthy People 2020: Vision.* Retrieved April 12, 2016, from https://www.healthypeople.gov/2020/About-Healthy-People.

U.S. Department of Labor Bureau of Labor Statistics. (2016). *Occupational outlook handbook, 2012–13 Edition. Health education.* Retrieved June 5, 2013, from http://www.bls.gov/ooh/community-and-social-service/health-educators.htm.

Wellness Council of America. (2006). Planning wellness: Getting off to a good start—part 1. *Absolute Advantage, 5* (4). Retrieved June 3, 2013, from http://www.welcoa.org/freeresources/index.php?category=8.

Agencies, Associations, and Organizations Associated with Health Education/Promotion

T here are many health agencies, associations, and organizations with which health education specialists interact. Most of these agencies/associations/organizations were created to help promote, protect, and maintain the health of individuals, families, and communities. For many health education specialists, these agencies/associations/organizations will be places of employment. These groups regularly hire health education specialists to plan, implement, evaluate, and coordinate their educational efforts. Health education specialists not employed by these groups will find them to be valuable sources of up-to-date information and materials. This chapter classifies the agencies/associations/organizations into three major categories: governmental, quasi-governmental, and nongovernmental. Because information on most of these agencies/associations/organizations that support the efforts of health education/promotion is available elsewhere (e.g., McKenzie & Pinger, 2015) and because this text was written primarily as an introduction to the profession, the primary emphasis of this chapter is on the professional health education associations/organizations.

▷ Governmental Health Agencies

Governmental health agencies are health agencies that have authority for certain duties or tasks outlined by the governmental bodies that oversee them. For example, a **local health department (LHD)** has the authority to protect, promote, and enhance the health of people living in a specific geographical area. Authority is given by the county, city, or township government that oversees the local health department. Governmental agencies, which are primarily funded by tax dollars (they may also charge fees for services rendered) and managed by government employees, exist at four governmental levels: international, national, state, and local (city and county). **Table 8.1** provides examples of governmental agencies and their governing bodies.

▷ Quasi-Governmental Health Agencies

Quasi-governmental health agencies (see **Figure 8.1**) are so named because they possess characteristics of both governmental health agencies and of nongovernmental agencies. They obtain their funding from a variety of sources, including community fund-raising efforts such as the United Way, special allocations from government bodies, fees for services rendered, and donations. They carry out tasks that are often thought of as services of governmental agencies, yet they operate independently of governmental supervision.

TABLE 8.1 **Governmental agencies and their governing bodies**

Level/Agency	Governing Body
International Level	
World Health Organization (WHO)	United Nations (UN)
Pan American Health Organization (PAHO)	An independent agency
National Level	
Centers for Disease Control and Prevention (CDC)	U.S. government, Department of Health and Human Services (HHS)
Food and Drug Administration (FDA)	U.S. government, Department of Health and Human Services (HHS)
State Level	
State health department	Individual state governments
State environmental protection agency	Individual state governments
Local Level	
Local health department	City, county, or township governments
Local school district	Local school boards

▶ **Figure 8.1** The American Red Cross is one of the best examples of a quasi-governmental agency.

Probably the best known quasi-governmental health agency is the **American Red Cross (ARC)**. Clara Barton founded it in 1881 as an outgrowth of her work during the Civil War. Today, the ARC has several "official" responsibilities given to it by the federal government, such as providing relief to victims of natural disasters (Disaster Services) and serving as the liaison between members of the active armed forces and their families during family emergencies (Services to the Armed Forces and Veterans). The ARC also provides many nongovernmental services such as its blood drives and safety services classes such as water safety, first aid, and CPR.

▷ Nongovernmental Health Agencies

Nongovernmental health agencies operate, for the most part, free from governmental interference as long as they comply with the Internal Revenue Service's guidelines for their tax status (McKenzie & Pinger, 2015). They are primarily funded by private donations, or, as is the case with professional and service groups, membership fees. The nongovernmental agencies can be categorized into the following subgroups: voluntary, philanthropic, service, religious, and professional.

Voluntary Health Agencies

Voluntary health agencies are some of the most visible health agencies in a community. Voluntary health agencies are a U.S. creation and grew out of unmet needs in communities. When governmental or quasi-governmental agencies were not in place to meet the needs of communities, interested citizens came together to form voluntary agencies. Such was the case with the American Cancer Society, the American Heart Association, the American

▶ **Figure 8.2** Nongovernmental health, philanthropic and service agencies meet important health-related needs in the community.

Note: The Rotary International logo is reprinted by permission of Rotary International.

Lung Association, the Alzheimer's Association, and the First Candle (formerly SIDS Alliance). The number of voluntary agencies seems endless, with agencies for about every disease and part of the body impacted by a disease or an illness. Most voluntary agencies have four primary purposes: (1) raise money to fund research and their programs, (2) provide education to both professionals and the public, (3) provide service to individuals and families affected by the disease or health problem, and (4) to advocate for beneficial policies, laws, and regulations that impact the work of the agency and in turn the people it is trying to help. Some of these organizations obtain their money from community fund-raising efforts like the United Way, but most raise their money through writing successful grant proposals, carrying out specific special events (e.g., dance-athons and golf outings), conducting door-to-door solicitation or direct-mail campaigns, and other means of receiving donations.

Philanthropic Foundations

Philanthropic foundations play an important role by funding programs and research on the prevention, control, and treatment of diseases and other health problems. *Philanthropy* means "altruistic concern for human welfare and advancement, usually manifested by donations of money, property, or work to needy persons, by endowment of institutions of learning and hospitals, and by generosity to other socially useful purposes" (Random House, 2010, ¶ 1). Although many philanthropic foundations accept charitable contributions, they differ from voluntary health agencies in two primary ways. First, they were created with an endowment and, thus, do not have to raise money. Second, they are able to finance long-term projects that may be too expensive or risky to be funded by other agencies. Examples of some philanthropic foundations that have supported work by health education specialists are the Ford Foundation, the Robert Wood Johnson Foundation, and the Rockefeller Foundation.

Service, Fraternal, and Religious Groups

Many different service, fraternal, and religious groups have also been important to health education specialists. Even though none of these groups has the primary purpose of enhancing the health of a community, they often get involved in health-related projects. Health education specialists commonly interact with these groups as part of community coalitions or when they are seeking resources to fund or enhance their programs. Examples of service and fraternal groups (and their health-related projects) include Rotary International (worldwide polio eradication), Lions (Lions Quest and preservation of sight), Shriners (children's hospitals), and American Legion (community recreation programs) (see **Figure 8.2**).

Religious groups also have contributed to the work of health education specialists' projects, both on a global level (e.g., the Protestants' One Great Hour of Sharing, the Catholic Relief Services, and the United Jewish Appeal) and on a local level (e.g., food pantries, sleeping rooms, and soup kitchens).

Professional Health Associations/Organizations

As noted earlier, the primary focus of this chapter is the professional health associations/organizations. The mission of **professional health associations/organizations** is to promote the high standards of professional practice for their respective profession, thereby improving the health of society by improving the people in the profession (McKenzie & Pinger, 2015). The mission is carried out by advocating for the profession; keeping the members up to date via the publication of professional journals, books, and newsletters; and providing the members with an avenue to come together at professional meetings. At these meetings, members have the opportunity to share and hear the new research findings, network with fellow professionals, and find out more about the latest equipment and published materials in the field. In addition, professional associations/organizations provide their members with benefits such as continuing education opportunities, networking, participation in tax-deferred annuity programs, discounts (annual national conventions, professional development sessions, publications), job placement, and a variety of other associated items (see **Box 8.1**).

Professional associations/organizations are member driven and composed, for the most part, of professionals who have completed specialized education and training and who are eligible for certification/licensure in their respective professions. These associations/organizations are funded primarily by membership dues, but it is becoming more common for them to

---

BOX 8.1

Benefits of Joining a Professional Association/Organization as a Student Member

- Opportunity to interact, collaborate, and network with other professionals in the profession
- Opportunity to meet and interact with health education/promotion students and faculty from other colleges and universities
- Develop professional colleagues
- Have a professional identity
- Professional guidance and mentoring
- Leadership development
- Learn more about how the profession and the association/organization operate
- Keep up to date on happenings in the profession and new health information
- Opportunity to participate in the association's/organization's electronic listserv, e-newsletters, Web chats, Webinars, and e-learning communities
- Advocacy alerts and updates
- Opportunity to grow professionally and personally while being supported and encouraged by others

- Be exposed to current research and pedagogy of the profession through meeting attendance and reading the publications of the association/organization
- Make professional contacts for future practicums, internships, or jobs
- Get connected to job banks and internship opportunities
- Opportunity to make a presentation at a professional meeting
- Opportunity to serve the profession through an association/organization
- Discounted registration fees for professional meetings and publications
- If certified, opportunity to earn continuing education contact hours (CECHs) for recertification of the Certified Health Education Specialist and Master Certified Health Education Specialist credentials and other licensures

Source: Adapted from Society for Public Health Education, Inc. and from Young & Boling (2004).

seek grant funds (*soft money*) to help promote their missions. Most of these associations/organizations hire staff for day-to-day operations, but the officers are usually elected professionals.

In the remaining portions of this chapter, we present information on the national professional associations/organizations that help promote the health education/promotion profession. The reader should also be aware that many of these national associations/organizations have affiliates and other related groups at the regional and/or state level. For example, the American Public Health Association is a national organization, but there are also state associations such as the Ohio Public Health Association or the Indiana Public Health Association. In addition, there are also some state-only organizations that are not affiliated with any national organization. (Ask your instructor if there are any such organizations in your state.) Often it is these regional or state affiliates/organizations that health education/promotion students become members of first because of their proximity to campus, opportunities to get involved in the professional organization, less expensive membership dues, and local networking benefits. **Table 8.2** contains information about the following organizations.

AMERICAN PUBLIC HEALTH ASSOCIATION

The **American Public Health Association (APHA)** "champions the health of all people and all communities" (APHA, 2016a, ¶ 1). APHA was founded in 1872 "as a result of the public health movement to combat yellow fever and other diseases in the 1870s" (APHA, n.d., p. 3). The mission of APHA is to "improve the health of the public and achieve equity in health status" (APHA, 2016a, ¶ 2). The association works toward this mission by bringing together the public health disciplines to collaborate on priority issues, publishing research and reports to improve public health science, providing a collective voice to advocate for laws and regulations that will advance public health while encouraging equity and access to care (APHA, 2016b).

Membership in APHA is open to professional, student, and retired health professionals, as well as agencies and voluntary organizations engaged in public health work. APHA currently has about 25,000 members. In addition, the organization represents another 25,000 individuals who are members of their affiliated state and regional health associations who are committed to creating a healthy global society (Galant, E., personal communication, May 17, 2016). Once individuals become members, they have the opportunity to join one of the subgroups of the organization—called Sections. The 31 Sections "represent major public health disciplines or public health programs. These Sections allow members with shared interests to come together to develop scientific program content and policy papers in their areas of interest or fields of practice, and they provide for professional and social networking, career development and mentoring" (APHA, 2016c, ¶ 2). Members can engage in a Section based on their area of work, such as health administration, or the area of emphasis of their work, such as food and nutrition.

The primary publication of APHA is the *American Journal of Public Health* (*AJPH*). This peer-reviewed journal is published monthly and is dedicated to the publication of original work in public health research, research methods, and program evaluation. The *AJPH* regularly includes editorials and commentaries and serves as a forum for health policy analysis. The association also publishes *The Nation's Health* 10 times per year. This newspaper includes reporting on current and proposed legislation, policy issues, news of actions within the federal agencies and Congress, or global issues. The publication also includes association and section news, job openings, and information on upcoming conferences. In addition to the *AJPH* and *The*

TABLE 8.2 **Information about key professional associations/organizations**

The American Academy of Health Behavior

Address:

17 Indian Creek Drive

Rudolph, OH 43462

Telephone: 419/760-6020

Website: http://www.aahb.org/

American College Health Association (ACHA)

Address:

1362 Mellon Road, Suite 180

Hanover, MD 21076

Telephone: 410/859-1500

Website: http://www.acha.org

American Public Health Association (APHA)

Address:

800 I Street, NW

Washington, DC 20001

Telephone: 202/777-APHA (2742)

Website: http://www.apha.org

American School Health Association (ASHA)

Address:

7918 Jones Branch Drive, Suite 300

McLean, VA 22102

Telephone: 703/506-7675

Website: http://www.ashaweb.org

Eta Sigma Gamma (ESG)

Address:

2000 University Avenue

Muncie, IN 47306

Telephone: 800/715-2559; 765/285-2258

Website: http://www.etasigmagamma.org

International Union for Health Promotion and Education (IUHPE)

Address:

42 Boulevard de la Libération

93203 Saint-Denis Cedex, France

Telephone: 33 1 48 13 71 20

Website: http://www.iuhpe.org

continued

TABLE 8.2 *continued*

National Wellness Institute, Inc. (NWI)

Address:
1300 College Court
PO Box 827
Stevens Point, WI 54481
Telephone: 715/342-2969

Website: http://www.nationalwellness.org

Society for Public Health Education (SOPHE)

Address:

10 G Street, NE, Suite 605
Washington, DC 20002
Telephone: 202/408-9804

Website: http://www.sophe.org

Society of Health and Physical Educators (SHAPE America)

Address:
1900 Association Drive
Reston, VA 20191
Telephone: 800/213-7193 or 703/476-3400

Website: http://www.shapeamerica.org/

Nation's Health, APHA also publishes books and other media on a variety of public health topics. Examples include the best-selling title *Control of Communicable Disease Manual* (Heymann, 2009) and the recent publication *Our Communities, Our Sexual Health: Awareness and Prevention for African Americans* (Sutton, Valentine, & Perkins, 2015). The most recent addition to the APHA's publications is its online newsletter called *Inside Public Health*. This e-newsletter highlights current happenings in the field of public health (APHA, 2016d).

There are other professional health associations that have a more focused mission. Some of those include the American College Health Association (ACHA), the American School Health Association (ASHA), the National Wellness Institute, Inc. (NWI), the SOPHE, the American Academy of Health Behavior, and SHAPE America (Society of Health and Physical Educators).

AMERICAN COLLEGE HEALTH ASSOCIATION

The **American College Health Association (ACHA)** was founded originally as the American Student Health Association in 1920. In 1948, the name of the association was changed to its current name. ACHA's mission is to "serve as the principal leadership organization for advancing the health of college students and campus communities through advocacy, education, and research." (ACHA, 2016a, ¶ 2). The association has three distinct types of memberships. One is for institutions of higher education. Currently, there are more than 800 such members.

ACHA also serves nearly 2,800 individual members who are interested in college health—that is, the health of college students. Included in the members are administrators, physicians and physicians' assistants, nurses and nurse practitioners, health education specialists, pharmacists, dentists, support staff who care for this special group of young adults, and students who are dedicated to health promotion on their campus. Most of these individual members are associated with the health service facilities on their respective campuses. The third type of membership is called sustaining members. This group is made up of nonprofit organizations and corporations interested in being more connected with the college health field (ACHA, 2016b).

Like some of the other associations/organizations, ACHA also has affiliates across the United States. ACHA is divided into 11 affiliates, each providing regional leadership and annual meeting opportunities. ACHA members receive concurrent membership in the affiliate organization at no additional cost (ACHA, 2016c). In addition, ACHA has nine membership sections, which are defined by the disciplines of college health. The Health Promotion Section, previously called the Health Education Section, was formed in 1958.

ACHA publishes several newsletters, numerous health information brochures, and other special publications. The members-only newsletter, *College Health in Action*, is available online at the Association's Web site. The professional journal of the ACHA is the *Journal of American College Health*, which is published bimonthly and is the only journal devoted entirely to the health of college students. The journal publishes articles encompassing many areas of college health, "including clinical and preventive medicine, health promotion, environmental health and safety, nursing assessment, interventions, and management, pharmacy, and sports medicine. The journal regularly publishes major articles on student behaviors, mental health and health care policies, and includes a section for discussion of controversial issues" (ACHA, 2016d, ¶ 4).

AMERICAN SCHOOL HEALTH ASSOCIATION

The **American School Health Association (ASHA)** began on October 27, 1927, as the American Association of School Physicians. The organization began to use its current name in 1936 (ASHA, 1976). The mission of ASHA "is to transform all schools into places where every student learns and thrives" (ASHA, 2014a, ¶ 4) (see **Figure 8.3**).

▶ **Figure 8.3** The American School Health Association focuses on the health of the school-aged child.

► **Figure 8.4** Professional development and continuing education are important benefits of membership in a professional organization.

Membership in the association comprises individuals and organizations, including schools and school districts that are supportive of an alignment with the advancement of school health programs and the mission of ASHA. ASHA is a multidisciplinary organization with nearly 650 members. Included in its membership are administrators, counselors, dieticians, nutritionists, health education specialists, physical educators, psychologists, school health coordinators, school nurses, school physicians, and social workers. ASHA members are provided a host of networking and professional development opportunities (see **Figure 8.4**) in the following four broad areas that impact school health: administration, coordination and leadership; programs and services; research and emerging issues; and teaching and learning (A. Dowling, personal communication, May 18, 2016).

The *Journal of School Health* (JOSH), which is published 12 times a year, is the primary publication of the ASHA. The journal is recognized widely and "is committed to communicating information regarding the role of schools, school personnel, or the school environment in facilitating optimal growth and development of children and youth" (ASHA, 2014b, ¶ 1). The readership of the journal includes researchers, school administrators, educators, nurses, physicians, dentists, psychologists and counselors, social workers, nutritionists, dietitians, and other health professionals. These individuals work cooperatively with parents and the community to achieve the common goal of providing youths with programs, services, and environment needed to promote health and to improve learning (ASHA, 2014b).

NATIONAL WELLNESS INSTITUTE, INC.

The **National Wellness Institute (NWI)**, founded in 1977, "was formed to realize the mission of providing health promotion and wellness professionals unparalleled resources and services that promote professional and personal growth" (NWI, 2016a). The mission of NWI "is to serve the professionals and organizations that promote optimal health and wellness in individuals and communities" (NWI, 2016a, ¶ 2). The mission is accomplished by

- Identifying quality resources
- Providing quality continuing education and resources

- Promoting opportunities for life-long learning
- Providing new and innovative professional development programs
- Developing effective educational lifestyle assessments
- Serving professionals and organizations that promote health and wellness (NWI, 2016a, ¶ 2)

There are three types of membership in NWI: individual, organizational, and student. The organizational membership allows five individuals at the same location to receive full NWI benefits. With each type of membership there is regular membership or a plus membership option, which includes a subscription to the *American Journal of Health Promotion*. With membership comes a number of publications including *Wellness Management*, a newsletter that includes information about successful programs, programming tips, resources, research, events, career opportunities, professional development, and more; *Wellness News You Can Use*, a collection of downloadable, reproducible consumer-oriented news stories, new research, and fun facts; *Well-Being Practitioner*, a magazine providing innovative and practical ideas in an easy-to-read format; and *International Wellness Connection*, which includes a series of monthly essays for wellness professionals across the world (NWI, 2016b).

One of the most visible components of the NWI is its National Wellness Conference. The conference is open to members and nonmembers alike and is a unique conference because it is a week of immersion into a wellness experience.

SOCIETY FOR PUBLIC HEALTH EDUCATION

The Society of Public Health Educators (SOPHE), founded in 1950, promotes healthy behaviors, healthy communities, and healthy environments through its membership, local chapters, and various partnerships. In 1969, the organization changed its name to the **Society for Public Health Education (SOPHE)**. The mission of SOPHE "is to provide global leadership to the profession of health education and health promotion and to promote the health of society" (SOPHE, 2016a, ¶ 3). At the national level, SOPHE's membership includes nearly 4,000 professionals from throughout the United States and 25 international countries. Members work in a variety of places, including K–12 schools, universities, healthcare settings, worksites, voluntary organizations, and local/state/federal government agencies. There are currently 20 SOPHE chapters covering 29 states (SOPHE, 2016a) (see **Box 8.2**). Like several of the other associations or organizations, SOPHE members have the opportunity to associate with one or more smaller working groups. In SOPHE the smaller groups are called Communities of Practice (CoP). CoPs "promote continuing education, networking, information exchange and advocacy among SOPHE members interested in specific topics and/or work settings. Members share a similar role or a passion about a health topic or area of practice and a desire to exchange ideas, resources, research, or solutions to common problems" (SOPHE, 2016b, ¶ 1). Additionally, the CoPs maintain listservs throughout the year to encourage dialogue and exchange (SOPHE, 2016b).

SOPHE has three premier peer-reviewed journals: *Health Education and Behavior, Health Promotion Practice,* and *Pedagogy in Health Promotion: The Scholarship of Teaching and Learning. Health Education and Behavior,* published bimonthly, is a well-respected journal that provides empirical research, case studies, program evaluations, and discussions of theories and health behavior (SOPHE, 2016c). *Health Promotion Practice* is published quarterly to "stimulate and accelerate communication between basic health promotion science and practice" and is devoted to the implementation of health education and promotion (SOPHE, 2016d, ¶ 4).

BOX

8.2

Practitioner's Perspective

STAFF ANALYST Melissa E. Shelton

CURRENT POSITION/TITLE: Staff Analyst

EMPLOYER: Houston Health Department

DEGREE/INSTITUTION/YEAR: M.P.A., Troy University, 1997 Ph.D. Student, Walden University, 2016

MAJOR: Public Health

SPECIALIZATION: Community Health Education Master Certified Health Education Specialist

Becoming a public health education professional: When I started my public health professional career, it began from a nontraditional approach; I first started an undergraduate program, and then I served active duty in the United States Navy (USN) as an enlisted medical specialist, also known as a hospital corpsman. I gained my experience in a public health role by providing health care and health education to Navy and Marine Corps members and their families. While serving in the USN, I completed my undergraduate degree in resources management and continued my education to obtain a master of public administration with a specialization in healthcare administration. During the time in the USN, I enjoyed being around and serving the military families. After completing my military obligation with the USN, I relocated to Houston, Texas. My first civilian professional job was with a local city health department in the Bureau of HIV/AIDS. My role as a community involvement coordinator involved coordinating, developing, and providing health education on HIV prevention to grades kindergarten through 12th. During this period, the topic of HIV/AIDS was still taboo and challenging, but this experience increased my passion for public health. I wanted to grow professionally and obtain more experience in the public health education field. I received an opportunity to expand my skills by working in the private sector at a health maintenance organization (HMO) associated with a hospital system through my job as a Health Education/Texas Health Steps Coordinator with the HMO's Medicaid program. This program

allowed me to provide health education and health promotion services and resources to women and children. The concept for the program was similar to working in a governmental public health education program but in a private sector setting. At this time, I had a wonderful opportunity to be commissioned as an Army Reserve officer and serve in the medical service corps. My career changed again as I was hired with a local county health department as a health communication specialist in their public health preparedness program. This position entailed developing a public health preparedness communication plan that outlined how to outreach to a diverse community in the event of a disaster. The communication plan served as a standard operating procedure (SOP) that included various components such as health education, public information, outreach team, etc. This opportunity also allowed me to take additional courses at a local university. These courses were used to help me qualify to take the certified health education specialist exam. I had another opportunity to be promoted to a health communications coordinator at the local county health department, which allowed me to work across the entire health department's divisions, such as environmental health. While working for the county health department, I was able to be in the first class to receive a Master of Certified Health Education Specialist (MCHES). My career track has continued by returning to a local city health department working as a staff analyst in adolescent health and injury prevention.

Serving in a professional association: A previous assistant director of health education for a county health department suggested that I join and become involved in the Society for Public Health Education (SOPHE). This discussion took place after my local county health department

continued

responded to the 2005 Hurricane Katrina event. Many of the residents from Louisiana had evacuated to the Harris County/Houston, Texas, area for refuge. I had a fantastic opportunity to work in the Harris County Office of Emergency Management Unified Command Joint Information Center (JIC) that was composed of various agencies throughout the Houston, Texas, area. Working in the JIC afforded me an opportunity to see firsthand what was going on with the new residents who relocated temporarily to the Astrodome. Through my observations and discussions with the new residents, I noticed that there was not a newsletter that was keeping everyone informed. I approached my supervisor about creating a newsletter that would inform, provide health education information, and provide updates to residents in the Astrodome. Several of the health education messages consisted of the importance of handwashing before eating, after eating, after going to the bathroom, and after changing a baby's diaper. The reason was to help reduce gastrointestinal problems that had occurred. After this event, I had my first opportunity to co-present with my assistant director in the health education division at the local county health department at the Society for Public Health Education (SOPHE). I also had the honor to be appointed and serve as Co-Editor of SOPHE's "News & Views." During my appointment, I had the opportunity to update the newsletter guidelines, provide input on the format, and made recommendations to the editorial board about the submission of articles. Also, I provided insight on how SOPHE members could tap into advanced leaders in the profession; highlighting professional development programs with an emphasis on global health issues; and the promotion of the health education advocacy summit by highlighting the use of social media platforms. In addition, I served as a SOPHE Abstract Reviewer for two past conferences, and I served on the Texas Society for Public Health Education (TSOPHE) board for five years. My

first active role as TSOPHE Secretary allowed me to learn TSOPHE's structure, goals, and how it relates to SOPHE's strategic plan. When elected as President–Elect and President of TSOPHE, my goals were to enhance the profession through recruiting of and mentoring students as members and to assign them projects with my health department. I also served as TSOPHE Communications Chair with the opportunity to redesign the TSOPHE newsletter to allow for TSOPHE members to be highlighted and have continuing education opportunities be spotlighted.

Being able to serve in the SOPHE arena allowed me to grow tremendously professionally. During my Ph.D. program in Community Health Education, I had an excellent opportunity to humbly serve as the elected 2015 Student Trustee, which allowed me to bring 14 years of professional and student experiences to the table. As a Ph.D. student, SOPHE allowed me to provide some unique perspectives on integrating academic pedagogy, research, and practice as it relates to advancing health promotion, health education, and new public health. I had the opportunity as the Student Trustee to work collaboratively with SOPHE to help refine the pathway for students to enter the evolving Health Education/Health Promotion profession. My goal was to facilitate the development of my peers, encourage them to be an active voice in the profession, and to advocate for the profession. My passion for health promotion and health education has continued to grow throughout my education and career journey.

Recommendation for those preparing to be public health education specialists: First, get involved in SOPHE and your local SOPHE chapter. Opportunities for personal growth involve more than going to work. If you want to serve in a leadership role, SOPHE is the best place to start. You can take the first step by joining SOPHE as

BOX

8.2

continued

a student and sign up for a committee of your interest. SOPHE allows you the opportunity to grow, learn various group dynamics, develop leadership, and have an opportunity to learn a new skill. Second, develop your brand through relationships with leaders and having a mentor who can guide your direction. You can start at your school with your professor. Professors have diverse backgrounds and a wealth of information about the health education specialist field. Third, be open minded. We are now working in an environment in which a health education specialist must be flexible. Check out the opportunities on SOPHE's Web site where you can have the opportunity to obtain continuing education to enhance your skills and learn about internships and fellowships that will jump-start your career.

Pedagogy in Health Promotion: The Scholarship of Teaching and Learning (PHP) is a quarterly journal focusing on such areas as curriculum and course/program design, assessment, and administration relevant to teaching and learning (SOPHE, 2016e).

SOPHE members can keep current with the latest health education news through two newsletters, *News U Can Use* and *News & Views*. *News U Can Use* is delivered electronically biweekly and includes legislative updates, meeting information, funding opportunities, resources, and reports. *News and Views* is a quarterly newsletter that features spotlights on members, profession updates, and news from SOPHE chapters, committees, and ambassadors (SOPHE, 2016f).

Like several of the other associations/organizations, SOPHE holds an annual meeting that provides members and health education professionals the opportunity to share and receive the most recent research findings, to earn continuing education contact hours, and to network with other professionals. The Advocacy Summit is another professional development opportunity SOPHE supports. The Advocacy Summit provides an opportunity for health education specialists to receive training in advocacy techniques and apply their new knowledge on a trip to Capitol Hill in Washington, D.C., to discuss health-related issues with staffers from key legislative subcommittees and representatives of their congressional districts.

INTERNATIONAL UNION FOR HEALTH PROMOTION AND EDUCATION

Though all of the professional associations/organizations noted already in this chapter have members from countries other than the United States, there is one professional association that is truly worldwide: the **International Union for Health Promotion and Education (IUHPE)**. There are over 2,000 members worldwide in approximately 150 countries. The IUHPE, founded in 1951 in Paris, is a global association with a mission "to promote global health and to contribute to the achievement of equity in health between and within countries of the world" (IUHPE, 2016a, ¶ 4). IUHPE fulfills its mission by "building and operating an independent, global, professional network of people and institutions to encourage the free exchange of ideas, knowledge, know-how, experiences, and the development of relevant collaborative projects, both at global and regional levels" (IUHPE, 2016a, ¶ 5). Membership includes government bodies, including universities and institutes, nongovernmental organizations, and individuals across all continents working to advance public health. IUHPE is involved in advocacy efforts as well as capacity-building, education, and training initiatives. The IUHPE has four priority areas: social determinants of health, health promotion in sustainable development, noncommunicable disease prevention and control, and health promotion systems. An obvious distinctiveness of IUHPE is its global reach in every continent (IUHPE, 2016b).

Every three years IUHPE holds a World Conference on Health Promotion as well as regional conferences, which have become important gatherings of health promotion experts and practitioners worldwide. The most recent one was held in Curitiba, Brazil, in May 2016. IUHPE has a "family" of journals. The official membership journal, which is published quarterly, is *Global Health Promotion* (formerly called *Promotion & Education*). "It is a multilingual journal, which publishes authoritative peer-reviewed articles and practical information for a worldwide audience of professionals interested in health promotion and health education" (IUHPE, 2016c, ¶ 1). All IUHPE members receive *Global Health Promotion* and can purchase, at a reduced rate, any of the other five journals (*Critical Public Health, Health Promotion International, Health Education Research, International Journal of Mental Health Promotion,* or the *International Journal of Public Health*) published in association through collaborative agreements with their respective publisher (IUHPE, 2016c).

AMERICAN ACADEMY OF HEALTH BEHAVIOR

The **American Academy of Health Behavior (AAHB)** is a professional organization unlike those presented so far in this chapter. Founded in 1997, the AAHB, or just The Academy, as it is referred to, is a society of researchers and scholars in the areas of health behavior, health education, and health promotion. The Academy "was created to improve the stature of health educators by supporting and promoting quality health behavior, health education, and health promotion research conducted by health educators" (Werch, 2000, p. 3). The mission of The Academy "is to serve as the 'research home' for health behavior scholars and researchers whose primary commitment is to excellence in research and the application of research to practice to improve the public's health" (AAHB, 2014, ¶ 2).

Individuals must apply for membership in The Academy, and acceptance is based on one's area of academic preparation and level of scholarly activity. The specific qualifications for membership are listed on The Academy's Web site (see **Table 8.2**). Currently, The Academy has 200 members. In summer 2016, The Academy started a new journal, *Health Behavior Research*. This will be an online, open-access publication featuring articles focused on theory and conceptual issues in health behavior research (J. Sommers, personal communication, May 20, 2016).

SHAPE AMERICA

(Society of Health and Physical Educators) is the newest professional organization. SHAPE America is the nation's largest membership organization of health and physical education professionals—preK–12 educators to university professors. Their mission is to "advance professional practice and promote research related to health and physical education, physical activity, dance, and sport (SHAPE America, 2016a).

SHAPE America publishes four signature journals for professionals in health education, physical education, and related fields. The *American Journal of Health Education* (AJHE) is published six times a year and includes research findings, community learning strategies, and recent health promotion trends. The other journals SHAPE America publishes are *Journal of Physical Education, Recreation & Dance* (JOPERD), *Strategies: A Journal for Physical and Sport Educators*, and *Research Quarterly for Exercise and Sport* (RQES) (SHAPE America, 2016b).

▶ **Figure 8.5** Seal of Eta Sigma Gamma

Source: National Office of Eta Sigma Gamma, 2000 University Ave., Muncie, IN 47306. Used with permission.

Professional development is one important membership benefit of SHAPE America. They offer workshops, webinars, online toolboxes for teachers and coaches, and various newsletters. A national convention brings nearly 5,000 health and physical education professionals together annually.

ETA SIGMA GAMMA

Founded in 1967, **Eta Sigma Gamma (ESG)** is the national health education honorary. The idea for the organization was born when three professors from Ball State University, Drs. William Bock, Warren E. Schaller, and Robert Synovitz, were on their way to a professional conference and were talking about the need for an honorary for the discipline. Their discussion led to the formation of the organization, which has had, from its beginning, the primary purpose of furthering the professional competence and dedication of individual members of the health education/promotion profession (ESG, 1991). The ideals of the honorary are symbolized in its seal. The seal (see **Figure 8.5**) "is divided into four equilateral triangles, each carrying a symbol. A lamp of learning is in the center triangle, surrounded by an open book representing teaching, a microscope signifying research, and an outstretched hand representing service. These three elements form the basic purposes of the organization and profession; teaching, research, and service. The unifying element of these purposes is symbolized by the lamp of learning, since it is through the learning process that each purpose is achieved" (ESG, 1991, p. 2).

As noted in **Table 8.2**, the national office of Eta Sigma Gamma is located in Muncie, Indiana, on the campus of Ball State University in the Department of Nutrition and Health Science. This is also where the Alpha Chapter (the first chapter of the honorary) is located. There have been 136 chapters installed on university/college campuses throughout the United States and more than 7,000 active members (J. Soules, personal communication, May 20, 2016). Chapters are awarded to colleges/universities based on a review and vote by the National Executive Committee of ESG on an application prepared by personnel at the petitioning college/university. From its beginnings, ESG has focused on the student members. Most individuals join the honorary when they are either undergraduate or graduate students. Membership is open to those who have a major or minor in health education and a grade point average equivalent to at least a *B–*. In fact, students can achieve membership only by affiliating through a collegiate chapter. Through their affiliation with the collegiate chapters, they are eligible to apply for the awards and scholarships of the honorary. Professionals active in the discipline of health education/promotion and holding a degree can affiliate through the Chapter-At-Large (ESG, 1991) (see **Box 8.3**).

ETA SIGMA GAMMA Sheridan Stanley

CURRENT POSITION/TITLE: Student & President of the Epsilon Nu Chapter of Eta Sigma Gamma

DEGREE/INSTITUTION: B.S. Public Health Studies anticipated Summer, 2016, University of North Carolina Wilmington

MAJOR: Public Health Studies with Concentration in Health Education

Becoming a public health major: Like many students I did not always know that I wanted to be involved in health, and I certainly did not know I wanted to be a public health educator. When I first started college, I was pursuing a career in civil engineering. It quickly became apparent that engineering was not the career for me. At that time, I enrolled in a local community college to take my general education classes while trying to discern what major I wanted to pursue. I struggled with this decision until I started thinking about what I enjoyed and what would bring me the most satisfaction. I realized that I had an interest in health and that I wanted to make a difference in the lives of those around me, but not in a traditional clinical setting. After doing research on various health careers, I was really attracted to public health. I applied to the Public Health Studies program at the University of North Carolina Wilmington. That was one of the best decisions I have ever made.

Getting involved in health education: I quickly learned that it was not enough just to learn about health education in the classroom, but that I needed to get involved in the community to gain practical experience. Through one of my classes, I was able to participate in an event that brought together an at-risk community in Wilmington and the local police department. My role in this event was to plan and implement a health-related activity for children in the community. My activity focused on the importance of a healthy environment and emphasized the need to recycle and not litter. This event gave me the opportunity to be active in the community and see what it would be like to be a public health educator.

Soon after, I began looking for further opportunities to get more involved, but I was struggling to find an organization on campus that mirrored my values and would provide me with the experience I needed for a career in health education. Several of my professors had been working to establish a chapter of Eta Sigma Gamma (a health education honorary) at UNCW. They had developed the application and had submitted it to the National Eta Sigma Gamma organization for approval. After looking into what the organization was about, I was determined to do whatever I could to play a role in the installation of a new chapter on the UNCW campus. Thanks to the perseverance of the public health faculty at UNCW, we were able to install our chapter of Eta Sigma Gamma on September 18, 2015. It was a memorable occasion with a representative from the national office present to install the chapter and induct the first group of students into the chapter.

Why I decided to join Eta Sigma Gamma: I decided to join Eta Sigma Gamma as a resource to acquire hands-on practical experience with health education. My goal was to focus on my professional development so that I could better market myself to future employers. UNCW did not offer any clubs or organizations that catered strictly to public health education until Eta Sigma Gamma was formed. I realized that such an organization would be my best option to get involved and build relationships with community partners as well as my fellow peers.

My involvement in Eta Sigma Gamma: Once we had our chapter installed, I knew I wanted to play a role in getting our organization off the ground. I was elected vice president during the fall 2015 semester and we began taking care of the tasks that accompany starting a new chapter. We also began to focus on

BOX 8.3 *continued*

service projects that would get us out into the community. One project I was involved with was the formulation and implementation of a lesson plan to be implemented at a local middle school. I used the skills I learned in program planning to develop a lesson plan on the dangers of tobacco products. I then participated in implementing the finished product during the students' health class. I found this experience to be immensely beneficial because it gave me the opportunity to develop a lesson plan and to present that lesson in a school setting.

I became president of our chapter of Eta Sigma Gamma at the beginning of the spring semester of 2016. We are currently working to provide our members with great opportunities to gain practical experience and build relationships with fellow ESG members as well as people in the community. Our chapter has adopted an at-risk community in the Wilmington area in conjunction with The Blue Ribbon Commission of New Hanover County as one avenue to gain those experiences. I have faith that our chapter of Eta Sigma Gamma will quickly grow into a high-functioning organization that can act as a catalyst for the students in whatever they pursue.

Recommendations for those preparing to be health education specialists: I would highly recommend joining Eta Sigma Gamma to any student pursuing a degree in health education. It is a great organization that will get you out of the classroom and into the field. Students who are preparing to be health education specialists really need to be involved on campus and in their communities. There are plenty of opportunities to apply the skills one has gained to better market oneself to potential employers. You must take advantage of every opportunity to gain firsthand experience while in school. These experiences will help you develop a better résumé to take to employers or for admission into graduate school programs. I would also recommend taking advantage of the time you have while in school to try different things and discover what really interests you. Public health can be very broad and the possibilities are endless. Make sure that you explore every avenue to find the career that is right for you.

Future plans: I am currently in the process of finishing my undergraduate degree in public health with a concentration in health education. I have applied to East Carolina University where I hope to continue my education and obtain a master's degree in public health with a concentration in health behavior. If I am accepted, I intend to become involved in the local chapter of Eta Sigma Gamma as well as any other organizations that may help me gain leadership experience that I can use in the future. I also plan to obtain a graduate assistantship to provide me with valuable research experiences within the program. The possibilities are endless, and I have a lot of excitement to discover what the future holds. I hope that you find as much joy while pursuing a degree in health education as I have.

ESG regularly produces four publications: its journal, *The Health Educator; The Health Education Monograph Series;* and *The Vision,* an online newsletter. Each of these publications is distributed twice a year. Like the publications of the other associations/organizations, the publications include the current works of the professionals in the field. However, unlike the others, only individuals who are current members of ESG can write articles for *The Health Educator* and *The Health Education Monograph Series.* Another unusual characteristic of the publications of ESG is that one entire issue of the *Monograph Series* each year is composed of articles written only by student members. This is another indication that the honorary is concerned about the preservice professional.

ASSOCIATIONS FOR DIRECTORS

There are two other professional groups that have ties to health education. They are the (1) **Directors of Health Promotion and Education (DHPE)** and (2) Society of State Leaders of Health and Physical Education. Unlike all the other professional groups discussed, membership in these organizations is tied to one's employment. The individuals who belong to these organizations are employees of their respective state/territorial/Indian Health Service departments of health or education. There are two types of membership available in the Directors of Health Promotion and Education (DHPE): voting membership and associate membership. The number of DHPE voting members is limited to the state or territorial level director of health promotion or public health education, Indian Health Services (IHS) director, or the equivalent. In states or territories where no such designation exists, the state, territorial, or IHS health official shall appoint an individual. Associate membership is open to individuals employed in the area of health education/promotion who support the purpose of the Association (DHPE, 2016b). The primary mission of the Directors of Health Promotion and Education (DHPE), which was formed in 1946, is to strengthen "public health capacity in policy and in systems change to improve the health of all and achieve health equity" (DHPE, 2016a, ¶ 2).

The **Society of State Leaders of Health and Physical Education** was founded in 1926 and is "a professional association whose members supervise and coordinate programs in health, physical education, and related fields of coordinated school health programs within state departments of education" (The Society, 2016a, ¶ 1). The mission of The Society is to use "advocacy, partnerships, professional development and resources to build capacity of school health leaders to implement effective health education and physical education policies and practices that support success in school, work and life" (The Society, 2016b, ¶ 1).

COALITIONS

Because of the large number of professional health education/promotion associations, there are times when there is a need to have a common voice for the profession. To help provide such a voice, coalitions of health associations/organizations have been created. The most prominent coalition is the Coalition of National Health Education Organizations, USA.

The **Coalition of National Health Education Organizations, USA (CNHEO)** is a nonprofit federation of organizations dedicated to advancing the health education/promotion profession. The coalition is composed of representatives (delegates and alternates) from seven national associations/organizations with identifiable health education specialist memberships and ongoing health education/promotion programs. The associations/organizations include the American College Health Association, American Public Health Association, American School Health Association, Directors of Health Promotion and Education, Eta Sigma Gamma, Society of State Leaders of Health and Physical Education, and the Society for Public Health Education (CNHEO, 2016b).

CNHEO was formed on March 1, 1972, after a series of three meetings in 1971 and 1972 to determine the feasibility of such an organization. The primary mission of the coalition is "the mobilization of the resources of the Health Education Profession in order to expand and improve health education, regardless of the setting" (CNHEO, 2016a, ¶ 1).

The work of CNHEO is financed by funds obtained from coalition member organizations, public and private agencies, and contributions and gifts from individuals. Over the years, the working relationship of the member organizations has been outlined in the *Working*

Agreement of the CNHEO. Also included in this document are the purposes of the coalition (CNHEO, 2016c, ¶ 2):

1. To strengthen communications among the member organizations as well as between the health education profession and policymakers, other professions, and consumers.

2. To develop, implement, and evaluate a shared vision and strategic plan for health education and the health education profession.

3. To educate policy-makers on the need for federal and state public policies that support healthy behaviors and healthy communities.

4. To collaborate on common issues, problems, and concerns related to health education.

5. To increase the visibility of the health education profession and its member organizations.

Unlike the other organizations and groups discussed in this chapter, the CNHEO functions with no paid staff members or permanent location. "The CNHEO carries on business by means of email communication, monthly conference calls, and periodic face-to-face meetings during member organization conferences. Through these means it has made significant progress in addressing its purposes and priorities" (Capwell, 2004, p. 13). Since its inception, the CNHEO has operationalized its purposes in a number of ways, contributing to the growth of the profession. Below is a list of some of the recent activities and accomplishments in which the CNHEO has been involved:

- Creation of position papers on topics of importance to the profession (e.g., preparation of elementary school teachers in the area of health education, and the strengthening of health education in the public health arena).

- Cosponsoring three invitational conferences in 1995 (NCHEC & CNHEO, 1996), 2002 (CNHEO, 2003), and 2016 to examine the status and future of the health education/promotion profession. These conferences led to the creation of goals and recommendations for the profession for the 21st century and commitments by member organizations to lead or assist in addressing the recommendations (CNHEO, 2003).(See Chapter 10 for more on the future of health education/promotion.)

- Creation of a unified "Code of Ethics for the Health Education Profession" (see Chapter 5 and Appendix A).

More information about CNHEO can be obtained by contacting the office of any of the member organizations or by logging on to the CNHEO Web site. The URL for this site is presented in the Weblinks at the end of the chapter.

▷ Joining a Professional Health Association/Organization

Becoming a member of a professional organization is not difficult. With the exception of a few of the associations/organizations previously noted (CNHEO, AAHB, ESG, and DHPE and The Society), membership in a professional organization can be obtained by completing an application form (available from any of the organizations, included in many of the official publications, or found at the organization's Web site [see **Table 8.2**]) and sending the money with the desired length and category of membership (different rates apply to different types of membership—for example, student, professional, retired) to the association/organization of choice. Most individuals join a professional association/organization for a year at a time. Some associations, however, provide multiple-year memberships at a reduced rate or even a lifetime membership. In general, the cost of a membership in a state or regional association/ organization is separate from and less than a membership in a national association/organization. If you are interested in joining a state or local association/organization, you can usually contact its national office to find out whom to contact locally.

▷ The Certification Body of the Health Education/ Promotion Profession: National Commission for Health Education Credentialing, Inc.

NCHEC (pronounced N-check) is unlike any other organization that has been discussed in this chapter. NCHEC is not a professional organization that health education specialists join, but rather the organization responsible for the individual credentialing of health education specialists; thus, it has no members. The history of the development of NCHEC was presented in Chapter 6, while the information presented here is to give the reader an understanding of how NCHEC operates.

"The mission of NCHEC is to enhance the professional practice of health education by promoting and sustaining a credentialed body of health education specialists. To meet this mission, NCHEC certifies health education specialists, promotes professional development, and strengthens professional preparation and practice" (NCHEC, 2016a, ¶ 1). The charge of NCHEC "is to develop and administer national competency-based examinations; develop standards for professional preparation; and promote professional development through continuing education for health education professionals" (NCHEC, 2016a, ¶ 2). Four boards and the NCHEC staff carry out the work of NCHEC. The boards include the Board of Commissioners [BOC], the Division Board for Certification of Health Education Specialists, the Division Board of Professional Development, and the Division Board for Professional Preparation and Practice. The four boards meet monthly via conference calls and have one or two face-to-face meetings each year.

The BOC, which is composed of 11 commissioners, is the governing board and the board responsible for all NCHEC activities (NCHEC, 2016a). The three division boards address the three activities noted in NCHEC's mission statement: certification, professional development, and professional preparation. Those who hold either the CHES or the MCHES credential elect the directors and commissioners of the various boards, with the exception of one. The lone exception is the public member of the BOC, who is appointed by the BOC after a call for nominations. In addition, the elected directors and commissioners are volunteers and must hold an active CHES or MCHES credential (NCHEC, 2016a).

The primary responsibility of the Division Board for Certification of Health Education Specialists (DBCHES) is to create the two examinations of NCHEC—the CHES exam and the MCHES exam. More specifically, DBCHES, which is currently composed of 11directors, along with the guidance of Professional Examination Services (PES) ensures a periodic review and evaluation of certification and examination processes, recommends policies and procedures for administering the CHES and MCHES examinations, writes the examination questions, creates the exams, determines the pass point (i.e., minimum score on the examinations required to obtain the certification), and ensures that NCHEC's competency testing meets acceptable standards (NCHEC, 2016a).

The work of the Division Board for Professional Development (DBPD), which is composed of seven directors, is to oversee the recertification and annual renewal procedures (NCHEC,

2016a). "More specifically, the DBPD recommends policies and procedures related to the designation of continuing education providers, recertification and the annual renewal of CHES; recommends fees for recertification, annual renewal and provider designation; and assures that the processes are monitored and periodically evaluated" (NCHEC, 2016a, ¶ 7).

The Division Board for Professional Preparation and Practice (DBPPP), which is also composed of seven directors, is responsible for promoting professional preparation (NCHEC, 2016a). "More specifically, the DBPPP works with colleges, universities and accrediting agencies to improve professional preparation programs and promote best practices in health education settings; and monitors and updates the certification application and eligibility review process" (NCHEC, 2016a, ¶ 8).

The CHES examination was given for the first time in 1990. The first MCHES examination was offered in 2011. Both examinations are offered twice a year—one in April and one in October—at approximately 130 locations throughout the United States. The examinations are each 165 questions long, and candidates have three hours to complete the exam. The eligibility criteria to take the examinations are presented in **Box 8.4**.

BOX 8.4

Eligibility Criteria to Sit for the CHES and MCHES Examinations

CHES Examination

Eligibility to take the CHES examination is based exclusively on academic qualifications. An individual is eligible to take the examination if he or she has the following:

A bachelor's, master's, or doctoral degree from an accredited institution of higher education; AND one of the following:

- An official transcript (including course titles) that clearly shows a major in health education (e.g., Health Education, Community Health Education, Public Health Education, School Health Education, etc.). Degree/major must explicitly be in a discipline of "Health Education." OR

- An official transcript that reflects at least 25 semester hours or 37 quarter hours of course work (with a grade "C" or better) with specific preparation addressing the Seven Areas of Responsibility and Competency for Health Educators

MCHES Examination

The MCHES exam eligibility includes both academic and experience requirements.

For CHES: A minimum of the past five (5) continuous years in active status as a CHES.

For Non-CHES or CHES with fewer than five years active status AND five years experience:

- A master's degree or higher in Health Education, Public Health Education, School Health Education, Community Health Education, etc.

- OR a master's degree or higher with an academic transcript reflecting at least 25 semester hours (37 quarter hours) of course work in which the Seven Areas of Responsibility of Health Educators were addressed.

- Five (5) years of documented experience as a health education specialist

To verify, applicants must submit:

1. Two verification forms from a current or past manager/supervisor, and/or a leader in a health education professional organization

2. A current curriculum vitae/ résumé

Source: The National Commission for Health Education Credentialing, Inc. (NCHEC). By permission.

NCHEC produces a number of different publications. The *NCHEC News* is NCHEC's newsletter for all CHES and MCHES (NCHEC, 2016c). The newsletter is published three times a year and is mailed to each current certification holder. Past issues of the newsletter are available online at the NCHEC Web site (NCHEC, 2016c). NCHEC also publishes documents that are useful for those working in professional preparation programs, those offering continuing education opportunities, and those individuals preparing to take either the CHES or the MCHES examination. Included in these publications are a companion guide for the examinations (NCHEC, 2016b) and the competency-based framework (NCHEC, 2016b). In reviewing the publications, these documents were generated from the findings of the Health Education Specialists Practice Analysis (HESPA) project (NCHEC, 2016b).

More information about NCHEC can be obtained by contacting the NCHEC office, 1541 Alta Drive, Suite 303, Whitehall, PA 18052-5642, Phone: (484) 223-0770, Toll-Free: (888) 624-3248, Facsimile: (800) 813-0727 or by logging on to the NCHEC Web site. The URL for this site is presented in the Weblinks at the end of the chapter.

▶ Summary

This chapter discussed the various health agencies, associations, and organizations with which the profession of health education/promotion interacts. The agencies/associations/organizations were presented within three major categories: governmental, quasi-governmental, and nongovernmental. The primary emphasis of the chapter was to present information about a subcategory of the nongovernmental associations/organizations, the professional associations/organizations. Those discussed included the American Academy of Health Behavior; the American Public Health Association; the American College Health Association; the American School Health Association; the National Wellness Institute, Inc.; the Society for Public Health Education; the Society of Health and Physical Educators; the International Union for Health Promotion and Education; Eta Sigma Gamma; and associations for directors (Directors of Health Promotion and Education and The Society of State Leaders of Health and Physical Education). Also, information about a coalition—the Coalition of National Health Education Organizations—and information on how to become a member of a professional association/organization was presented. The chapter concluded with an overview of the National Commission for Health Education Credentialing, Inc. and the eligibility criteria for taking the CHES or MCHES examination.

▶ Review Questions

1. Define and explain the differences among the following types of agencies: *governmental health agency, quasi-governmental health agency,* and *nongovernmental health agency.*

2. At what levels do governmental agencies exist? Provide an example of an agency at each level.

3. What are the four primary activities of most voluntary health agencies? Give an example of each.

4. What are the purposes of a professional association/organization?

5. What are the benefits derived from membership in a professional association/ organization? Why should students become members?

6. What is the oldest and largest professional health association in the United States?

7. Name two professional health associations/organizations that focus their efforts on work settings for health education specialists. Name two other professional health associations/organizations that are not as focused on a work setting.

8. What is the name of the health education honorary? Where was it founded and where is the national office located? In general, where are the chapters of the honorary found?

9. What makes the AAHB different from the other professional organizations/associations presented in this chapter?

10. What is a coalition? Name one health education coalition. What is the primary purpose of this coalition? What are some of the recent activities of the coalition?

11. How does a person become a member of a professional organization?

12. What is the NCHEC? How is it different from the other organizations presented in the chapter?

▷ Case Study

Hilary has been employed by the XYZ voluntary health organization for almost a year now. The job has really gone well. She enjoys the work, likes her coworkers, and has been able to use much of what she learned during her health education/promotion professional preparation program. Recently, the organization received word that it had been awarded a $15,000 grant to conduct a health education/promotion program for a local senior citizens group on living a healthier life. Her supervisor, Ms. Denison, has given Hilary the responsibility to take the leadership for the project. One restriction on the use of the money is that the program must be planned by a representative group from local voluntary and governmental health education/promotion organizations. Therefore, Hilary's first task is to invite local groups to send a representative to the initial planning meeting. Hilary has set the goal of having seven different health voluntary and governmental agencies involved. If you were Hilary, which organizations would you invite to the initial meeting? Justify why you would select these seven.

▷ Critical Thinking Questions

1. For a number of years, many practicing health education specialists have pushed for a single professional health education/promotion association that would bring together many of the existing associations (i.e., ACHA, ASHA, SOPHE) so that health education/ promotion would have a single professional association voice. Would you be in favor of or against combining all the health education/promotion professional associations into a single association? Defend your response. As part of your response, indicate what you think are the strengths and weaknesses of your position.

2. In this chapter you have read about a number of different professional health education/promotion associations. On graduating from college, few new professionals have enough money to join several different professional groups. Assuming that you have enough money to join one national professional group on graduation, what association/organization would it be? Explain the reasoning you would use to select the one organization to join.

3. One of the major issues facing many professional health education/promotion associations is retaining members from year to year. Some members do not renew their membership because of cost. Others do not renew because they do not feel that they receive enough benefits. After conducting a membership survey, a professional health association has decided to revamp the benefits provided to members. Assume that you have been appointed as a student member to the executive committee of the professional association and that the president of the association has charged the committee with revamping the membership benefits package. Each member of the executive committee has been asked to create a list of benefits. What would be on your list? Explain why you selected each item.

4. Throughout this book you have been introduced to the work of health education specialists. This chapter focused on the different professional organizations of our profession. We also presented information on the NCHEC. We stated that being a member of a professional organization is different than becoming certified as a health education specialist. Compare and contrast what you see to be the benefits of membership in a professional organization and becoming a CHES or MCHES. Aside from the financial costs, do you see any drawbacks of membership and certification?

▷ Activities

1. Closely examine one professional health association/organization and prepare a PowerPoint presentation, poster, or other visual presentation on the history of that association/organization.

2. Interview two health education/promotion faculty members at your school and ask them the following:
   - Do they belong to any professional health education associations/organizations?
   - If they belong, why?
   - What benefits do they see in belonging to them?
   - What association/organization would they recommend that you join?

3. Does your school have a chapter of ESG? If not, make an appointment with the department head/chairperson to inquire about the possibility of starting one on your campus.

4. Write a one-page paper using the following two sentences to start the paper: "If I could join one professional health association/organization, it would be _____. My reasons for choosing that association/organization are _____."

5. Visit the Web site of the Coalition of National Health Education Organizations (CNHEO) (http://www.cnheo.org). Once at the site, read the "21st Century" reports: (1) *The Health Education Profession in the Twenty-First Century Progress Report 1995–2001* and (2) *Coalition of National Health Education Organization's 2nd Invitational Conference: Improving the*

Nation's Health Through Health Education—A Vision for the 21st Century. After reading the reports, create your own list of five activities that you feel the profession should engage in during the next 10 years to move the profession forward. Provide a brief (i.e., a couple of paragraphs) rationale for why you included each activity on your list.

 # Weblinks

1. **http://www.astho.org**

   The Association for State and Territorial Health Officials (ASTHO)

   This is the Web site for the ASTHO, which is the national nonprofit organization representing the state and territorial public health agencies of the United States, the U.S. territories, and the District of Columbia. Among other items, this site includes links to each of the state and territorial health departments.

2. **http://www.cancer.org/**

   American Cancer Society (ACS)

   This is the home page for the ACS. The site presents the most up-to-date information on cancer, including treatment and prevention. The site also provides information about the ACS and the resources it can provide for cancer survivors and program planners.

3. **http://www.cnheo.org**

   Coalition of National Health Education Organizations (CNHEO)

   This is the home page for the CNHEO. At the site, you will find information about all the member organizations, as well as the coalition's mission, goals, *Working Agreement*, the "Code of Ethics for the Health Education Profession," and the "21st Century" reports.

4. **http://www.heart.org/HEARTORG/**

   American Heart Association (AHA)

   This is the home page for the AHA. The AHA provides health education specialists with a wealth of information and materials about many of the cardiovascular diseases and stroke.

5. **http://www.lungusa.org**

   American Lung Association (ALA)

   This is the home page for the ALA. The ALA provides information about various lung diseases, including asthma, chronic obstructive pulmonary disease (COPD), and lung cancer, and resources for stopping smoking.

6. **http://www.welcoa.org**

   The Wellness Council of America (WELCOA)

   This is the home page for the WELCOA. This site provides a variety of resources for those interested in work-site wellness programs.

7. **http://www.cdc.gov/**

   Centers for Disease Control and Prevention (CDC)

   This is the home page of the CDC. This Web site includes information for the lay public (e.g., traveler's health and emergency preparedness) as well as information to assist health education specialists (e.g., health topics A–Z, CDC recommendations, *MMWR*, and special funded initiatives).

8. http://www.healtheducationadvocate.org/

Health Education Advocate

This is the homepage of the Health Education Advocate that is sponsored by the CNHEO. This site provides up-to-date advocacy information for health education specialists, as well as links to other advocacy sites.

9. http://www.nchec.org

National Commission for Health Education Credentialing, Inc.

This is the homepage for NCHEC. At this site you can find out more about the CHES and MCHES examinations, order publications to help you prepare for the examinations, and get up-to-date on individual credentialing.

(Note: See Table 8.2 for the URLs of the various professional associations or organizations discussed in this chapter.)

References

American Academy for Health Behavior (AAHB). (2014). *About the Academy*. Retrieved May 20, 2016, from http://www.aahb.org/About_the_Academy.

American College Health Association (ACHA). (2016a). *About ACHA*. Retrieved May 17, 2016, from http://www.acha.org/ACHA/About/.

American College Health Association (ACHA). (2016b). *Membership*. Retrieved May 17, 2016, from http://www.acha.org/ACHA/Membership/.

American College Health Association (ACHA). (2016c). *Regional affiliates*. Retrieved May 17, 2016, from http://www.acha.org/ACHA/Networks/Regional_Affiliates.aspx.

American College Health Association (ACHA). (2016d). *ACHA publications*. Retrieved May 17, 2016, from http://www.acha.org/ACHA/Resources/Publications/ACHA/Resources/Publication.aspx?hkey=7c6f174f-ea50-4102-947e-38c2de3b7d53.

American Public Health Association (APHA). (2016a). *About APHA*. Retrieved on May 17, 2016, from https://www.apha.org/about-apha.

American Public Health Association (APHA). (2016b). *Our work*. Retrieved on May 17, 2016, from https://www.apha.org/about-apha/our-work.

American Public Health Association (APHA). (2016c). *Member sections*. Retrieved May 17, 2016, from https://www.apha.org/apha-communities/member-sections.

American Public Health Association (APHA). (2016d). *Publications & periodicals*. Retrieved May 17, 2016, from https://www.apha.org/publications-and-periodicals.

American Public Health Association (APHA). (n.d). *The American Public Health Association: Keeping public health in the public eye for more than a century*. Washington, DC: Author.

American School Health Association (ASHA). (1976). *History of the American School Health Association, 1926–1976*. Kent, OH: Author.

American School Health Association (ASHA). (2014a). *ASHA*. Retrieved May 17, 2016, from http://www.ashaweb.org/.

American School Health Association (ASHA). (2014b). *Journal of School Health*. Retrieved May 17, 2016, from http://www.ashaweb.org/resources/journal-of-school-health/.

Capwell, E. M. (2004). Coalition of national health education organizations. *Californian Journal of Health Promotion, 2* (1), 12–15.

Coalition of National Health Education Organizations (CNHEO). (2003). *21st century report*. Retrieved May 20, 2016, from http://www.cnheo.org/publications.html.

Coalition of National Health Education Organizations (CNHEO). (2016a). *About us*. Retrieved May 20, 2016, from http://www.cnheo.org/index.html.

Coalition of National Health Education Organizations (CNHEO). (2016b). *Members*. Retrieved May 20, 2016, from http://www.cnheo.org/member_organizations.html.

Coalition of National Health Education Organizations (CNHEO). (2016c). *Working agreement*. Retrieved May 20, 2016, from http://www.cnheo.org/working_agreement.html.

Director of Health Promotion and Education (DHPE). (2016a). *About DHPE.* Retrieved May 20, 2016, from http://www.dhpe.org/?page=About_Main.

Director of Health Promotion and Education (DHPE). (2016b). *Membership.* Retrieved May 20, 2016, from http://www.dhpe.org/?page=Membership_Main.

Eta Sigma Gamma (ESG). (1991, November). *Eta Sigma Gamma.* Muncie, IN: Author.

Heymann, D. L. (Ed.). (2009). *Control of communicable diseases manual* (19th ed.). Washington, DC: American Public Health Association.

International Union for Health Promotion and Education (IUHPE). (2016a). *Mission.* Retrieved May 20, 2016, from http://www.iuhpe.org/index.php/en/iuhpe-at-a-glance/mission.

International Union for Health Promotion and Education (IUHPE). (2016b). *Projects.* Retrieved May 20, 2016, from http://www.iuhpe.org/index.php/en/projects.

International Union for Health Promotion and Education (IUHPE). (2016c). *Publications.* IUHPE. Retrieved May 20, 2016, from http://www.iuhpe.org/index.php/en/publications.

McKenzie, J. F., & Pinger, R. R. E. (2015). *An introduction to community & public health* (8th ed.). Sudbury, MA: Jones & Bartlett Publishers.

National Commission for Health Education Credentialing, Inc. (NCHEC). (2016a). *Mission and purpose.* Retrieved May 20, 2016, from http://www.nchec.org/mission-and-purpose.

National Commission for Health Education Credentialing, Inc. (NCHEC). (2016b). *Publications.* Retrieved May 20, 2016, from http://www.nchec.org/publications.

National Commission for Health Education Credentialing, Inc. (NCHEC). (2016c). *The NCHEC NEWS bulletin.* Retrieved May 20, 2016, from http://www.nchec.org/nchec-news-bulletins.

National Commission for Health Education Credentialing, Inc., & Coalition of National Health Education Organizations, USA (NCHEC & CNHEO). (1996). The health education profession in the 21st century: Setting the stage. *Journal of School Health, 66* (8), 291–298.

National Wellness Institute (NWI). (2016a). *About NWI.* Retrieved May 17, 2016, from http://www.nationalwellness.org/?page=About_NWI.

National Wellness Institute (NWI). (2016b). *National Wellness Institute member benefits.* Retrieved May 17, 2016, from http://www.nationalwellness.org/?page=MemberBenefits.

Random House, Inc. (2010). Philanthropy. In Dictionary.com *Unabridged.* Retrieved August 30, 2010, from http://dictionary.reference.com/browse/philanthropy.

SHAPE America (Society of Health and Physical Educators). (2016a). *About SHAPE America.* Retrieved May 20, 2016, from http://www.shapeamerica.org/about/.

SHAPE America (Society of Health and Physical Educators). (2016b). *SHAPE America journals.* Retrieved May 20, 2016, from http://www.shapeamerica.org/publications/journals/.

Society for Public Health Education (SOPHE). (2016a). *About SOPHE.* Retrieved May 17, 2016, from http://sophe.org/about.cfm.

Society for Public Health Education (SOPHE). (2016b). *Communities of practice.* Retrieved May 20, 2016, from http://www.sophe.org/Communities_Practice.cfm.

Society for Public Health Education (SOPHE). (2016c). *Health education & behavior journal.* Retrieved May 20, 2016, from http://www.sophe.org/Health_Education.cfm.

Society for Public Health Education (SOPHE). (2016d). *Health promotion practice.* Retrieved May 20, 2016, from http://www.sophe.org/Health_Promotion_Practice.cfm.

Society for Public Health Education (SOPHE). (2016e). *Pedagogy in health promotion: The scholarship of teaching and learning.* Retrieved May 20, 2016, from http://www.sophe.org/Pedagogy_in_HP.cfm.

Society for Public Health Education (SOPHE). (2016f). *Publications & resources.* Retrieved May 20, 2016, from http://www.sophe.org/Publications_Resources.cfm.

Society of State Leaders of Health and Physical Education (The Society). (2016a). *About us.* Retrieved May 20, 2016, from http://thesociety.org/Home/About.

Society of State Leaders of Health and Physical Education (The Society). (2016b). *Mission & history.* Retrieved May 20, 2016, from http://thesociety.org/About/Mission.

Sutton, M., Valentine J. A., & Perkins, W. (2015). *Our communities our sexual health: Awareness and prevention for African Americans.* Washington, DC: APHA Press.

Werch, C. E. (2000). Editorial: What use, the American Academy of Health Behavior? *American Journal of Health Behavior, 24* (1), 3–5.

Young, K. J., & Boling, W. (2004). Improving the quality of professional life: Benefits of health education and promotion association membership. *Californian Journal of Health Promotion, 2* (1), 39–44.

Chapter 9

The Literature of Health Education/Promotion

Chapter Objectives

After reading this chapter and answering the questions at the end, you should be able to:

- Describe the difference between a *primary*, a *secondary*, a *tertiary*, and a *popular press* literature source.

- Write an abstract or a summary of an article from a peer-reviewed journal.

- Critique a journal article using a logical sequence of questions.

- Become familiar with the most commonly used journals in the field of health education/promotion.

- Identify the most commonly used online computerized databases for finding health education/promotion information.

- Locate an article related to some aspect of health education/promotion using an online database.

- Conduct an Internet search for information about a health-related topic using one of the Web site URLs listed in the chapter.

- Critique the validity of the information obtained from searching a site on the Internet.

I n her work as a health education specialist, Georgia administers a federally funded statewide center that distributes prevention information on alcohol, tobacco, and other drugs. Materials in the center include monographs containing the results of research studies on possible treatment protocols and prevention interventions; prevention and education materials from a variety of federal, state, and nonprofit agencies; information on evidence-based practice in both prevention and treatment; and an extensive video library. Almost daily, she and her staff receive requests for information from law enforcement agencies, legislators and organizational policy makers, community groups, school personnel, counselors, nonprofit organizations, treatment professionals, state agencies, churches, and individual patrons.

Over the past three or four years, more university health education/promotion students have been visiting to acquire materials for class projects, research studies, or potential thesis topics. These students often request Georgia or her staff to recommend the most up-to-date primary and secondary source materials and the most reputable Web sites related to substance abuse prevention.

After reading and applying the information contained in this chapter, you should be able to address questions similar to those received by the staff of the center previously described. Serving as a resource for health information (Responsibility 6) is a critical skill that must be acquired by those practicing as health education specialists.

The amount of information about any given topic is growing at almost an exponential rate. Terms such as *information overload* and *information burnout* are being heard more and more. Arguably, the area in which information is growing fastest and in which there is tremendous public interest is health. People today seem obsessed with gathering information about such health topics as diet, exercise, stress management, vitamins, drugs, sexuality, depression, safety, disease, violence prevention, healthcare policies, health insurance options, and the cost of medical procedures or prescription drugs.

The increasing demand for information, coupled with the fact that data are being produced at an ever greater rate, creates added need for health education specialists (see **Box 9.1**). Two of the major responsibilities of a health education specialist, as discussed in Chapter 6, involve being a resource person for health information (Responsibility 6) and communicating to others about health education needs, concerns, and resources (Responsibility 7) (see **Figure 9.1**). When seeking out current and accurate information the health education specialist must be able to find and evaluate its credibility. Then the facts and ideas are disseminated to consumers through appropriate channels and explained in a manner that is meaningful to the intended audience. This chapter introduces prospective health education students to the most common sources of health-related information used by health education specialists. It also describes how to access the subject matter from these sources. When searching for valid and reliable materials, it is always wise to seek the assistance of a reference librarian should questions arise.

▶ **Figure 9.1** Health education specialists often make presentations to community groups.
Source: Health Medical Wellbeing Proper Care Concept, Shutterstock, 450296554 RF

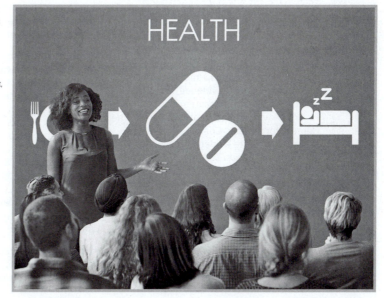

ADOLESCENT HEALTH EDUCATOR Janet Kamiri

CURRENT POSITION: Adolescent Health Educator

DEGREE/INSTITUTION: B.A., 2010, School Health Education, Ball State University

EMPLOYER: Social Health Association of Indiana

How I obtained my job: My career began as a health teacher in a public school system. During my time as a school health teacher, I had a lot of guest speakers in my classroom from outside nonprofit health education agencies. I was always so impressed with their presentations. When I decided to leave the classroom, I submitted letters of interest and followed up with the executive directors of the different agencies. I informed people in my network that I was looking for a position. I continued to look for job postings and when a position was finally listed, I submitted my application and followed up. I was invited for an interview and hired later in the week!

How I utilize health education and the literature in health in my job: In my job as an Adolescent Health Educator, I use health literature on a regular basis to inform curriculum and program development as well as my teaching. I teach primarily human growth and development (puberty) and teen pregnancy and STD prevention. This is a highly sensitive, very political topic. People have a lot of personal values and opinions around this content. Because of this, it is even more important to make sure all programming is informed by current research, good evidence, and best practices in health education.

We heavily rely on information from the Centers for Disease Control and Prevention in addition to evidence-based programs like the Teen Pregnancy Prevention programs from the Office of Adolescent Health. We also seek out other evidence-based programs with proven success in similar populations and use these programs or adapt them to meet the needs of our target population.

I find it extremely helpful to subscribe to email lists from credible sources such as the CDC and email blasts from various departments of health and universities. I get key word alerts from various search engines that identify journal and newspaper articles to make sure that I am aware of trending health issues. Additionally, both I and the agency subscribe to multiple academic professional journals.

What I love most about my job: I love working with students and seeing their excitement when they learn something new or have a question answered. I feel good about the work that I am doing knowing that all of the curricula and programs are based on good quality research and best practices.

What I like least about my job: I'm very fortunate to work in a setting where most days I love my job. Like any job, however, there are days that it is hard. Working in a nonprofit setting means that there are a lot of different stakeholders' perspectives and requirements to take into consideration. Meeting the requirements of funders and the needs of communities and schools while still implementing evidence-based programming with fidelity can be a lot to balance, and it can be frustrating trying to find the best approach.

Recommendations for those preparing to be health education specialists: Read as much as you can! Read journal articles, reports, news articles—anything related to your area of work. Being informed on current events and trends in health is extremely helpful and important for you and your agencies' credibility. Social media platforms are a great resource, too. Follow as many different agencies as you can. Listen to podcasts from trendsetters and thought leaders and become the best informed expert you can be in whatever setting you work.

The role of the health education specialists in the future: The landscape of health education is ever changing. The health

BOX

9.1

continued

education specialist can influence trends in health care and prevention. As prevention is emphasized, the health education specialist will become an even more highly sought after and respected position. Health education specialists are unique in that they are able to work closely with communities and individuals. As a result, they are able to plan and implement programs that can affect behavior change and prevent many long-term health consequences.

▷ Types of Information Sources

When accessing information, it is important to note whether the source is primary, secondary, or tertiary. **Primary sources** of data or information are published studies or eyewitness accounts written by the people who actually conducted the experiments or observed the events in question. A journal that publishes original manuscripts only after they have been read by a panel of experts in the field (peer-reviewers) and recommended for publication is termed a **peer-reviewed journal**. Examples of primary sources are research articles written by the researcher(s); personal records (autobiographies); podcasts or video/audio recordings of actual lectures (which may also be secondary sources depending on whether the information presented is the speakers' own work [primary] or a compilation of the works of self and others [secondary]); speeches, debates, or events; official records of legislative sessions or minutes of community meetings; newspaper eyewitness accounts; and annual reports.

Of note is the fact that some peer-reviewed journals now are published only in electronic format. Some of these electronic journals follow the subscription-only format of their print counterparts. Other electronic journals are **open access journals** that come in a variety of reader access levels. Some articles are immediately available to individual subscribers or subscribing institutions, others allow delayed access to articles for anyone with an Internet connection, and some of the publishing sites have a mixture of the two availability types. The "open access" designation means that the article is copyrighted but generally can be used more liberally than articles with more traditional copyrights. Databases such as BioMed Central (biomedcentral.com) are repositories of these types of journals, many of which are new and most of which use scientists who have been editorial board members on highly prestigious paper-based journals for their editorial review boards. The increased cost of paper-based journals and publishing company charges will undoubtedly expand the number of electronic-only primary sources of information in the future.

Secondary sources are usually written by someone who was not present at the event or did not participate as part of the study team. The value of these sources is that they often provide a summary of several related studies or chronicle a history or sequence of events. The writers of secondary sources may also provide editorial comments or alternative interpretations of the study or event. Secondary sources often provide a bibliography of primary sources. Examples of secondary sources are journal review articles, editorials, and non-eyewitness accounts of events occurring in the community, region, or nation.

Although peer-reviewed journals usually publish primary source articles, they occasionally contain secondary source articles. The types of secondary source articles most likely to be found in a peer-reviewed journal are articles summarizing the results of several studies, editorials, or positions deemed important enough (by a panel of expert reviewers) to be interesting and useful to those who read the journal.

Tertiary sources contain information that has been distilled and collected from primary and secondary sources. Examples include handbooks, informational pamphlets or brochures from governmental organizations (or hospitals, or national nongovernmental agencies such as the American Cancer Society or March of Dimes), newsletters such as the University of California's Berkeley Wellness Letter, almanacs, encyclopedias, fact books, dictionaries, abstracts, and other reference tools. At this stage, information from such sources is accepted as fact by the scientific community. The operative word in the preceding sentence is *fact*. Information that has no documentation and is laced with opinion or intended for marketing a service or product is not considered a tertiary source; publications of that type are classified as popular press sources.

A fourth source of health information, **popular press publications**, is probably the most difficult to check for credibility. Popular press publications range from weekly summary-type magazines (e.g., *Time, Newsweek,* and *U.S. News & World Report*), regular articles in newspapers (e.g., Dr Oz's column), and newspaper supplements (e.g., *Parade*) to monthly magazines (e.g., *Shape, Self,* and *Men's Health*) and tabloids (e.g., *The Star, People,* and *Us*). At times, any of these may contain a primary source of information (as in an interview). Most often, however, they are secondary sources at best. Often, articles in the popular press include opinions or editorials that express the bias of the author or the editor of the publication. Popular press articles should be heavily scrutinized as to the source of the information before being cited as authentic and accurate.

Before concluding this discussion, it is important to note that, with the exception of open access journals, no Web site references were included in the literature types described. This is because Web sites are generally not peer reviewed. Just about anyone can publish an article on the Web without an impartial reader or group of readers reviewing it beforehand. To be sure, Web pages are often wonderful sources of information, but they can just as often be replete with bad information. A discussion of methods to determine the accuracy of material on the Web is included later in this chapter. Sorting through the maze of health information can be a daunting task, even for the most skilled health education specialist. To equip the health education specialist for assuming the responsibilities of providing and disseminating information, several tasks need to be mastered. The next several sections of this chapter are designed to provide background for the student in (1) identifying the components of a research article; (2) critically reading a research article; (3) ascertaining the accuracy of the information in articles that are non-research-based or are from secondary or popular press sources; (4) writing an abstract or a summary of a journal article; (5) identifying and locating primary and secondary sources most commonly used by health education specialists using indexes, abstracts, and computerized databases; and (6) retrieving health-related information on the Internet.

▷ Identifying the Components of a Research Article

A research article usually begins with an abstract, which is a brief description of the study's results. The abstract describes the research questions that were tested, outlines the study design, and lists one or two major findings from the study. The abstract is meant to communicate essential information, so that readers will know whether the study has information related to the topic they are interested in. An example of an abstract (Hibbard and Greene, 2013) follows:

> Patient engagement is an increasingly important component of strategies to reform health care. In this article we review the available evidence of the contribution that patient activation—the skills and confidence that equip patients to become actively engaged in their health care—makes to health outcomes, costs, and patient experience. There is a growing body of evidence showing that patients who are more activated have better health outcomes and care experiences, but there is limited evidence to date about the impact on costs. Emerging evidence indicates that interventions that tailor support to the individual's level of activation, and that build skills and confidence, are effective in increasing patient activation. Furthermore, patients who start at the lowest activation levels tend to increase the most. We conclude that policies and interventions aimed at strengthening patients' role in managing their health care can contribute to improved outcomes and that patient activation can—and should—be measured as an intermediate outcome of care that is linked to improved outcomes. (p. 207)

The introduction section, which sometimes is divided into subsections, follows the abstract. Its purpose is usually threefold: (1) to give readers a more detailed description of the research question(s) or hypotheses being tested, (2) to review related literature, and (3) to explain the need for or the significance of the study. This section communicates the rationale behind the researchers' decision to conduct the study.

The methodology section comes directly after the introductory material. In this section, there is usually a description of (1) the research design used, (2) the subjects who took part in the research, (3) the instruments used to gather the data necessary to answer the research questions, and (4) any administrative procedures involved in conducting the research, such as methods used to select the subject(s), gather the data, or protect the rights of the subject(s).

Following the methodology section are the results and discussion sections. The results section gives the research findings by describing the results of the statistical procedures used in analyzing the data (in the case of studies involving quantitative methods—methods involving the analyses of numerical data) and provides an overall answer to the research questions or hypotheses that were described in the introductory section. The discussion section provides a forum for the researcher to interpret the conclusions and meanings and to comment on the implications of the data analyses. In addition, the researcher often includes a narrative about the limitations of the study and makes recommendations for further research on the topic.

▷ Critically Reading a Research Article

The volume of articles on any single health topic continues to escalate. It is important to be able to evaluate the information for accuracy and saliency from sources of all types. Research articles serve as primary sources of valuable information for health education specialists. Beginning students in the field of health education/promotion are not expected to be able to immediately understand every nuance in a research article. It is essential, however, to begin to frequently read scientific reports and journal articles to become familiar with their style. Often, pre-formulating generic questions suitable for critiquing any study can help when evaluating study results. Following is a sequence of questions found to be of help when such an evaluation is necessary. The list is adapted from *Studying a Study and Testing a Test: How to Read Medical Evidence* (Riegelman, 2005).

1. Were the goals/aims of the study defined in a clear manner?

2. Were the research questions/hypotheses clearly stated?

3. Was the description of the subjects clear? Did the article state how the subjects were recruited?

4. Were the design and location of the study described clearly?

5. Were the data collection instruments described?

6. Were reliability and validity reported for the instruments?

7. Did the results directly address the research questions or hypotheses?

8. Were the conclusions reasonable in light of the research design and data analyses performed?

9. Were the findings extrapolated to a population that is similar to the population studied?

10. Were the study implications meaningful to the population you serve?

The final test comes when students can read an article and begin to view themselves in the position of a reporter who has the task of describing the study, its findings, and its limitations to an audience in no more than five minutes. People who can restate study findings and limitations in their own words have accomplished much in becoming critical consumers of scientific and nonscientific literature as well as better resources for others.

▷ Evaluating the Accuracy of Non-Research-Based Sources

As with journal articles that are research based, it is important to be able to evaluate whether or not the information presented is reliable, regardless of the source. Cottrell (1997) conducted a search for instruments that could assist him in teaching his students to assess the accuracy of information found in almost any type of journal or magazine. The questions that emanated from the results of his search include the following:

1. What are the author's qualifications? Does the person have an academic degree in the field being written about? (A note of caution—a degree does not make someone absolutely qualified, but it provides evidence that *suggests* the person is qualified.)

2. What is the style of presentation? Look for health information written in a scientific style of writing, not a style that uses generalities or testimonials.

3. Are references included? A well-written article provides references to the primary sources used. Be aware when someone is writing about another person's research because that individual may be interpreting the results in a different way than the author did.

4. What is the purpose of the publication? Be aware of publications, news or otherwise, that contain advertisements designed to sell items discussed in the articles.

5. What is the reputation of the publication? Is it peer reviewed? Professional journals are good sources of information. Popular press publications can sometimes have poor information related to health issues.

6. Is the information new? When reading for the first time, be skeptical. Information must be validated over time. New information is newsworthy but may not be valid.

It is important to realize that becoming a skeptical, critical consumer of printed and Web-based health information is an important first step in being seen by others as credible. For the public to use the expertise and training of health education specialists to a greater degree, the health education specialist must develop a reputation for providing accurate and current information.

▷ Writing an Abstract or a Summary

Another valuable skill when reading and interpreting health-related literature of any kind (primary, secondary, tertiary, or popular press) involves learning to write an abstract or a summary of an article. Although abstracts and summaries are both short forms of describing a research study, the major differences lie in the extent of the content. Abstracts are short (usually 150–250 words). They are written to identify the purpose of the research, the study questions, the methods used by the researcher, and one or two major findings. Summaries, on the other hand, may be two to three pages in length and include all of the elements of the abstract. In addition, summaries are meant to reveal any secondary findings, to describe study limitations, and to provide a more detailed review of the researcher's conclusions and recommendations from the viewpoint of the summary's author.

It is recommended that beginning health education specialists practice writing both abstracts and summaries of the articles they read. Using this technique sharpens the ability of the health education specialist to discriminate between health-related articles that are reliable and credible for health education/promotion and those that contain erroneous or misleading claims or information.

▷ Locating Health-Related Information

Health education specialists serve as major health information resource persons for many constituencies. It does not matter if they are employed in the school, the clinic, the work site, or the community setting. In all cases, inquiries from a variety of people wanting to know about a health topic or wanting interpretation of the latest research findings are directed to health education specialists. Therefore, it is essential that the latter be knowledgeable about how to find the information requested. The next section identifies resources that health education specialists can use to locate information on health education/promotion and explains how to access it.

Journals

As has been previously mentioned, much of the evidence that health education specialists use to make decisions when planning, implementing, and evaluating health promotion programs can be found in journals that publish primary research articles and position papers about health topics and health programs. The following are examples of journals commonly used by health professionals. The list by no means includes all journals of benefit to the health education specialist.

1. *AIDS Education and Prevention.* An international journal designed to support the efforts of professionals working to prevent HIV and AIDS, *AIDS Education and Prevention* includes scientific articles by leading authorities from many disciplines, research reports on the effectiveness of new strategies and programs, debates about key issues, and reviews of books and video resources. The journal also covers a wide range of public health, psychosocial, ethical, and public policy concerns related to HIV and AIDS.

2. *American Journal of Health Behavior* (formerly *Health Values*). Articles feature research about the impact of personal behavior patterns and practices on health promotion. The journal emphasizes efforts at fostering a better understanding of the multidisciplinary interface of systems and individuals as they impact behavior. Examples of successful multidisciplinary approaches to improving health at the community level are featured. Only available online after 2009.

3. *American Journal of Health Education.* Includes research findings, community health intervention and learning strategies, and health promotion strategies. Some articles are designed as self-study courses.

4. *American Journal of Health Promotion.* This journal features original research articles, the testing of health behavioral theory on selected populations, and program evaluation. It is an excellent source of work-site health promotion articles.

5. *American Journal of Public Health.* Published by the American Public Health Association, this journal features reports related to health research, program evaluations, and health policy analysis, as well as articles on special topics on the health of selected groups and communities.

6. *Evaluation and the Health Professions.* Articles generally focus on practitioner-friendly research related to the development, implementation, and evaluation of community-based health programs. Healthcare researchers and evaluators can find examples of state-of-the-art tools and methods for conducting meaningful evaluations.

7. *Family and Community Health.* Presents creative, multidisciplinary perspectives and approaches for effective public and community health programs. Issues focus on a single topic and address problems of concern to a wide variety of population groups with diverse ethnic backgrounds, including children and the elderly, men and women, and rural and urban communities.

8. *Health Affairs.* This journal is published bimonthly and features health policy–related articles of national concern or interest. The journal serves as a major source of primary research concerning healthcare coverage, health economics, health reform, and the impact of policy on the health of the populace.

9. *The Health Educator: The Journal of Eta Sigma Gamma.* Published by Eta Sigma Gamma, the health education honor society, this journal includes articles related to most health education/promotion topics in a variety of settings. Many of the studies and commentaries are submitted by students in health education/promotion and/or public health programs.

10. *The Hastings Center Report.* This journal focuses on the ethical, social, legal, and economic factors in health policy, medicine, health care delivery, and public health.

11. *Health Education & Behavior* (formerly *Health Education Quarterly*). The official publication of the Society for Public Health Education, Inc. (SOPHE), its articles center on health behavior and education, case studies in health, program evaluation,

and strategies to improve social and behavioral health. Each submission includes a commentary on the application of findings to the practice setting.

12. *Health Education Research*. Official publication of the International Union for Health Promotion and Education and features articles concerning health promotion program planning, implementation, and evaluation. Articles focus on application of results in the practice of health promotion.

13. *Health Promotion International*. The majority of research studies and commentaries are on issues related to health promotion in schools, clinics, worksites, and communities located outside the United States. Unique to this journal is the fact that submissions describing spontaneous activities, organizational change interventions, and social and environmental development are featured too.

14. *Health Promotion Practice*. Publishes articles devoted to the practical application of health promotion and education in a variety of settings including community, health care, educational, worksite, and international. Articles focus on best practices and their application to health policies that promote health and disease prevention.

15. *Global Journal for Health Education and Promotion (GJHEP)* (formerly *The International Electronic Journal of Health Education*). Features articles on nearly every aspect of health education, including school health, community health, worksite health promotion, the ethical implications of health education, and the philosophy of health education. Published by Sagamore Publishing.

16. *The Journal of American College Health*. Published by the American College Health Association in cooperation with Heldref Publications, its articles are limited to those that relate to health promotion or health service provision in the college or university environment. This is the *only* journal written by college health professionals for college health professionals.

17. *Journal of Community Health*. This journal features articles relating to the practice, teaching, and research of community health; preventive medicine; and analysis of delivery of healthcare services.

18. *Journal of Health Communication*. This journal is published eight times a year. It presents the latest developments in the field of health communication, including research in risk communication, health literacy, social marketing, communication (from interpersonal to mass media), psychology, government, policy making, and health education around the world.

19. *Journal of Nutrition Education and Behavior*. The official publication of the Society of Nutrition Education and Behavior, this journal publishes articles that are germane to the interface between nutrition education and behavior as practiced worldwide. It serves as a resource for anyone interested in nutrition education or diet and physical behavior.

20. *Journal of Rural Health*. Published by Wiley-Blackwell Publishing, Inc. for the Rural Health Association, this journal's articles focus on professional practice, research, theory development, and policy issues related to health in the rural setting.

21. *Journal of School Health*. Published for the American School Health Association, articles in this journal are related to the public or private school setting from pre-K through grade 12. Articles generally focus on children's health issues but may include information related to other aspects of coordinated school health programs.

22. *Global Health Promotion*. This is an official publication of the International Union for Health Promotion and Education (IUHPE), published by Sage Publications. Most issues are topical in nature (e.g., environmental health, population health, and infectious disease prevention) and feature articles related to the application of public health and health promotion in countries around the globe. Articles are published in several languages.

23. **Pedagogy in Health Promotion: The Scholarship of Teaching and Learning**. A quarterly journal first published in 2016. Curriculum and course design, assessment, and administration relevant to teaching and learning are topics that provide focal points for articles in this publication.

24. *Public Health Reports*. Published by the Association of Schools of Public Health, this journal reports findings from many avenues of research related to health services acquisition, health policy development, and health promotion at the community level.

25. *Health Behavior and Policy Review*. A bi-monthly journal that was first published in January 2014. The journal features articles on policy development impacting health behaviors that are population rather than individual focused. Research guiding policy development and prioritizing health policy choices is also a focus.

Indexes and Abstracts

Indexes and **abstracts** provide links to articles from many peer-reviewed journals, books, and research reports. An index references articles from journals, books, and reports pertaining to topics that fall under the subject headings for which the index was created (e.g., health behavior, physical activity, methamphetamine treatment, or corporate health education/ promotion programs). An abstract provides somewhat similar information but also includes short summaries of the article's content to help the researcher determine whether the article contains the information she or he is seeking.

Although some indexes and abstracts can still be found in hard copy, many of them are migrating to online or electronic formats. The cost of publishing paper versions plus the ease of user access to online materials is reducing the number of paper version editions of either indexes or abstracts. *Index Medicus*, an abstract that has been printed for more than a century, is an example of a publication that is no longer available in paper copy because of the high cost of printing the volumes. In its place, the National Library of Medicine and the National Institutes of Health have created a site (http://www.ncbi.nlm.nih.gov/pubmed/) that combines the information formerly available in *Index Medicus* with many other sources to create a database that is accessible to anyone with a computer.

Government Documents

The U.S. Government Printing Office (GPO) publishes volumes of materials of use to health education specialists. This section (adapted from the University of Akron library Web site [University of Akron, 2013]) is meant to provide a generic description of the types of documents that can be accessed in the government documents section of an academic library. Because each library has slightly different procedures for finding these documents, students are encouraged to communicate with the government documents librarian at their university for the specifics on locating documents. It should be noted that the U.S. government is shifting away from issuing paper copies and is increasing the number of documents available online.

Government publications range from official documents including laws, court decisions, and records of congressional actions to the results of government-sponsored technical and scientific studies. Information on topics such as obesity, water treatment, or exercise can also be found in a government documents section.

Government documents are not organized under the same classification scheme as a traditional general collection. Instead, they are organized and shelved according to Super-intendent of Documents (SuDocs) numbers. The SuDocs number is unique in that it has a colon. For example, A1:1 is an annual report from the Agriculture Department. Numbers of the documents are arranged alphabetically by agency, and the numbers are whole numbers, not decimals (e.g., HE 1.6 comes before HE 1.9). The letter that begins the SuDocs number signifies the publishing agency, as noted:

A   Agriculture Department

C   Census Bureau

D   Department of Defense

E   Department of Energy

HE   Health and Human Services

X–Y   Congress

Government documents contain a storehouse of valuable and current information and should not be overlooked when seeking information on a health topic of interest. Most librar-ies have online search capabilities for government documents, so as with many traditional sources of information, accessing them has become much less labor intensive.

Electronic Databases

Electronic databases often provide a preferred alternative to manually searching indexes or abstracts (see **Figure 9.2**). As mentioned previously, most, if not all, of the publishers of the hard-copy abstracts and indexes either have converted or are converting their documents to an online format. Much like an index or abstract, each database has a general subject area (e.g., medicine, education, psychology, and community health). The electronic database pro-vides access via the Internet. Computer searches using databases are significantly faster than manual searches, and they have the advantage of enabling the user to link several concepts together to provide focus for a search.

For example, if a person wanted to search for articles about "health behavior" and the in-fluence of "health communication" on behavior, an electronic database would allow the user to enter both terms into the computer and connect them by placing the word *and* between them. The result will be to eliminate any articles that do not have both *health behavior* and *health communication* as key terms. Other terms can be used to further narrow a search to be as specific as desired. The main concern the computer database user faces is to accurately specify the key terms associated with the information desired, so the resulting list of references that is generated will be of use. Computerized searches require little computer knowledge; however, it is always advisable to seek the assistance of a librarian when beginning to seek informa-tion. Users should also know that just because the information is readily available online, it is not free. Academic libraries spend hundreds of thousands of dollars per year to ensure that

▲ **Figure 9.2** Electronic databases such as the National Library of Medicine (NLM) provide ready access to information on a particular topic.

students and faculty have access to the free or low-cost materials they need. The databases most used by health education specialists are

1. **ERIC (Education Resource Information Center)**. It includes the *Current Index to Journals in Education (CIJE)* and *Resources in Education (RIE)*. ERIC is an information clearinghouse that collects, sorts, classifies, and stores thousands of documents on topics pertaining to education and allied fields of study. An advantage to using ERIC is that many types of documents are contained in the database that are not journal articles—for example, proceedings of meetings, teaching strategies, lesson plans, commentaries, and policy documents.

2. *MEDLINE*. This is the premier biomedicine database indexing more than 3,000 journals. It covers the fields of medicine, nursing, dentistry, veterinary medicine, and preclinical sciences. MEDLINE is also the commercial version of PubMed. The major differences between the two versions are that PubMed goes back further into the literature, has several small databases not included in the commercial version, and uses a different search platform.

3. *ScienceDirect*. This is one of the largest full-text scientific databases in the world covering physical sciences, life sciences, health sciences, and engineering material. It indexes more than 2,500 peer-reviewed journals and more than 11,000 books. More than 9.5 million journal articles and book chapters are contained in this database.

4. **CINAHL with Fulltext**. It contains more than 300,000 citations from 1983 until the present. It references journal articles and book chapters, pamphlets, audiovisuals,

educational software, and conference proceedings in the areas of nursing, health education, health services, and healthcare administration.

5. *ETHXWeb*. This database covers the years 1974–2009 and is no longer being updated. Topics include ethical, legal, and public policy issues surrounding health care and biomedical research. Citations are derived from the literature of law, religion, ethics, social sciences, philosophy, the popular media, and the health sciences.

6. *PsycINFO*. This is the largest database of peer-reviewed literature in the areas of mental health and behavior sciences.

7. **Ovid Healthstar**. Ovid Healthstar includes data from the National Library of Medicine's (NLM) MEDLINE and former HealthSTAR databases. As such, it contains citations of the published literature in health services, technology, administration, health policy, health economics, and research. It focuses on both the clinical and nonclinical aspects of healthcare delivery.

8. *PubMed*. A service of the National Library of Medicine that contains more than 17 million citations from MEDLINE and other life science journals for biomedical articles dating back more than a half-century. The database includes links to full text articles and other related resources.

9. *Physical Education Index*. This database includes references to more than 400 periodicals on physical education, health education, dance, physical therapy, and sports medicine.

10. *Google Scholar*. Covers scholarly research from books, theses, dissertations, journal articles, government documents, etc. It indexes professional societies, online repositories, university sites, government Web sites, etc. If you use settings, you can customize it to link to your university library's resources.

Application Scenario

Assume you are a newly employed health education specialist in a hospital outpatient clinic. One of your jobs is to provide information to patients after they have seen the physician. A skeptical Ms. X has just been diagnosed with coronary artery disease, and the physician has sent her to you to discuss the impact of lifestyle on her condition. Using the Internet, find several sources of information that you could give her to read that might assist you with the education process. Make certain to evaluate the accuracy of the information you retrieve using the criteria in the section that follows because it is highly likely Ms. X will need some assurance that the information you are providing her is accurate.

▷ Evaluating Information on the Internet

Previously in the chapter, directions were given for evaluating the accuracy and validity of information from journal and popular press sources. Today, largely because of the massive amount of information available on the Internet and because nearly anyone can publish on the Web, it is equally imperative that the health education specialist know how to evaluate material obtained via an Internet search. T. J. Madden, a health sciences reference specialist in the Albertson Library at Boise State University, suggests using CRAAP test which was originally developed at California State University, Chico (personal communication, April 2013). See **Figure 9.3** for an example of information from an Internet search. You can use the criteria below to evaluate the credibility of the information on the website shown.

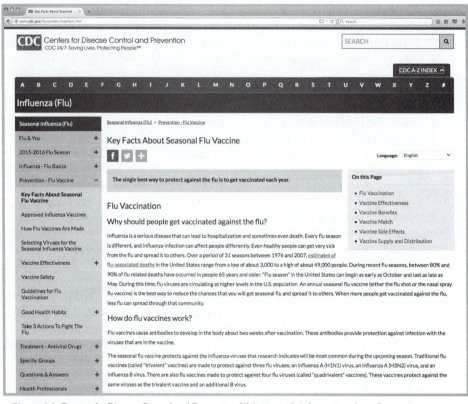

▲ **Figure 9.3** Centers for Disease Control and Prevention Web site with information about flu vaccine.

Evaluation Criteria

Currency: *The timeliness of the information*.

- When was the information published or posted?
- Has the information been revised or updated?
- Does your topic require current information or will older sources work as well?
- Are the links functional?

Relevance: *The importance of the information for your needs*.

- Does the information relate to your topic or answer your question?
- Who is the intended audience?
- Is the information at an appropriate level (i.e., not too elementary or advanced for your needs)? Have you looked at a variety of sources before determining this is one you will use?
- Would you be comfortable citing this source in your research paper?

Authority: *The source of the information*.

- Who is the author, publisher, source, or sponsor?
- What are the author's credentials or organizational affiliations?

- Is the author qualified to write on the topic?
- Is there contact information, such as a publisher or email address?
- Does the URL reveal anything about the author or source (examples: .com, .edu, .gov, .org, or .net)?

Accuracy: *The reliability, truthfulness, and correctness of the content.*

- Where does the information come from?
- Is the information supported by evidence?
- Has the information been peer reviewed?
- Can you verify any of the information in another source or from personal knowledge?
- Does the language or tone seem unbiased and free of emotion?
- Are there spelling, grammar, or typographical errors?

Purpose: *The reason the information exists.*

- What is the purpose of the information?
- Is it to inform, teach, sell, entertain, or persuade?
- Do the authors or sponsors make their intentions or purpose clear?
- Is the information fact, opinion, or propaganda?
- Does the point of view appear objective and impartial?

▶ Summary

This chapter has presented an overview on accessing and evaluating health-related information. An increasing demand for health knowledge, coupled with the fact that the information is being produced at an ever greater rate, creates added responsibility for health education specialists. Two of the major roles of health education specialists as discussed in Chapter 6 involve being resource people for health information and communicating to others about health education/promotion needs, concerns, and resources. To perform these tasks, the health education specialist must have the skills to find information, must evaluate the source of the information to determine its credibility, and must disseminate the information through the appropriate channels to consumers. In addition, the health education specialist must be able to explain the information effectively. Becoming familiar with the tools found in this chapter is a necessity for all students wanting to enter the field of health education/promotion.

▶ Review Questions

1. Describe the difference between primary, secondary, tertiary, and popular press sources.
2. How do an article abstract and an article summary differ in content?
3. What are the questions you should ask yourself when critiquing a journal article? What are the differences between the questions asked when evaluating a primary research article and those asked when evaluating a secondary source or popular press article?

4. Pick any three of the previously listed journals that focus on the field of health education/promotion. What types of information would you expect to find in each of the journals you named?

5. What advantage might the information from a government document have over another source on the same topic?

6. How does one go about evaluating information retrieved from the Internet?

▷ Case Study

As a health education/promotion major, you have just finished studying about the Responsibilities and Competencies for Entry-Level Health Education Specialists (found in Appendix B of this text). During this unit the instructor invited a group of practicing health education specialists to the class to participate in a panel discussion on the validity of the various roles in the real-life practice of health education/promotion.

Following the presentation, each of the panelists offered to host two to three students from the class for four hours per week for three weeks at his or her place of work. This opportunity resulted from student questions to the panelists concerning their desire to transfer the classroom learning to the work setting. Several of the students expressed frustration at what they perceived to be the emphasis on theory and the lack of application in their courses and coursework. The panelists readily conceded that the 12-hour block of time each student would spend at the worksite with them would not totally solve theory-practical application problems, but they hoped it might help the students to see that, at least in the case of the majority of the responsibilities and competencies, what they studied about in class was what the health education specialist was doing.

After a quick meeting between the instructor and the panel members, placement assignments were made for the students. Because of your interest in becoming a health education specialist in a clinical setting, you were assigned to a community health clinic to shadow a physician to see what kind of health education is given to patients.

On your first day, the physician to whom you are assigned requests that you accompany her into the examination room as she sees patients. During the first two hours, she sees three patients for colds or influenza, two patients for hypertension, one patient for emphysema, one patient for diabetes, one for a broken hand, and two teenage patients for sports physicals. After these appointments, she takes some time to visit with you and discuss your initial perceptions. During the conversation, she asks if you are aware of any good health education/promotion information sites for teens on the Internet. You promise to do some research on this question and bring the information on your next visit. What information do you think would be of benefit to teens? Which two or three sites would you recommend and why?

▷ Critical Thinking Questions

1. Assume that all information about any topic is available on the Internet. If that were true, would there be any need for health education specialists? Defend your answer.

2. Make a list of two advantages and two disadvantages of the Internet from your perspective. Assuming that your answers reflect universal truths about the Internet, how might you persuade someone who is not computer literate to use a computer to search for health information?

3. Given that so much information is available online, under what circumstances does it make sense to use the library?

4. If the Internet had been developed in the early 1900s, how might the U.S. healthcare system and the role of health education specialists differ from what they are today?

 ## Activities

1. You are employed as a health education specialist in a district health department and have just received a call from a member of a local coalition wanting to know where to find some peer-reviewed studies that summarize the content and effectiveness of available school-based sexuality education curricula. Use an index to find a reference to an article that meets those criteria.

2. Was the article you located in Activity 1 a primary or secondary source of information? Provide a rationale for your answer.

3. Using a database (CINAHL, MEDLINE, PsycINFO, or ERIC), find a primary research article relating to motorcycle safety (e.g., the use of a helmet, wearing protective gear, or road surfaces). Critique the article by applying the questions found in the "Critically Reading a Research Article" section of this chapter.

4. Use your choice of a browser and look up the term *endometriosis*. Then evaluate at least two of the sites that appear using the CRAAP methodology.

5. Perform an Internet search on the topic of breast cancer. Compare the results of your findings from a primary source, a government publication, and a popular press publication.

 ## Weblinks

EPIDEMIOLOGICAL AND STATISTICAL INFORMATION

1. http://wonder.cdc.gov

   CDC WONDER

   Wide-ranging online data for epidemiological research—an easy-to-use, menu-driven system that makes the information resources of the CDC available to public health professionals and the public at large. It provides access to a wide array of public health information.

2. http://www.cdc.gov/nchs/

   National Center for Health Statistics (NCHS)

   NCHS is the nation's principal health statistics agency. Their Web site offers access to an extensive collection of health statistics intended to guide those working to improve public health.

3. http://www.cdc.gov/mmwr/index.html

   Morbidity and Mortality Weekly Report (MMWR)

   MMWR is a weekly report prepared by the CDC. State health departments report their findings to MMWR. The site offers access to studies and reports and also provides useful information on a wide range of diseases.

4. **http://www.census.gov**

   U.S. Bureau of the Census

   The Web site of the U.S. Census Bureau allows the user to access specific data for his or her state, county, or city. View results from Census 2000 and Census 2010 and access analytical reports on population change, race, age, family structure, and more.

INFECTIOUS DISEASES

5. **http://www.cdc.gov/DataStatistics/**

   Centers for Disease Control and Prevention—Data and Statistics

   With the mission of preventing illness, disability, and death, the CDC conducts epidemic investigations, laboratory research, and public education programs to attempt to prevent and control diseases and disorders of all types.

CHRONIC DISEASES

6. **http://www.cdc.gov/chronicdisease/index.htm**

   CDC Chronic Disease Prevention and Health Promotion

   This section of the CDC is dedicated to chronic diseases and provides links to a variety of helpful sites, including a diabetes public health resource and sites discussing heart disease, nutrition, and physical activity.

7. **http://www.cancer.gov/**

   National Cancer Institute (NCI)

   The NCI's Web site covers information on a variety of cancer topics, discussing treatment, prevention, research, and much more. The NCI supports prevention and treatment of cancer, rehabilitation, and continued care of cancer patients and their families.

8. **http://www.diabetes.org**

   American Diabetes Association (ADA)

   The ADA provides diabetes research, scientific findings, information, and advocacy. The site contains helpful information for people with diabetes, their families, health professionals, and the public.

DISEASE CONTROL AND PREVENTION

9. **http://store.samhsa.gov/home**

   Substance Abuse and Mental Health Services Administration

   This site features links to ordering government materials online that focus on professional and research topics; issues in the field of treatment, prevention, and recovery; and information on conditions and disorders.

10. **http://www.samhsa.gov/about-us/who-we-are/offices-centers/csap**

    Center for Substance Abuse Prevention (CSAP)

    CSAP is funded by the Substance Abuse and Mental Health Services Administration (SAMHSA) and is responsible for improving the access to and quality of substance abuse prevention services to the public. CSAP provides national leadership in the development of policies, programs, and services to prevent the onset of illegal drug use and underage alcohol and tobacco use, and to reduce the negative consequences of using substances.

11. https://www.whitehouse.gov/ondcp

    Office of National Drug Control Policy (ONDCP)

    With the goal of reducing illicit drug use, substance abuse-related crimes, drug trafficking, and drug-related health problems, the ONDCP is working to establish a national strategy to fight these dilemmas. The site contains national priorities, annual reports, and a tremendous amount of drug information.

12. http://www.cdc.gov/hiv/dhap/about.html

    CDC's Division of HIV/AIDS Prevention

    With a mission to prevent HIV infection and reduce the incidence of HIV-related illness, the CDC's Division of HIV/AIDS Prevention Web site provides useful information for those working in the health field. The site includes such topics as prevention tools, research, brochures, and fact sheets.

13. http://www.childrenssafetynetwork.org

    Children's Safety Network

    The Children's Safety Network, funded by the Maternal & Child Health Bureau (MCH) and the U.S. Department of Health and Human Services, provides technical assistance, training, and resources to MCH and other injury prevention professionals in an extensive effort to reduce the burden of injury and violence to our nation's children.

14. http://www.fda.gov/Food/default.htm

    Food and Drug Administration (FDA)

    This site not only outlines national programs intended to increase food safety awareness, but it also contains information concerning the laws enforced by the FDA and provides helpful tips on preventing food-related illness.

15. http://oncolink.com

    OncoLink

    OncoLink, provided by the Abramson Cancer Center of the University of Pennsylvania, is the Web's first cancer resource. The site provides up-to-date cancer news and research. Locate information on the causes of cancer, screening and prevention, clinical trials, and other resources on cancer.

16. http://www.cdc.gov/travel/

    Travelers' Health

    Locate health information for specific destinations, stay up to date on outbreaks throughout the world, and learn how to avoid illness from food and water.

17. http://www.cdc.gov/tb/

    CDC's Division of Tuberculosis Elimination

    With the mission of "preventing, controlling and eventually eliminating tuberculosis from the United States," the Web site of the CDC's Division of Tuberculosis Elimination contains useful information to aid that mission. Learn all there is to know about tuberculosis, locate statistics on its occurrence, and obtain education and training materials on it.

18. http://www.healthywomen.org/

    National Women's Health Information Center

    The National Women's Health Information Center, sponsored by the Department of Health and Human Services Office on Women's Health, provides health information for women across the country. It offers information on heart disease, body image, breastfeeding, screening and immunization schedules, and more.

19. http://www.menshealthnetwork.org

    Men's Health Network

    The Men's Health Network is an informational and educational organization recognizing men's health as a specific social concern.

20. http://www.kidshealth.org/

    KidsHealth

    KidsHealth is the largest and most visited site on the Web, providing doctor-approved health information about children from before birth through adolescence. Created by the Nemours Foundation's Center for Children's Health Media, the award-winning KidsHealth provides families with accurate, up-to-date, and jargon-free health information they can use.

21. http://www.nsc.org

    National Safety Council

    The National Safety Council is focused on providing safety and health information to reduce the number of injuries and deaths from preventable accidents. Their Web site contains information on new policies and laws enacted to prevent unintentional injuries. It also provides statistics and helpful tips regarding this health topic.

22. http://ctb.ku.edu/en

    Community Tool Box

    The goal of the Community Tool Box is to support work in community health promotion and development. The Tool Box provides multiple pages of practical skill-building information on more than 250 different topics related to community development. Topic sections include step-by-step instruction, examples, checklists, and related resources.

NATIONAL AGENCIES

23. http://www.cdc.gov

    CDC—Centers for Disease Control and Prevention

    The CDC is recognized as the leading federal agency for protecting the health and safety of the public, providing credible information to enhance health decisions and promote health. The Web site of the CDC includes a variety of helpful health and safety topics. The information covers everything from health promotion to vaccines to traveler's health. Data, statistics, publications, and products are also available.

24. http://www.hhs.gov

    USDHHS—Department of Health and Human Services

    The Department of Health and Human Services is the U.S. government's principal agency for health protection and the provision of human services. Its site is divided into health topics such as Safety & Wellness, Diseases & Conditions, and Families & Children. Readers can also use the Resource Locator and Reference Collections to find such things as healthcare facilities and publications.

25. http://www3.epa.gov/

    EPA—Environmental Protection Agency

    The EPA is focused on protecting human health and the environment by working for a cleaner, healthier environment. The site provides air quality reports, current environmental news stories, and tips on how the public can make the environment healthier. The QuickFinder allows fast and easy access to a variety of environmental topics.

26. http://www.ihs.gov/

IHS—Indian Health Service

Indian Health Service is the Federal Health Program for American Indians and Alaska Natives. IHS is focused on improving the health of these groups while attempting to ensure they have access to culturally acceptable health services.

27. http://www.ama-assn.org

American Medical Association

This Web site is divided into a section for physicians and medical students and a section for patients. The patient section allows the user to search for a doctor and obtain health information and resources. The physician section provides information on such topics as medical education, legal issues, and advocacy.

28. http://www.nih.gov

National Institutes of Health (NIH)

The Web site of the NIH is loaded with a wide variety of great health information. It contains an A–Z index of health resources, a wealth of grant information, and a section dedicated to scientific resources.

29. https://www.govinfo.gov/

Government Publications Office (GPO)

This is a beta test site from the GPO that was activated in February 2016. It is designed to offer free online access to official publications from all three branches of the Federal Government.

INTERNATIONAL AGENCIES

30. http://www.who.int/en

WHO—World Health Organization

The Web site of WHO is an incredible resource. The site includes a tremendous listing of pages, organized by health and development topics that contain links to WHO projects, initiatives, activities, information products, and contacts.

31. http://www.paho.org

PAHO—Pan American Health Organization

PAHO, affiliated with WHO, focuses on a multitude of public health topics, with the mission of promoting health in the Americas.

32. http://www.un-ilibrary.org/

The United Nations Library

Includes health-related information on diseases, policies, legislation, and the health status of countries around the globe.

INTERNET-BASED MEDLINE SEARCH SYSTEMS

33. http://www.pubMed.gov/

PubMed

PubMed is a service of the NLM. It includes literally millions of citations for biomedical articles going back to the 1950s. The citations are from MEDLINE and additional life science journals. PubMed includes links to many sites providing full-text articles and other related resources.

34. http://www.medscape.com/px/urlinfo

    Medscape from WebMD (free access to MEDLINE)

    Medscape allows the user to register for free access to MEDLINE, continuing medical education (CME) courses, medical journals, medical news, and more. Medline's database of medical abstracts may be searched by title or author.

35. http://www.nlm.nih.gov

    National Library of Medicine (NLM)

    The NLM, on the campus of the NIH in Bethesda, Maryland, is the world's largest medical library. Excellent central source of current information on results of health research for the lay person, the practicing health professional, the health researcher, and health librarians. Updated daily.

36. https://www.nlm.nih.gov/medlineplus/

    MedlinePlus

    Health professionals and the general public alike can easily access information on MedlinePlus that is accurate and up to date. MedlinePlus has extensive information from the National Institutes of Health and other trusted sources on more than 650 diseases and conditions.

PUBLIC HEALTH PRACTICE

37. http://www.cdc.gov/stltpublichealth/

    Office of State, Tribal, Local and Territorial Support (OSTLTS)

    This office resulted from a reorganization at the CDC. The priority of the OSTLTS is to improve the capacity and performance of the public health system at all levels. The office works both within CDC and in the field to identify gaps, opportunities for collaboration, and the strategies needed to support growth and enhancement of public health work.

38. http://www.apha.org

    American Public Health Association (APHA)

    The APHA is the world's largest and oldest organization of public health professionals. Useful sections include Continuing Education, Newsroom, and Science and Programs.

STATE AND LOCAL PUBLIC HEALTH DEPARTMENTS

39. http://www.astho.org/

    Association of State and Territorial Health Officials (ASTHO)

    ASTHO is the national nonprofit organization representing the public health agencies of the United States, the U.S. Territories, and the District of Columbia, as well as the 120,000 public health professionals these agencies employ. ASTHO members, the chief health officials of these jurisdictions, are dedicated to formulating and influencing sound public health policy and to ensuring excellence in state-based public health practice.

40. http://www.healthguideusa.com/index.htm

    Health Resource Guide USA

    Health Guide USA provides quick reference to a tremendous listing of healthcare-related resources throughout the United States. It provides locations of state and local health departments, as well as medical schools and medical licenses.

GENERAL HEALTH INFORMATION

41. http://www.google.com

Google

Google's keyword search engine is pop-up free and a great tool for finding anything on the Web. Google has several specialized search features such as Blog Search and Alerts. Many people and organizations have a health-related blog, and you can use Blog Search to find these blogs. If you want to receive email updates on various health topics, you can set up an Alert and content will be sent directly to your inbox.

42. https://www.optum.com/individuals-families/get-healthy-stay-healthy.html

OPTUM

Provides MD-reviewed information on a variety of health topics. The information is easy to understand and can be used by a health education specialist to research background information related to all aspects of health.

43. http://www.WebMD.com

WebMD

Site devoted to providing current and relevant consumer health information on a variety of topics. Medical facts are reviewed by physicians prior to posting.

44. http://www.yahoo.com/Health/

Yahoo! Health

Get in-depth coverage on a variety of health issues, including a directory of the most popular Web sites related to a particular health topic.

45. http://www.mayoclinic.com

Mayo Clinic

The Mayo Clinic offers a wealth of health information developed and reviewed by more than 2,000 physicians and scientists. The site also allows access to healthy living tools, such as a personal health card and a first-aid and self-care guide.

46. http://www.berkeleywellness.com

Cal Berkeley Wellness Letter

The Wellness Letter relies on the expertise of the School of Public Health and other researchers at UC Berkeley, as well as other top scientists from around the world. It translates this leading-edge research into practical advice for daily living—at home, at work, while exercising, and in the market or health-food store.

47. http://www.healthfinder.gov

Healthfinder®

Healthfinder, developed by the Department of Health and Human Services, directs the user to various health resources depending on his or her needs. Resources include such things as online publications, clearinghouses, support groups, government agencies, and Web sites.

48. https://www.usa.gov/health

USA.gov-Health

The Health and Nutrition section of the U.S. Government's Official Web portal is filled with great health information. The Healthfinder link enables access to the Personal Health Tools link, which features tools for calculating body mass index (BMI) and taking an online checkup. The site also features health topics for population groups and helps the user locate health services in his or her area.

49. http://www.foundationcenter.org

Foundation Center

The Foundation Center has free online grant-writing guides and tutorials and fee-based grant-writing courses for new and experienced grant writers. The Foundation Finder search is a good way to find funders in your area.

50. http://www.goaskalice.columbia.edu/

Go Ask Alice!

Go Ask Alice's Q&A database houses numerous health-related questions and answers. It is produced by Columbia University's Health Education Program.

51. http://www.health.gov/nhic

National Health Information Center (NHIC)

The NHIC is a health information referral service. NHIC puts health professionals and consumers who have health questions in touch with organizations that are best able to provide answers.

NEWS STORIES

52. http://www.reutershealth.com

Reuters Health Products and Services

Reuters is the premier supplier of health and medical news on the Internet. The Health eLine is a wonderful section for the general public.

53. http://www.usatoday.com/news/health/default.htm

USA Today Health

This section of *USA Today* provides some of the most current news stories related to health.

54. http://www.nlm.nih.gov/medlineplus/newsbydate.html

MedlinePlus—Health News by Date

The news section of MedlinePlus provides current health-related articles from the past 30 days from the New York Times Syndicate, Reuters Health Information, and others.

HEALTH EDUCATION/HEALTH PROMOTION JOBS

55. http://www.hpcareer.net

HPCareer.Net

This is the official career resource site for the American Kinesiotherapy Association (AKTA), the Medical-Fitness Association (MFA), and the National Commission for Health Education Credentialing (NCHEC).

56. http://sph.emory.edu/careers/index.html

Rollins School of Public Health at Emory—Careers

Includes a section titled Public Health Jobs.

HEALTH POLICY

57. http://www.nashp.org

National Academy for State Health Policy

The National Academy for State Health Policy conducts policy analysis; provides training and technical assistance to states; produces informational resources; and convenes state, regional, and national forums. This site enables the user to access these services and the results of policy studies that have been completed.

58. http://www.heritage.org

    The Heritage Foundation

    This site provides access to well-written and well-documented health policy research and analysis papers in which the conclusions often reflect a more conservative perspective.

59. http://rwjf.org/

    The Robert Wood Johnson Foundation

    The Robert Wood Johnson Foundation has a goal of funding projects that improve the health and health care of all Americans. This site features many of the foundation's policy papers, current and future studies, and projects that the foundation is or will consider funding. The organization is considered nonpartisan.

60. http://kff.org/

    The Henry J. Kaiser Family Foundation

    The Henry J. Kaiser Family Foundation is a nonprofit, privately operating foundation focusing on the major healthcare issues facing the nation. The foundation is an independent voice and source of facts and analysis for policy makers, the media, the healthcare community, and the general public.

61. http://www.commonwealthfund.org/

    The Commonwealth Fund

    This site contains policy briefs and full-text health policy papers that are well written and well documented and are often from a more liberal perspective.

62. http://www.statecoverage.org/

    State Coverage Initiatives (SCI)

    The SCI program is a national initiative of The Robert Wood Johnson Foundation that works with states to plan, execute, and maintain health insurance expansions, as well as to improve the availability and affordability of healthcare coverage. The site includes the results of many states' initiatives to increase health insurance coverage for their residents.

GENERAL

63. http://findarticles.com/p/articles/tn_health

    Find articles

    Provides free access to millions of articles from many top publications.

64. https://scholar.google.com/

    Google Scholar

    This site provides another alternative to search through scholarly literature across many disciplines and sources, including theses, books, abstracts, and articles. Use the "More" link, choose "Settings", then click on Library links to link to electronic materials at libraries where you have borrowing rights.

References

California State University Chico. (2013). Evaluating information applying the CRAAP test. Retrieved February 16, 2016, from http://www.csuchico.edu/lins/handouts/eval_websites.pdf

Cottrell, R. R. (1997). *A guide to evaluating a journal article*. Unpublished manuscript.

Hibbard, J. H., & Greene, J. (2013). What the evidence shows about patient activation: Better outcomes and health care experiences; fewer data on costs. *Health Affairs, 32* (2), 207–214.

Riegelman, R. K. (2005). *Studying a study and testing a test: How to read medical literature* (5th ed.). Philadelphia: Lippincott Williams & Wilkins.

University of Akron. (2013). *Government documents*. Retrieved May 27, 2013, from http://www.uakron.edu/libraries/services/services-detail.dot?inode=360659&title=Government%20Documents.

Future Trends in Health Education/Promotion

Chapter Objectives

After reading this chapter and answering the questions at the end, you should be able to:

- Identify a setting in which health education specialists will practice in the next five years to a greater degree than they do today.

- Describe four major societal changes that will influence the practice of health education/promotion in the next 10 years.

- Explain at least one major implication of credentialing for future health education specialists.

- Compare and contrast the roles of health education specialists in the four practice settings.

- Identify several reasons that health education specialists should be optimistic about future employment opportunities.

- Evaluate the role of the health education specialist in addressing the increasing costs of health care.

I t is said that one of the few constants in life is change. Societal trends are having an increasing impact on the profession of health education/promotion. The topic of health is consistently of interest to the populace in the United States. With increasing numbers of citizens interested in health information, spiraling healthcare costs, a reliance on technology for information delivery and acquisition, rapidly changing demographic patterns, a heightened skepticism of the medical establishment and health insurance companies, the passage of the Affordable Care Act, and a more interconnected world, the environment that will confront health education specialists in the next 20 years is quite different from that of only a decade ago. These changes present the health education specialist with enormous opportunities. The focus of this chapter is to explore future developments in the discipline of health education/promotion, and we hope, to create a sense of excitement and anticipation about the challenges that lie ahead.

Imagine that you have just arrived in the United States from another planet. The year is 1995. Assume that the first thing you see is a one-hour television news program. Based solely on that program and the commercial messages during the station breaks, how would you describe the lives of people on the planet you are visiting? Now, transport yourself ahead to today and repeat the exercise. Although it is not the purpose of this chapter to dwell on comparative history, it is noteworthy that, in a brief span of 20-plus years, the communication methods and patterns in the United States and many other countries have changed dramatically. For example, in the early 1990s there was effectively no online access to information of any sort. In 2010, up to 80 percent of all U.S. adults using the Internet reported using it to seek information about health (Fox, 2011). Several of the aforementioned societal shifts have profound implications for the way health education/promotion will be practiced as the 21st century continues its second decade.

The first section of this chapter discusses changing demographic patterns. Societal trends that are predicted to play a role in the practice of health education/promotion in future decades will be featured. Issues related to credentialing and preparation will follow. Using this information as a foundation, the chapter concludes by postulating about the impact of these changes for the health education specialist in the school, public health, work-site, and medical care settings. One caveat is in order before this discussion: Obviously, no one knows exactly what the future will hold. The information presented is meant to stimulate thinking about the role health education specialists will play from now until the years 2020–2030.

▷ Demographic Changes

Over the past 30 years, the population growth rate in the United States has increased at about 1 percent per year. Although this stable growth pattern is probably manageable for the long term, a more in-depth study of the **demographic profile**—the breakdown of the U.S. population by age group, sex, race, and ethnicity—shows a dramatically altered picture from that of just 10 years ago. This consistently changing demographic profile—specifically, a greater percentage of minority residents and an ever aging population—has important implications for the future practice of health education specialists (see **Figure 10.1**).

▶ **Figure 10.1** Health promotion for the elderly will be in increasing demand in the next century.

Minority Population Changes

Clark's (1994) comments, written midway through the last decade of the 2?? century, remain cogent today. She states, "We are undergoing a massive change in cult??? ??? society. We are literally looking different as a nation and the conventional majority ??? ??? norms are being challenged as we become a more diverse, more ethnic, more ??? culture. Health educators have long prided themselves with working across culture??? ??? cultural changes are . . . greater than we have experienced previously" (p. 137).

It seems that the increased racial and ethnic diversity in the United State??? ??? major causes. In the 1800s and early to mid-1900s, the bulk of immigrants to the ??? ??? came from Western Europe. Hale (2000) mentions that worsening economic con??? ??? Mexico and Central America over the decade from 2000 to 2010 are largely respon??? ??? the large number of immigrants from those areas. Gheisar and Clark (2000) write th??? ??? e populations streaming to the United States from war-ravaged regions of Asia, A??? ??? Eastern Europe are presenting new challenges (and opportunities) for the public h??? ??? munity. This wave of new immigration, coupled with the fact that, regardless of ??? ??? origin, immigrants have higher rates of fertility than native-born peoples, mean??? ??? hifts in culture and the challenges to majority norms alluded to by Clark are likel??? ???.

Statistics from a report by Colby and Ortman (2015) indicate that o??? ??? opulation grew by 3.3 percent since 2010. The 2010 census found that the U.S. ??? ??? ation was composed of 12.4 percent African American, 16.3 percent Hispanic, ??? ??? an or Pacific Islander, and 0.9 percent Native American. **Table 10.1** shows the ??? ??? ntage figures for each of these population groups by the year 2060 (U.S. Census ??? ???).

From Table 10.1 it is readily apparent that the greatest percentage incr??? ??? ext 45 years will come from the Hispanic and Asian/Pacific Islander groups. Th??? ??? rcentage increase of Hispanics and Asians from 2015 until 2060 is 115 perce??? ??? rcent, respectively. During this same time period, the percentage of non-Hisp??? ??? in the population will fall from 62.2 percent in the year 2015 to about 43.6 percen??? ??? r 2060, a decrease of about 8.2 percent of the overall 2060 U.S. all-races population.

At least one ramification of these changes, increasing numbers of ethnic m??? ??? students in public school, is already being felt in the classrooms of our nation. In 2012, approximately 49 percent of the children in public schools in the United States were minorities as reported by the National Center for Education Statistics (2015). According to the U.S. Census Bureau, in 2012 the majority 50.4 percent of children under one year of age in the United States are

TABLE 10.1 **Projected U.S. population percentages of African Americans, Hispanics, Native Americans, and Asians or Pacific Islanders: 2010 and 2060**

Race	2010 (%)	2060 (%)
African American	12.4	14.3
Hispanic	16.3	28.6
Native American	0.9	0.7
Asian/Pacific Islander	5.0	11.7

Source: U.S. Census Bureau (2012)

minority children (U.S. Census Bureau, 2012). From schools in Caldwell, Idaho, with a student population of nearly 65 percent Hispanic, to Chicago, Illinois, with a Hispanic and other minority race student population of more than 80 percent, the escalating minority population makes an already diverse nation even more so. This trend presents health education specialists with an ever-widening array of opportunities and challenges as the 21st century continues to unfold.

Aging

Another demographic factor that will impact the practice of health education/promotion in the future is the aging population. A report from the Pew Research Center (2014) lists persons age 65 or older as currently representing 13.0 percent of the U.S. population. Between the years 2010 and 2050, the population older than 65 is expected to grow to equal 22.0 percent of the total. To further illustrate this trend, the median age of the U.S. population in 2010 was 37.2. In the year 2020, it is estimated to be 38.3; and in 2050, it will be 41.

One of the major reasons for the aging trend is that older Americans are living longer than ever before. Other causative factors accentuating changes in age demographics are that married couples in the United States are having fewer children, and the oldest of the baby boomers (those born between 1946 and 1964) are now beginning to retire. This group's massive size causes it to have a dominant effect on U.S. population statistics.

▷ Societal Trends

There probably has not been a time when societal change was as rapid as in the latter decades of the 20th century. For example, since 1960, there have been changes in societal mores and practices, such as more openness to cohabitation, a greater tolerance for premarital sex, more vocal and open gay relationships including the legalization of gay marriage, a greater number of single-parent households, an increase in child abuse, more violence, an increase in the amount and availability of pornographic materials, massive changes in the number of ethical issues related to medicine, alterations in the way the medical establishment is organized and medical care is delivered, a decreasing respect for authority of any kind, declining state and federal support for K–12 public schools and higher education institutions, an infusion of and a reliance on technology, and a distrust of the political establishment in general. All of these factors play a big role in shaping the structure of society in the future. This section discusses several of the major societal trends that experts agree will impact health education/promotion in the new millennium.

Technology

Certainly, the boom in **technology** has affected, if not transformed, the lives of many people around the globe. Many of the advances in communication, transportation, medicine, engineering, and ease of access to information have created an enhanced quality of life for people worldwide. The increased availability and use of technology also creates myriad opportunities for the prospective health education specialist in the planning, design, implementation, and evaluation of programs and materials.

Today, it is impossible to find a campus that does not feature student computer labs in numerous locations and wireless technology in all buildings. In today's environment, many courses and even entire degree programs are offered using Web-based technologies, enabling the student to participate in class sessions in "real time" no matter where he or she resides. The constantly expanding technological capabilities in the field of education have created a learning environment in which information is readily available and lessons can be easily structured to require a greater degree of critical thinking and be more interactive than was possible only a few years ago. An increasing number of journals are published only in electronic form; no printed hard copy is available, and projects are under way to digitize entire collections of books and monographs, making the information contained in those publications not only more readily accessible but also content searchable. There is no doubt that the knowledge explosion trend fueled by new innovations in educational technology will continue and accelerate.

What does this rapid acceleration mean for health education specialists? Gold and Atkinson (2006) offer several intriguing considerations on how the advances in technology can and will revolutionize the delivery of health education/promotion:

- Extending our traditional health education/promotion delivery systems by reaching out across time and space, as well as literacy and language
- Allowing both synchronous and asynchronous communications in pictures, sounds, movement, and virtual reality
- Individualizing and personalizing communication and instruction through tailored messages and interventions based on the variables we know are likely to influence interest, ability, readiness, and a host of other relevant variables
- Extending the way we internalize, understand, individualize, and use massive amounts of data through instant access to even the minutest detail in a large data repository
- Enhancing opportunities to provide new services and interventions by creating new practices and strategies (p. 46)

The increased use of Web 2.0 and the expanding number and use of social media Internet sites and messaging protocols over the past five to ten years have elevated the possibilities for health promotion much as Gold and Atkinson postulated. Research by Thackery and colleagues (2008), Korda and Itani (2013), and Neiger and colleagues (2012) on methods to effectively use social media for health promotion has demonstrated that these media can work to not only inform and change attitudes but to alter behavior. As with most "in person" interventions, however, crafting the messages using behavioral theory and making certain that the message is designed in such a manner that two-way communication is achieved greatly increase the chances of success.

Clearly technology will greatly shape the face of the delivery of health education/promotion into the future. Students of health education/promotion must become familiar with the various media methods available to gather and deliver information including the creation of messages across multiple platforms such as tablets, laptop computers, and phones and, perhaps, in multiple languages. Social media such as Twitter, Facebook, Pinterest, and Google+ are all ways to communicate around specific health conditions. IMS Institute for Informatics looked at patient and consumer use of health apps and found there are over 165,000 health-related software programs or apps that allow people to track their health. Individuals can wear fitness trackers, and the data connects to other digital devices to track steps, sleep, calories, and water. Apps can send alerts to move more, provide health information, and people can join groups for support (Chen et al., 2016). There may be a time in the not too distant future when health education specialists will be able to personalize messages (e.g., oncologists personalizing treatments based on DNA tests) (D. Zuckerman, personal communication, 2013).

Family Structure

The U.S. family structure has changed dramatically since the 1960s (see **Figure 10.2**). The **traditional family** (two parents and their children) is becoming less and less common because of factors such as high rates of divorce, smaller families, postponed marriage and childbearing, teenage and nonmarital childbearing, stepfamilies, homosexual couples, and dual-earner marriages (Acock & Demo, 1994). According to the Pew Research Center (2015), only 61 percent of households fit the definition of a family having both a married male and female at home, and one fourth of those homes are in a remarriage situation. Thirty-two percent of families have children younger than 18 living with them.

▶ **Figure 10.2** An awareness of different family structures, such as extended families or single parents, is an important consideration when planning prevention messages.

In addition, about 33 percent of Americans live alone or in nonfamily combinations, such as with housemates, friends, or partnerships outside legal marriage.

In 1970, 85 percent of children younger than the age of 18 lived with both parents, and 18 percent lived with the mother only. In 2012, 64 percent of those younger than 18 lived with both parents, and 24 percent lived with the mother only. Of note is the fact that slightly more than 6 percent of 0- to 17-year-olds in 2012 lived with grandparents, other relatives, or in the homes of nonrelatives (Child Trends Data Bank, 2013).

The impact caused by these new structures is being felt throughout our society. Children are the most affected. The Pew Research Center (2015) reported that 31 percent of children under 6 today have experienced a major change in their family structure including parental divorce, separation, marriage, cohabitation, or death (p. 17).

With the high cost of goods and services in the United States, the number of mothers in the workforce with children under 18 has changed dramatically. A 2015 Pew Research Center study found that 71 percent of those mothers are now in the workforce—an increase of nearly 80 percent since 1980. This places a strain even on nuclear families with two parents; affordable daycare services for the children must be obtained. For many low-income and single-parent families, the choice is no care or supervision at all—a situation that puts children at risk. Under the Affordable Care Act (ACA), more people have health insurance through the state health exchanges, Medicaid expansion, and employers. In 2014, the first year people were required to purchase insurance under the ACA, 89.6 percent of people had health insurance coverage for part or all of the year (Smith & Medalia, 2015). Currently, there are 19 states that have chosen not to expand Medicaid so there are still millions of people without health insurance who typically work in service-oriented positions that often pay minimum wage and are a major source of employment for many low-skilled workers (Garfield & Damico, 2016). As a result, nearly 32 percent percent of children under 18 in the United States are living in poverty. This is the highest rate in the industrialized world and most poor children are Latino, black, and American Indian (Yang, Ekono, and Skinner, 2016). The linkage between these factors may be a predisposing condition leading to an increased rate of child abuse (McKenzie, Kotecki, & Pinger, 2008). Finally, it is no secret that the economic downturn since 2008 has contributed significantly to increasing the number of families and children under economic stress as a result of job loss or underemployment. Although the number of people employed in 2016 has actually exceeded the number of persons employed prior to the downturn, the type and often the pay scale of available jobs differs greatly from the job mix before 2008, further exacerbating the problem of economic distress (B. Parrish, personal communication, 2016).

The changes previously noted have significant implications for health education specialists. Family structures will likely remain diverse in the coming years and will probably operate on a new set of norms. In other words, new methods of reaching individuals, families, and communities will need to be created to improve the health of all family members in accordance with their needs.

Political Climate

As was mentioned previously, there remains little doubt that today there is an increasing frustration with politics and politicians in general. Whether a person is a **conservative**, one who generally distrusts governmental regulations and tax-supported programs for addressing social or economic problems; a **moderate**, one who usually acts in a more situationally specific manner in regard to using tax-supported programs to solve societal problems; or a **liberal**, one who generally supports government programs to attack social and economic problems, there seems to be no end to the bickering and infighting among and between members of various political parties. Many of the political issues considered in Congress relate to health. For example, the landmark agreement between the tobacco industry and the states over the sale and marketing of tobacco products to minors; the addition of prescription drug benefits to Medicare; determination of Medicaid eligibility and Medicaid expansion; the repeal of a motorcycle helmet law in Texas; the passage of physician-assisted suicide laws in California, Oregon, Washington, Montana, and Vermont; the escalating cost of prescription drugs; debates as to whether to allow health insurance companies to offer coverage across state lines; immigration reform and whether to offer healthcare coverage for those undocumented immigrants currently in the United States; climate change; pornography as a public health issue; minimum wage; timely physical and mental health care for veterans returning from wars in Iraq and Afghanistan; passage of and stages of implementation of the Affordable Care Act; community health center legislation; gun control; and the debate as to whether to increase spending on school lunches at the expense of Supplemental Nutrition Assistance Program (SNAP) aka food stamp allotments are examples of political issues that directly impact the health of the populace.

Politics and health seem to be inextricably linked. Some governmental officials and legislators worry that public health professionals infringe on personal autonomy by advocating for seat belt laws, tobacco laws, work-site wellness programs, helmet laws, air bags, environmental protection, healthier options in fast foods and public schools, gun control laws, and health insurance for all. Others believe that legislation fostering a social climate that enhances the health of the population as a whole is worth the sacrifice of some personal choice and autonomy.

As citizens and professionals, the involvement of health education specialists in the political process is important. O'Rourke (2006) states, "Health education not only seeks to change lifestyles, but to create public understanding of the political issues involved in public health programs" (p. 9). He goes on to challenge all health education specialists to assume a **macrolevel** view of health problems. Using this approach, health education specialists move from a position of assisting behavior change one person at a time to community-based interventions. In implementing the community-based programs, success often depends on the health education specialist having a working knowledge of the political process and how it impacts every decision. Hunter (2008) supports the fact that public health professionals can no longer be bystanders but must become passionate advocates for healthy change in individuals and communities. He believes that the collective advocacy of all public health practitioners is vital in moving governmental bodies to support and improve health.

There is little doubt that health education specialists must become participants in the political process. O'Rourke (2006) eloquently makes a case for enhancing the effectiveness of health education/promotion through an approach that

> encompasses collective responsibility and community involvement through participation in
> the political process and service on county health boards, city councils, and school boards. In
> these capacities, health educators can influence the health of entire communities and not rely
> on the 'one person at a time' model of improving health through individual responsibility. (p. 8)

To that end, a method for health education specialists to increase their visibility and political clout is advanced by McDermott (2000) when he challenges present and future health education specialists to consider the importance of research in the practice of health education/promotion. For interventions to be effective, health education specialists must use evidence-based practices when these practices are known. Future gains in the effectiveness and scope of prevention programs probably will be made only when health education specialists insist on pushing the research envelope to determine the factors that affect health and cause health disparities in populations, are components of effective intervention programs, and allow for dissemination of these programs across a variety of settings. Including community partners, community-based participatory research, and legislators in these research efforts is a strategy proven to gain trust and allies more welcoming to the benefit of macrolevel initiatives.

Medical Care Establishment and the Affordable Care Act

The healthcare system in the United States continues to be in need of an overhaul. Passage of the Affordable Care Act in early 2010 was a start in the right direction, but the exact impact of that legislation is far from certain as many of the provisions in the plan are set to be enacted from 2014 to 2020. Meanwhile, the cost of care continues to escalate, and the system seems stuck in an unsustainable model of reimbursement for procedures (fee-for-service) instead of a capitated reimbursement structure for helping people stay well. Citizens increasingly desire to be participants in their own care and to be provided with options. Enhancing the quality of life as opposed to simply increasing longevity is becoming a prevalent goal of U.S. healthcare consumers.

There are several reasons for this trend. Although few would deny that our medical care system has been responsible for saving countless lives, clearly health is largely a reflection of the nature of the environments in which a person resides, personal lifestyle choices, and standards of living, and not the medical care system. In the United States, medical care tends to concentrate on secondary and tertiary care and to ignore the value of primary prevention. In the United States, only three cents of every healthcare dollar are spent on prevention, and well more than 75 percent of healthcare costs are attributable to preventable disease conditions (Forsberg & Fichtenberg, 2012).

These points are substantiated by Williams, McClellan, and Rivlin (2010) and Goodarz and colleagues (2010) when they state that healthier lives are best fostered in a climate of a culture of health. What seems to be most important in creating and maintaining health are the actions taken by individuals and communities to select and support habits like choosing what food we eat, having healthy relationships, staying physically active, and investing in safe and environmentally friendly neighborhoods. Much of health is tied not to medical intervention but to primary prevention.

The Affordable Care Act has increased the opportunities for health education specialists. Koh and Sebelius (2010) document that this law "promotes wellness in the workplace, providing new health promotion opportunities for employers and employees" (p. 4). In addition, the act strengthens the community role in promoting prevention and serves to enhance partnerships between state and local government and community groups and nonprofits.

Professionals representing the Society for Public Health Education (SOPHE, 2013) have published a "must read" issue brief titled, "Affordable Care Act: Opportunities and Challenges for Health Education Specialists," which discusses the potential expanding roles for health education specialists in both the healthcare and community settings under healthcare reform. This document succinctly captures the positives and barriers inherent as health education specialists strive to become included as members of a health team that seeks to promote health in the whole person.

The Boise, Idaho–based nonprofit corporation, Healthwise, the provider of the Web-based health information found in WebMD and responsible for much of the health education/promotion content disseminated by major insurance companies and hospitals around the country, offers an example of the value of health education/promotion in a clinical arena. Healthwise professionals have developed a health information and education prescription format tailored for consumers so that they can obtain the information they need to make choices about their own care. In addition, the information equips them to ask for the care that they need and facilitates their saying no to care that they do not need. Thus, patient autonomy is enhanced.

This approach bodes well for enhanced opportunities for health education specialists who desire to practice in a healthcare setting in large part because of the myriad set of situations, policies, and approaches that seem to have no solution: high pharmaceutical costs, nearly 36 million Americans currently without health insurance (Marken, 2015), continuous federal tinkering with both the Medicare and Medicaid systems, lack of oversight for universal quality of care standards, high-cost care with limited emphasis on quality, lack of affordability of private pay insurance, inconsistent chronic disease management protocols, and frustration with a lack of emphasis on prevention. Given these circumstances, health education specialists can facilitate patient choice by helping patients understand their options regarding physician choice, healthcare insurance plan, type of care, and intensity of services. In addition, they can assist medical organizations by increasing patient satisfaction through contributing to more one-on-one contact, improving patterns of communication between patient and provider, evaluating outcomes, and enhancing patient compliance with treatment regimens (T. Epperly, personal communication, Family Medicine Residency of Idaho, Boise, May 2015).

▷ Professional Preparation and Credentialing

Although the issues of professional preparation and credentialing were extensively covered in Chapter 6, both have implications for the future practice of health education/promotion. Thus, the reasons why health education/promotion practice might be affected by these issues are of some importance.

Professional Preparation

In this discussion, it is not our intent to provide a list of courses that must be taken to become a "better" health education specialist. Coursework is by nature specific to the institution you are attending. Course titles and descriptions vary widely from one program to another. As you are aware, the coursework you will take in your degree program is interdisciplinary. We attempt to provide some ideas, concepts, and objectives for you to consider as you enter your preparation program.

The social changes previously discussed in this chapter are the challenges driving health education specialists of the future to be proactive in meeting the demands placed on them.

What tasks will a health education specialist need to be able to perform to be effective in the decades ahead? Clark (1994) helps answer this question by making several salient points about health education/promotion in the future:

1. The mission will be less providing factual information and more helping people become more analytical thinkers . . .

2. There will be . . . stronger partnerships with the medical establishment. . . .

3. Health education specialists will need . . . Long-term, not short-term, thinking . . .

4. A greater emphasis will be placed on values clarification. . . .

5. . . . Education at the community level will be the focus of most health interventions.

6. There will be an enhanced need for quality research . . .

7. Health education specialists must . . . use technology to help people learn.

8. . . . The gap between school and community services will close.

9. Environmental activism will continue to emerge . . .

10. . . . people will judge the success of health education/promotion by whether or not their quality of life has improved.

Several of Clark's thoughts echo those of O'Rourke (2006), who challenges health education specialists to be more macrolevel-oriented. In other words, there is an ever-growing need to facilitate health education/promotion interventions at the community level (as opposed to the individual level, or **microlevel**). Inherent in this charge is that those who reside in the community where the intervention occurs will be totally involved in the planning from the outset. English and Videto (1997) affirm these observations when they state, "Regardless of our place of practice, our ability to identify and meet the needs of our local communities and neighborhoods is likely to be the measure that will determine our success as health educators . . . successful programs use community involvement" (p. 4).

Three additional documents that provide information about the competencies health education specialists must possess into the future are described next. The first two can be found using the Weblinks at the end of this chapter. The first document features the deliberations by members of the Committee on Educating Public Health Professionals for the 21st Century. The workshop participants who wrote the article "Who Will Keep the Public Healthy? Workshop Summary" (Weblinks #3) identify eight new content areas that should be added to the curricula of individuals studying to practice public health: informatics, genomics, communication, community-based participatory research, global health, health policy, health law, and public health ethics. Although the report is largely directed at universities offering graduate programs, even a cursory glance finds several suggested content areas that are relevant to the practice of health education/promotion. The list also shows the rapidly expanding knowledge base the future health education specialist will need to have to successfully interact with health professionals from a variety of other fields. The more understanding a health education specialist has about the vocabulary and nature of the work of other health providers, the more likely she or he is to be an accepted and valued member of the healthcare community.

The second document is the Web site for the National Commission for Health Education Credentialing (NCHEC) (2016), which features the results of a study titled "2015 Health Education Specialist Practice Analysis (HESPA)" commissioned by the Society for Public Health

Education (SOPHE), and the National Commission for Health Education Credentialing (NCHEC). The findings report on changes in health education practice since the 2010 Health Educator Job Analysis (HEJA) study.

The third document, a cogent paper written by McKenzie (2004), cautions that those in charge of health education preparation programs must not assume that it is possible or even advisable to prepare "generic" health education specialists. The four practice settings to which he refers in the quote that follows are discussed later in this chapter. McKenzie states, ". . . even though the responsibilities and competencies of health educators are similar regardless of the settings, the work is indeed different and the preparation cannot be the same . . . " (p. 48).

In June, 2014, the Council on Education for Public Health released accreditation standards for Standalone Baccalaureate Programs (SBP). This allows for health education programs not associated with schools of public health to go through a nationally recognized accreditation process. The former approval process offered by SOPHE/AAHE Baccalaureate Program Approval Committee (SABPAC) ended in 2015 (Elaine Ault, personal communication, April 2016).

It is apparent that tomorrow's health education specialists must be able to respond rapidly to changes in all avenues of society. When planning, implementing, and evaluating programs and working in multidimensional settings, they must enter into collaborative relationships with healthcare professionals from other disciplines in a spirit of cooperation. Health education specialists who are not afraid to be innovative, who respect but do not fear change, who are not just purveyors of information but community builders and facilitators of learning, who are politically active, who continue to be curious and learn themselves, who have a sense of adventure, and who seek the truth through thoughtful research, study, and dialogue are the individuals who will lead our profession into the next several decades.

Credentialing

The history of and reasons for credentialing were thoroughly covered in Chapter 6. There are, however, several facets of credentialing that need reemphasis because they have profound implications for the future practice of health education/promotion.

The credentialing process as it now stands begins with the candidate's submitting a transcript of coursework in health education to the NCHEC. On verification by NCHEC that the candidate has completed coursework leading to a degree in health education and the coursework has focused on the responsibilities and competencies of an entry-level health education specialist, the applicant is permitted to sit for the certification exam. Exam questions are based on the seven responsibilities and competencies for entry-level health education specialists. Individuals who pass the exam are awarded a Certified Health Education Specialist (CHES) credential. Those individuals must then complete continuing education units on a regular basis to maintain their credential.

A question that is often asked is, "Should all individuals who seek a CHES certification complete the same process?" As mentioned previously, this tends to skew the credential in favor of creating a generic health education specialist (McKenzie, 2004). Some practicing health education specialists argue that the skills needed to teach health in a school setting differ from those needed to conduct a community program at a local American Cancer Society office or to direct health promotion programs at a worksite or clinical healthcare site. For example, school health education specialists often see the need to be content specialists, whereas community health education specialists may be more focused on process and skills.

Health education specialists practice in a variety of settings (e.g., school, worksite, community, and health care), they may work with different populations (e.g., adults, the aged, children, and minorities), they may be process specialists (e.g., program planners, program implementers, and program evaluators), or they may be content specialists (e.g., HIV/AIDS, cancer prevention, injury or violence prevention, and nutrition). Should there be a generic credential? Perhaps in the future there will be "practice-specific" credentials. A potential important consequence of having a CHES credential is that of eligibility for reimbursement for services rendered. As different care models are advanced with prevention as a focus (thanks to the Affordable Care Act), insurers are limiting the types of providers eligible for reimbursement. Without some external credential or license, it is highly unlikely that any health education services rendered in a medical care setting will be reimbursed (Idaho Blue Shield Human Resources Department, personal communication, April 2015).

The credentialing process is here to stay. The bottom line is that this certification program does establish a national standard for individual health education specialists. In the past, certifications could differ by state, and some states or regions had local certifications and registries. Having a national certification better ensures that health education specialists in every state or setting have the same training and academic requirements. The CHES process works well and is endorsed by prevention specialists and organizations nationwide. Potential changes to the credentialing process and necessary competencies that emanate from the 2015 Health Education Specialist Practice Analysis (HESPA) referenced in the previous section of this chapter will most likely occur. Students should stay abreast of developments in credentialing by visiting the NCHEC and SOPHE Web sites on a regular basis.

Caile Spear, literally the last president of the now disbanded professional organization, AAHE, posits that the joining together of the public health professions that focus on prevention will better make their voice more clearly heard and their message more uniform. She goes on to say that the joining of these professions will mimic what funding agencies are doing in that they would be soliciting projects that encompass holistic approaches to addressing health issues. Funding agencies are moving away from providing funds for specific health problems (e.g., substance abuse, child abuse, lack of physical activity, etc.) to funding more global strategies. Similarly, a united group of prevention professionals (including health education specialists), regardless of practice setting, will be more powerful in making a local and national case for the role of prevention in overall health than the current model in which prevention professionals often are members of several different professional organizations (personal communication, May 2013).

As the profession of health education/promotion continues to evolve and health education specialists become more visible partners in the delivery of health services, students considering careers in this field should seriously consider obtaining CHES certification. The CHES credential assists employers in identifying practitioners who have met national standards, and it assures the consumers of health education/promotion services that the health educators with whom they work are competent professionals.

It is important to note that several states now include health education specialists in the list of approved providers in Medicaid reimbursed programs such as weight loss clinics (Idaho Administrative Rules, 2016). Each health education specialist needs to check with her or his state to see if this action applies in their locale.

▷ Implications for Practice Settings

Chapter 7 detailed the variety of settings in which health education specialists can practice: the worksite, school, clinical/health care, and public health. Each setting has unique characteristics, and the practice set of skills or competencies may vary from one setting to another. However, the settings also are similar in that the goal of health education/promotion is to create a climate that facilitates the improvement of health status for every member of the population served by each entity. The first part of this chapter described various influences destined to impact the health of the populace into the next century. This section briefly summarizes the future role of the health education specialist in each setting.

School Setting

"Children don't learn as well when they are not healthy" (Seffrin, 1994, p. 397). "Schools are an integral part of the community, and, if we don't have high quality school health education we will pay the price later in higher costs to all of us. Health education specialists regardless of practice setting should support and be champions for well-funded, vigorous and vital school health programs" (Spear, personal communication, June, 2016). In 2015, Congress passed the Every Student Succeeds Act (ESSA), and for the first time health education has been included as a "core subject" (United States 114th Congress, 2015–16). Providing high-quality health education in schools means more students will learn how to increase positive health behaviors and reduce negative ones. These statements characterize the goal and importance of school health education and provide direction for school health education specialists.

If children's well-being is to be maintained or enhanced, a coordinated approach to providing health education is needed (Allensworth & Kolbe, 1987). The Centers for Disease Control and Prevention (CDC) has expanded the former Coordinated School Health model to The Whole School, Whole Community, Whole Child model. This new model "promotes greater alignment between health and education outcomes . . . creates a unified model that supports a systematic, integrated, and collaborative approach to health and learning" (Lewallen, Hunt, Potts-Datema, Zaza, & Giles, 2015). Model components include (1) health education, (2) nutrition environment and services, (3) employee wellness, (4) social and emotional school climate, (5) physical environment, (6) health services, (7) counseling, psychological, and social services, (8) community involvement, (9) family engagement, and (10) physical education and physical activity.

Should you choose to practice health education/promotion in a school setting, what skills and abilities must you possess if schools are to incorporate a coordinated health education/promotion program to address the health needs of children and adolescents, both now and in the future? In light of the information on influences on health in this chapter and that on settings for health education/promotion from Chapter 7, we think that the following skills are imperative. You must be able to

1. Create a logical scope and sequence to health content units that incorporate age-appropriate information.

2. Prepare and deliver lessons that are participatory in nature, stress skill development, and foster attitudes necessary for problem solving and informed decision making.

3. Use technology and social media to assist in both updating your own skills and delivering health education/promotion messages to your school and community.

4. Acquire sound oral and written communication techniques.

5. Apply behavior-change strategies and what is known about environmental influences on behavior to the classroom setting.

6. Teach and promote the enhancement of strategies to increase health literacy among the population served to reduce health disparities (Hasnain-Wynia & Wolf, 2010).

7. Use both qualitative and quantitative strategies to evaluate your lessons, your units, and the district health education/promotion program.

8. Assess the health needs of the students, faculty, and staff.

9. Ensure that health and counseling services are provided for students.

10. Read and interpret the findings of health research on effective health programs and practices.

11. Learn about the influence of culture on health, cultivate sensitivity toward it, and instill an awareness of it in your teaching.

12. Assist teachers at all grade levels in obtaining age-appropriate health education materials and help coordinate a classroom scope and sequence for all grade levels in your district.

13. Work both independently and as a member of a team.

14. Collaborate with health education specialists practicing in the community, work-site, or healthcare setting to coordinate the delivery of disease prevention and health promotion messages and programs.

15. Create or coordinate a parent/community health education/promotion advisory council.

16. Actively participate in local, state, regional, and national professional organizations.

17. Serve as resource person and liaison between the school health setting and other settings in which health education might occur.

School health educators who possess these skills will be well prepared to lead programs that enhance the health of the students, teachers, and staff in their schools.

Work-Site Setting

The workplace of today bears little resemblance to that of only 20 years ago. Because many employers want to attract the best employees and realize that employee satisfaction is key in productivity and retention, worksites have introduced programs for employees and their families that provide continuing education, recreational opportunities, health promotion, and financial planning. In particular, worksites have become an increasingly important setting for health education/promotion programs. Examples of programs offered include stress management, work-site safety, drug and alcohol abuse prevention, and tobacco cessation. As noted previously in this chapter, the Affordable Care Act also signals the advent of a renewed emphasis on work-site health promotion (Koh & Sebelius, 2010).

The influence of changing demographic patterns on health education/promotion in general was discussed previously. However, another factor must be taken into account when specifically anticipating the future direction of work-site health promotion. The greatest percentage of persons joining the workforce in the decades between 2015 and 2050 will be women and minorities.

The expansion of work-site health promotion programs bodes well for the future of health education/promotion and the concurrent need for an increasing number of trained health education specialists. This truth has broad implications for the future practice of work-site health education/promotion. Together with the information presented both earlier in this chapter and in Chapter 7, the following competencies represent a baseline for the future practice of health education/promotion in work-site settings:

1. Become familiar with the culture inherent in a business setting.

2. Use up-to-date technology to market programs to work-site supervisors, employees, and their families through newsletters, brochures, Internet chat groups, and social media.

3. Plan and manage a budget.

4. Acquire grant writing skills.

5. Implement programs in a manner consistent with management philosophy.

6. Coordinate needs assessments of work-site populace and conduct evaluations of program components.

7. Design and employ evaluation strategies that are outcome-based to assess program effectiveness.

8. Conduct fitness assessments and participate in health screenings.

9. Function as a resource person for health information for employees and their families.

10. Identify and work with aspects of the corporate organizational climate that facilitate or impede participation.

11. Recognize the importance of cultural and demographic influences on individual and group health behavioral choices.

12. Attain a working knowledge of epidemiological and statistical principles and applications.

13. Acquire sound oral and written communication techniques.

14. Gain a thorough understanding of current, relevant literature and well-designed research studies that influence health promotion practice in the work-site setting.

15. Work both independently and as a member of a team.

16. Teach and promote the enhancement of strategies to increase health literacy among the population served to reduce health disparities (Hasnain-Wynia & Wolf, 2010).

17. Prepare and conduct prevention presentations to work-site subgroups.

18. Coordinate employee coalitions and steering committees to maximize employee input into program components.

19. Be able to apply behavior-change strategies and what is known about environmental influences on behavior to the work-site setting.

Incorporating competencies such as those listed previously into the professional preparation program will help ensure that you are ready to begin practice as a work-site health education specialist.

Public Health Setting

The community setting (called the *public health setting* in this text) has a myriad of options for the practice of health education/promotion. For example, health education specialists are employed in many local, city, state, and federal health departments; in many federal agencies; in county extension agencies; in nonprofit and volunteer health organizations (e.g., American Cancer Society, American Heart Association, American Red Cross); in churches; in homeless shelters; in grassroots community organizations; and in prisons. One reason for the diversity of opportunities is that the mission, goals, and objectives of one community agency may differ dramatically from those of another. Some agencies might have a health education specialist serving as a coordinator of services or as a fund-raiser, whereas in another agency the educator might plan, conduct, and evaluate programs. Another, more obvious, reason for increased employment opportunities is that almost every locale in the United States has one of the aforementioned groups.

The purpose of community health organizations is to both monitor and improve the health of the public they serve. Goodman (2000) mentions that when health education specialists combine forces with people from other professional disciplines (e.g., ecologists, economists, anthropologists, communication specialists), the probability of reducing the health risks of populations is heightened. Consequently, collaboration with community organizations and with other professionals to address population health is a skill that all health education specialists must develop. In this era of using health education/promotion to help reduce healthcare costs while improving the quality of care, and with an increasing need for community-level programs, public health education specialists are well positioned to participate in improving the health of citizens from all regions of the United States.

With employment opportunities for health education specialists in the public setting on the rise, what skills will the public health education specialists of the future need to function effectively? Following is a list of basic competencies or attributes that will be critical to the effective practice of public health education. They are not listed in any specific order of importance.

1. Recognize the importance of cultural and demographic influences on individual and group health behavioral choices.

2. Maintain competence in the use of technology and social media to access and deliver health-related information.

3. Learn to be flexible because the job probably will involve changing and varied responsibilities.

4. Learn another language.

5. Learn and use strategies to seek information, guidance, and support from community members regarding their health needs.

6. Assess strengths of communities in building a plan to assist them in meeting their health needs.

7. Design and employ evaluation strategies that are outcomes based to assess program effectiveness.

8. Gain a thorough understanding of current, relevant literature and well-designed research studies that influence practice in the community setting (i.e., community-based participatory research).

9. Apply behavior-change strategies and what is known about environmental influences on behavior to the public health setting.

10. Learn and practice research-based, coalition-building strategies.

11. Actively participate in local, state, regional, and national professional organizations.

12. Work independently and as a member of a team.

13. Advocate policies that enhance the role of prevention and provide for universal access to health services when needed.

14. Foster the ability to work in a multidisciplinary and a multicultural environment.

15. Teach and promote the enhancement of strategies to increase health literacy among the population served to reduce health disparities (Hasnain-Wynia & Wolf, 2010).

16. Study and apply the fundamentals of obtaining extramural funding.

17. Use a variety of marketing strategies to reach diverse community constituencies.

18. Attain a working knowledge of epidemiological and statistical principles and applications.

19. Acquire excellent oral and written communication techniques.

A well-trained community health education specialist will undoubtedly make an increased contribution to the health of diverse populations. With the increasing health awareness of U.S. citizens and the multitude of cultural changes in society, community health education specialists have a bright and exciting future.

Clinical or Healthcare Setting

Healthcare settings employ health education specialists in a variety of institutions and a multitude of ways. Health education specialists can be employed in for-profit and public hospitals, health maintenance organizations (HMOs), health insurance corporations, medical care clinics, and home health agencies. They might be involved in conducting one-on-one patient education; planning and implementing education programs for enrollees or other medical providers; coordinating community education programs on a variety of health topics; conducting program evaluations; marketing the health services available through the hospital, clinic, or HMO; conducting health education/promotion activities for the employees; or serving as a member of a community health promotion team.

Epperly (personal communication, May 2013) feels that healthcare providers, insurance companies, and the public in general are becoming more receptive to the notion that accurate and timely health information is an important part of any treatment regimen. Lack of adequate health education/promotion can negate potential positive contributions in the prevention and management of disease. With no end in sight to the skyrocketing costs of health care, the word *prevention* is being incorporated into more care plans than ever before.

Yarnall and colleagues (2003) note that the evidence of preventive services is well established but the rate of the delivery of preventive services by medical providers is severely lacking. Their study of time burdens required to deliver preventive care concluded that the major reason for the lack of delivery is that, to fulfill the U.S. Preventive Health Services Task Force recommendations, a primary care physician with a "normal" practice would have to dedicate nearly 7.5 hours per day solely to the delivery of preventive services. Obviously, this time allocation is impossible because physicians need to spend most their time diagnosing and treating disease. Yarnall's study concludes with the following statement: "Our current system of preventive care delivery—provided by physicians . . . no longer meets national needs. New methods of preventive care delivery are required, as well as a clearer focus on which services can be best provided, and by whom" (p. 640).

The shift in practice norms by most clinical healthcare professionals requires trained personnel to ensure that education in the healthcare setting meets the needs of both the patient and the provider and motivates the patient to adopt a healthier lifestyle and comply with any treatment regimen. Given the medical community's acceptance of the value of health education/promotion in patient care, the outlook is positive for more employment opportunities for health education specialists in healthcare settings. What skills, competencies, and attributes will be absolutely necessary for the health education specialist of the future who seeks employment in a healthcare setting? Following is a list of suggested competencies in no particular order:

1. Learn to perform basic health screening techniques like blood pressure monitoring and pulse and respiration measurements.

2. Obtain a working knowledge of epidemiological and statistical principles and applications.

3. Maintain competence in the use of technology to access and deliver health-related information.

4. Acquire sound oral and written communication techniques.

5. Become familiar with the clinical disease process.

6. Learn a second language.

7. Obtain a working knowledge of the role of informatics in assisting in prevention at all vulnerable points in the causal chains leading to disease, injury, or disability (Davies, Smith, & Gustafson, 2001).

8. Recognize the importance of cultural and demographic influences on individual and group health behavioral choices. Health education specialists should be culturally competent.

9. Be able to apply behavior-change strategies and what is known about environmental influences on behavior to the healthcare setting.

10. Coordinate interdisciplinary teams or steering committees to maximize input into program components.

11. Teach and promote the enhancement of strategies to increase health literacy among the population served to reduce health disparities (Hasnain-Wynia & Wolf, 2010).

12. Provide training in health education/promotion theory to other members of the healthcare team.

13. Become familiar with technological innovations to provide better outreach to patients, employees, and their families through a variety of electronic and hard copy newsletters, brochures, Internet chat groups, Web sites, and social media.

14. Advocate policies that enhance the role of prevention and provide for universal access to health services when needed.

15. Work independently and as a member of a team.

16. Prepare and deliver lessons that are participatory in nature and research-based, that stress skill development and foster attitudes necessary for problem solving and informed decision making.

17. Learn to be flexible, as the job probably will involve changing and varied responsibilities.

18. Serve as a liaison between the healthcare setting and other settings in which health education might occur.

19. Function as a resource person for health information for patients and their families.

With rapid changes occurring in medical care delivery today, there is much reason for health education specialists to be optimistic about employment opportunities. As the public demands health education/promotion and disease prevention as a part of their medical care treatment plan, health education specialists will increasingly be identified as the best prepared to assist individuals in adopting healthy lifestyles.

▷ Alternative Settings

Besides the four traditional practice settings previously discussed, there are several other viable alternatives for the practice of health education/promotion into the next century. In this section, we briefly introduce these choices so that individuals who are interested can research them further.

The first alternative is to teach health education/promotion in a **postsecondary institution**, usually defined as an institution that educates people after they graduate from high school. There will continue to be a need for qualified instructors. Minimum standards for obtaining one of these positions is usually a master's degree in health education and two to five years of experience for a community college or vocational school position, and a doctorate and two to five years of experience for a college or university position.

Students who are interested in combining the fields of health education/promotion and journalism can find positions in both the print (traditional print media as well as using blogging, Twitter, and reporting for online sources) and TV media as health reporters for newspapers, magazines, and TV stations. A broad-based knowledge of health issues and a passion for writing or speaking are necessary qualifications.

Because of the increasing interdependence among nations and because there are many areas of the world in which health assistance is badly needed, health education specialist positions will continue to be available in foreign countries. Examples include positions with organizations such as the Peace Corps, Project Hope, the United Nations, the Pan American Health Organization, and the World Health Organization. Many national church organizations also send interdisciplinary health teams to international locations to improve the health of the populace. Often, the health education specialist must have a college degree, some experience, and ability to speak a foreign language.

Medical supply companies, pharmaceutical companies, sports equipment manufacturers, health topic curriculum developers or companies, health food stores, and textbook publishers often employ health education specialists in sales positions. A college degree is required.

In addition, willingness to travel, excellent oral and written communication skills, critical thinking, an ability to analyze research information (what is "real" and what is "hype"), and an ability to work with all types of people are necessary prerequisites.

Because of the aging of the U.S. population, demand for health education specialists in long-term care institutions and retirement communities is escalating. Elders are living longer and want to be active in their retirement years; thus, many employment opportunities are opening up. Usually, a college degree is required. Excellent oral and written communication skills are essential, as is a desire to listen and learn from the wisdom of individuals residing in these communities.

There continues to be an increasing number of opportunities for health education specialists in entrepreneurial and consultant roles. As self-employed persons, these individuals are free to set up their own practice, hiring out as consultants to organizations that temporarily need someone with expertise in grant writing, program planning and evaluation, software development, professional speaking, or technical writing. Other possibilities include contracting with several small businesses to conduct work-site health promotion, freelancing with HMOs and other insurance providers to offer health education/promotion services (reimbursement will be an issue), serving as a content specialist (e.g., stress management, eating disorders, substance abuse) to businesses and corporations, becoming a certified personal trainer, and teaching part-time in colleges, community colleges, or evening community education/promotion programs.

Now that we have explored the differences in the various practice settings, we reemphasize the fact that there are common tasks for health education specialists that transcend the individual practice settings. Dr. John Seffrin, director of the American Cancer Society, eloquently reminds us of the direction health education/promotion must take, no matter what the practice setting, if it is to realize its potential. His scholar's address (Seffrin, 1997), given to members of the AAHE, describes four actions for present and future health education specialists that still ring true today:

1. Look at ourselves as major players in keeping Americans healthy; to that end, work with policy makers to affect legislation that truly promotes health.

2. Collaborate with other health professionals in both the for-profit and the not-for-profit sectors.

3. Strive to exhibit greater professional solidarity; be an advocate for the profession of health education/promotion and the role that trained health education specialists can play as part of the healthcare team.

4. Advocate for those who do not have a voice; be a spokesperson in the political arena and work to ensure that health services and health education/promotion are available for all.

Summary

This chapter began with the notion of change as a constant. Although no one can actually "see" into the future, it is obvious that flexibility is imperative to adapt to ongoing change. This is an exciting time to become a health education specialist. Opportunities have never been greater, and the future has never looked brighter. The job outlook for health education specialists is anticipated to increase by 37 percent over the next 10 years (Bureau of Labor Statistics, 2013). There is little doubt that health education/promotion will continue to expand in all of the more traditional as well as some of the nontraditional settings. Health education specialists have the training and expertise to make a positive difference in enhancing the quality of life for all people. We wish you success as you begin your journey.

 ## Review Questions

1. Identify three work-site settings in which health education specialists will practice to a greater degree than they currently do.

2. How will each of the societal changes discussed in the chapter impact the practice of health education/promotion in the work-site setting? The clinical/medical care setting? The school setting? The public health setting?

3. What are the implications for health education/promotion graduates who choose not to become credentialed (CHES)?

4. Using the list of basic competencies listed under the section on practicing in the clinical care setting, which of the items in the list fit into the following categories: assessment, instruction, and collaboration? Which are the most difficult to classify?

5. What is meant by the statement "Health education specialists need to become enhanced advocates for the profession"?

6. How will the passage of the Affordable Care Act impact the practice of health education/promotion?

 ## Case Study

One day, while leaving the health education/promotion office on your campus, you notice an announcement posted on the message board that the health education/promotion program in which you are enrolled is seeking national accreditation. The announcement includes information from the department chair on the reasons for accreditation along with a request for student assistance in working with faculty to prepare the necessary self-study documentation before the visit from an outside review team. Because you are entering the second semester of your junior year, you decide that a great way to learn more about the health education/promotion program and the field of health education/promotion in general would be to volunteer.

You notify the department chair of your willingness to help, and she appoints you to one of the program study committees, specifically the committee dealing with the use of Web-based teaching in delivering the health education/promotion curriculum. You are excited about that committee because you have some opinions on the value of Web-based courses. Although you have never enrolled in a Web-based course yourself, you know people who have, and they seem to have mixed feelings about the courses they have taken. The ambivalence of your classmates has led you to believe that Web-based courses are not as rigorous as courses offered by more traditional methods, and they do not allow for as much interaction between students as do traditionally delivered courses.

At the first meeting of the study committee, the committee chair outlines tasks that will need to be accomplished and suggests a timeline for completion. One of the major tasks is to determine whether the Web-based courses offered by the department are meeting the goals for which they are designed. What key questions would you need to ask to obtain that information? What methods would you use to collect the data? How might the findings be used by health education/promotion programs in planning for the future?

Critical Thinking Questions

1. After reading the chapter and in your opinion, what major demographic trend will most impact the delivery of health education/promotion in the next several decades? Given your answer, describe the health education specialist in the year 2025.

2. Compare and contrast the lists of competencies noted in the chapter for the four major practice settings in which a health education specialist might practice. Use your findings to support or refute the claim made by some professionals that health education specialists will be much more effective if their preparation programs include coursework specific to the settings in which they will practice.

3. Read the 2015 HESPA report commissioned by SOPHE that was referred to in the chapter. Using the information from that report, what duties might you assign to health education specialists desiring to practice in the clinical setting? How might your choices influence the Centers for Disease Control and Prevention goal of eliminating health disparities in the United States within the next 10 years?

4. Assume that it is the year 2045 and you are retiring after many years as a practicing health education specialist. At your retirement banquet, you have been asked to spend five minutes summarizing the accomplishments of your profession. What will you say?

5. What are two ways in which the health education/health promotion community can make the message of prevention more palatable to the public? What are the major barriers you must address? How might you implement your ideas?

Activities

1. Make a list of your five strongest attributes. Make a second list of the five tasks you most like to do. Using these lists and what you know about health education/promotion, write a paragraph describing the "perfect" health education/promotion job for you.

2. Construct and administer a short survey to the health education/promotion faculty at your institution to determine their thoughts on the major factors influencing the current and future practice of health education/promotion. Compile your results.

3. Interview a graduate from your school's health education/promotion program who is now practicing in the field as a certified health education specialist. Try to ascertain his or her feelings about his or her position and the influences he or she feels will impact health education/promotion practice both now and in the future.

4. Write a job description that will be used to advertise for a new public health education specialist position in a work-site setting. In the document be sure to include necessary applicant qualifications and expected duties.

Weblinks

1. http://www.healthypeople.gov

   Healthy People 2020

   Web site of the national *Healthy People 2020* documents that describe U.S. goals and objectives for creating a healthier population by 2020.

2. http://www.kingcounty.gov/healthservices/health.aspx

   Seattle and King County Public Health Section

   This outstanding Web site was launched by the Seattle King County Health Department to help health education specialists and the public obtain current information on a variety of pertinent public health topics such as bioterrorism preparedness, family planning and reproductive health, diabetes, HIV/AIDS, and others.

3. http://www.nationalacademies.org

   "Who Will Keep the Public Healthy?"

   Search the National Academies Web site for a 2003 report from the Institute of Medicine of the National Academies that suggests specific ways to improve public health professionals' capabilities to address new and complex challenges. The report emphasizes that public health professionals in government health departments, other health services, community agencies, and universities have a shared responsibility to prevent illness and injury and keep communities healthy.

4. http://www.nchec.org/

   National Commission for Health Education Credentialing

   Provides information on the competencies to be a health education specialist including updated competencies as a result of the 2015 HESPA Study referenced earlier in the chapter.

5. http://www.kff.org

   The Henry J. Kaiser Family Foundation

   The Kaiser Family Foundation Web site highlights health policy issues and enables the user to access background information on several current health policy topics. Modules and slide tutorials explaining the policy issues are also included.

6. http://www.rwjf.org/

   Web site of the Robert Wood Johnson Foundation featuring papers on health policy, health issues analyses, grant opportunities, and research and commentaries on healthcare reform.

7. http://www.cdc.gov/healthcommunication/

   CDC Web site on health communications and marketing strategies for health promotion programs. Features examples of programs that have been successful. Also has a portal to the *Health Communication Science Digest* journal.

References

Acock, A. C., & Demo, D. H. (1994). *Family diversity and well-being*. Thousand Oaks, CA: Sage.

Allensworth, D. D., & Kolbe, L. J. (1987). The comprehensive school health program: Exploring an expanded concept. *Journal of School Health, 57* (10), 409–412.

Bureau of Labor Statistics. (2013). U.S. Department of Labor, Occupational outlook handbook, health educators. 2012–2013 edition. Retrieved on June 3, 2013, from http://www.bls.gov/ooh/community-and-social-service/health-educators.htm.

Chen, A., Ferlaino, V., El-Kaissi, S., Pan, S. H., Suduteh, T., et al. (2016). *mHealth: Customization and integration for merging data in healthcare.* Retrieved on April 21, 2016, from http://www.vcbeat.net/wp-content/uploads/2015/10/IIHI_Patient_Adoption_of_mHealth.pdf

Child Trends Data Bank. (2013). *Family structure.* Retrieved on September 4, 2013, from http://www.childtrendsdatabank.org/.

Clark, N. M. (1994). Health educators and the future: Lead, follow, or get out of the way. *Journal of Health Education, 25* (3), 136–141.

Colby, S. L., & Ortman, J. M. (2015). Projections of the size and composition of the U.S. population: 2014–2060. *Current Population Reports: U S. Census Bureau,* 1–13.

Davies, J., Smith, G., & Gustafson, D. (2001). Public health informatics transforms the notifiable condition system. *Northwest Public Health, Spring/Summer,* 14–17.

English, G. M., & Videto, D. M. (1997). The future of health education: The knowledge to practice paradox. *Journal of Health Education, 28* (1), 4–8.

Forsberg, V., & Fichtenberg, C. (2012). *The prevention and public health fund: A critical investment in our nation's physical and fiscal health.* American Public Health Association, Center for Public Health Policy Issue Brief, 1–52.

Fox, S. (2011). Health topics: 80% of users look for health information online. Pew Internet and American Life Project. Retrieved May 18, 2013, from http://www.pewinternet.org/Reports/2011/HealthTopics.aspx.

Garfield, R. & Damico, A. (2016). The coverage gap: Uninsured poor adults in states that do not expand Medicaid – An Update. *Henry J. Kaiser Family Foundation Issue Brief.*

Gheisar, R. E., & Clark, C. J. (2000). New immigrant and refugee communities mean new challenges for public health. *Washington Public Health, Fall,* 2. Retrieved August 23, 2013, from http://www.nwpublichealth.org/docs/wph2000/trends.pdf.

Gold, R. S., & Atkinson, N. L. (2006). Imagine this, imagine that. A look into the future of technology for health educators. *The Health Education Monograph Series, 23* (1), 44–48.

Goodarz, D., Rimm, E. B., Oza, S., Kulkarni, S., Murray, C. J. L., et al. (2010). The promise of prevention: The effects of four preventable factors on national life expectancy and life expectancy disparities by race and county in the United States. *PLoS Medicine, 7* (3), 1–13.

Goodman, R. M. (2000). On contemplation at 50: SOPHE presidential address. *Health Education and Behavior, 27* (4), 423–429.

Hale, C. (2000). Demographic trends influencing public health practice. *Washington Public Health, Fall,* University of Washington, 1–3.

Hasnain-Wynia, R., & Wolf, M. (2010). Promoting health care equity: Is health literacy a missing link? *Health Services Research, 45* (4), 897–903.

Hunter, D. J. (2008). Health needs more than healthcare: The need for the new paradigm. *European Journal of Public Health, 18* (3), 217–219.

Idaho Administrative Rules. (2016). Retrieved on April 20, 2016, from http://adminrules.idaho.gov/rules/current/16/0309.pdf.

Institute of Medicine. (2003). *Who will keep the public healthy? Educating public health professionals for the 21st Century.* Washington, DC: National Academies Press.

Koh, H. K., & Sebelius, K. G. (2010). Promoting prevention through the Affordable Care Act. *The New England Journal of Medicine,* 1–5. Retrieved on September 9, 2010, from http://healthpolicyandreform.nejm.org/?p=12171.

Korda, H., & Itani, Z. (2013). Harnessing social media for health promotion and behavior change. *Health Promotion Practice, 14* (1), 15–23.

Lewallen, T. C., Hunt, H., Potts-Datema, W., Zaza, S., & Giles, W. (2015). The whole school, whole community, whole child model: A new approach for improving educational attainment and healthy development for students. *Journal of School Health, 85,* 729–739.

Marken, S. (2015). U.S. uninsured rate at 11.4% in second quarter. *Gallup Research Group.* Retrieved on April 19, 2016, from http://www.gallup.com/poll/184064/uninsured-rate-second-quarter.aspx.

McDermott, R. J. (2000). Health education research: Evolution or revolution (or maybe both)? *Journal of Health Education, 31* (5), 264–271.

McKenzie, J. F. (2004). Professional preparation: Is a generic health educator really possible? *American Journal of Health Education, 35* (1), 46–48.

McKenzie, J. F., Kotecki, J. E., & Pinger, R. R. (2008). *An introduction to community health.* Boston, MA: Jones and Bartlett.

National Center for Education Statistics. (2015). Racial and ethnic enrollment in public schools. *The Condition of Education 2015.*

National Commission for Health Education Credentialing (NCHEC). (2016). Retrieved on April 17, 2016, from http://www.nchec.org/assets/2251/executive_summary.pdf.

Neiger, B. L., Thackery, R., Van Wagenen, S. A., Hanson, C. L., West, J. H., et al. (2012). Use of social media in health promotion: Purposes, key performance indicators, and evaluation metrics. *Health Promotion Practice, 13* (3), 159–164.

O'Rourke, T. (2006). Philosophical reflections on health education and health promotion: Shifting sands and ebbing tides. *The Health Education Monograph Series, 23* (1), 7–10.

Pew Research Center. (2014). Population change in the U.S. and the world from 1950–2050. *Global Attitudes and Trends, Chapter 4,* 1–15.

Pew Research Center. (2015). The American family today: Parenting in America. Retrieved on April 20, 2016, from http://www.pewsocialtrends.org/2015/12/17/1-the-american-family-today/.

Seffrin, J. R. (1994). America's interest in comprehensive school health education. *Journal of School Health, 64* (10), 397–399.

Seffrin, J. R. (March 1997). *AAHE scholar's address.* St. Louis: American Alliance for Health, Physical Education, Recreation, and Dance Convention.

Smith, J. C., & Medalia, C. (2015). *Health insurance coverage in the United States: 2014. U.S. Census Bureau.* Retrieved on April 21, 2016, from https://www.census.gov/content/dam/Census/library/publications/2015/demo/p60-253.pdf

Society for Public Health Education (SOPHE). (2013). *Affordable Care Act: Opportunities and challenges for health education specialists.* Retrieved on May 22, 2013, from http://www.sophe.org/Sophe/PDF/ACA-Opportunities-and-Challenges-for-Health-Educators-FINAL.pdf.

Thackery, R., Neiger, B. L., Hanson, C. L., & McKenzie, J. F. (2008). Enhancing promotional strategies within social marketing programs: Use of web 2.0 social media. *Health Promotion Practice, 9* (4), 338–343.

United States 114th Congress. (2015–16). Every Student Succeeds Act (ESSA). Retrieved on April 21, 2016, from https://www.congress.gov/bill/114th-congress/senate-bill/1177/text.

U.S. Census Bureau. (2012). *Most children younger than 1 are minorities.* Retrieved June 2, 2013, from http://www.census.gov/newsroom/releases/archives/population/cb12-90.html.

Williams, D. R., McClellan, M. B., & Rivlin, A. M. (2010). Beyond the Affordable Care Act: Achieving real improvements in Americans' health. *Health Affairs, 29* (8), 1481–1488.

Yang, J., Ekono, M., & Skinner, C. (2016). *Basic facts about low income children: Children under 18 in 2014. National Center for Children in Poverty.* Retrieved on April 20, 2016, from http://www.nccp.org/publications/pub_1145.html.

Yarnall, K. S. H., Pollack, K. I., Østbye, T., Krause, K. M., & Michener, L. (2003). Primary care: Is there enough time for prevention? *American Journal of Public Health, 93* (4), 635–641.

DEVELOPMENT OF A UNIFIED CODE OF
ETHICS FOR THE HEALTH EDUCATION
PROFESSION[1]

The earliest code of ethics for health educators appears to be the 1976 Society for Public Health Education (SOPHE) Code of Ethics, which was developed to guide professional behaviors toward the highest standards of practice for the profession. Following member input, Ethics Committee Chair Elizabeth Bernheimer and Paul Mico refined the code in 1978. Between 1980 and 1983 renewed attention to the code of ethics resulted in a revision that was to be reviewed by SOPHE chapters and, if accepted, then submitted to other health education professional associations to serve as a guide for the profession (Bloom, 1999). The 1983 SOPHE Code of Ethics was a combination of standards and principles but no specific rules of conduct at that time (Taub, Kreuter, Parcel, & Vitello, 1987).

Following the previous recommendation of SOPHE president, Lawrence Green, that SOPHE, the American Association for Health Education (AAHE), and the Public Health Education section of APHA consider appointing joint committees, a SOPHE–AAHE Joint Committee was appointed by then-AAHE president Peter Cortese and then-SOPHE president Ruth Richards in 1984. This committee was charged with developing a profession-wide code of ethics (Bloom, 1999). Between August 1984 and November 1985 the committee, chaired by Alyson Taub, carried out its charge to (1) identify and use all existing health education ethics statements, (2) determine the appropriate relationship between the code of ethics and the role delineation guidelines, including recommendations for enforcement, and (3) to prepare an ethics document for approval as a profession-wide code of ethics. The joint committee found that the only health education organization to work on ethics, other than SOPHE, was the American College Health Association, which included a section on ethics in their *Recommended Standards and Practices for a College Health Education Program.* The committee concluded that it was premature to describe how the code might relate to the role delineation guidelines and further recommended that individual responsibility for adhering to the Code of Ethics be the method of enforcement. Finally, the joint committee recommended that, in the absence of resources to retain expert consultation in development of ethical codes of conduct, the 1983 SOPHE Code of Ethics be adopted profession-wide and serve as a basis for the next step involving development of rules of conduct (Taub et al., 1987). Although SOPHE accepted the joint committee's recommendation, there was no similar action by AAHE (Bloom, 1999). The AAHE board chose not to accept the suggestion of adopting the SOPHE code on behalf of the profession because they realized that the membership of AAHE needed to be more completely involved in discussing and formulating a Code of Ethics before the AAHE

---

[1] This introduction was prepared through the joint efforts of Ellen Capwell (SOPHE), Becky Smith (AAHE), Janet Shirreffs (AAHE), and Larry K. Olsen (ASHA). Prepared 11/14/99.

board could adequately represent the interests and needs of AAHE members in collaborative work on ethics with other professional societies.

In September of 1991, an ad hoc AAHE ethics committee, chaired by Janet Shirreffs, was charged by president Thomas O'Rourke to develop a code of ethics that represented the professional needs of the variety of health education professionals in the membership of AAHE. They were to review the literature, including other professional codes of ethics, and conduct in-depth surveys of AAHE members. For the next two years, the AAHE ethics committee executed its charge through a variety of venues, including correspondence, surveys, face-to-face meetings, presentations, and discussion sessions at the national conventions of the American Association for Health Education (AAHE), The American School Health Association (ASHA), and the American Public Health Association (APHA), and through conducting focus group sessions at strategic locations around the country. Based on the work of this committee, an AAHE Code of Ethics was adopted by the AAHE Board of Directors in April 1993 (AAHE, 1994). Subsequently, both AAHE and SOPHE continued to focus on ethical issues. SOPHE has promoted programming in ethics through its annual and midyear meetings. In December 1992, a summary of the 1983 SOPHE Code of Ethics was prepared by Sarah Olson and distributed as a promotional piece. The SOPHE Board of Trustees supported the summary Code of Ethics in 1994. Since 1993, AAHE has had a standing committee on ethics that recently proposed convention programming and publications in the area of ethics. Recognizing the need to work with other organizations toward a profession-wide code of ethics, the SOPHE Board requested that the Coalition of National Health Education Organizations (CNHEO) propose a strategy for accomplishing this goal. In July 1994, the board adopted a motion that SOPHE support a profession-wide code of ethics based on ethical principles and that AAHE should be contacted for support in the effort (Bloom, 1999).

In 1995, the National Commission for Health Education Credentialing, Inc. (NCHEC) and CNHEO cosponsored a conference, The Health Education Profession in the Twenty-First Century: Setting the Stage (Brown, Cissell, DuShaw, Goodhart, McDermott, et al., 1996). During that conference, it was recommended that efforts be expanded to develop a profession-wide code of ethics.

Shortly thereafter, delegates to the CNHEO pledged to work toward development of a profession-wide code of ethics using the existing SOPHE and AAHE codes as a starting point (Bloom, 1999). A National Ethics Task Force was subsequently developed, with representatives from the various organizations represented on the coalition. It was decided that the coalition delegates would not be the task force. As a result, the various member organizations of the coalition were asked to recommend individuals for inclusion on this important task force.

During the November 1996 APHA meeting, Larry Olsen, who was the coordinator of the CNHEO and delegate to the coalition from ASHA, William Livingood (SOPHE), and Beverly Mahoney (AAHE) led a session on ethics sponsored by the CNHEO. At that meeting, the basic conceptual plan that had been developed by the coalition's Ethics Task Force was presented. Those attending the session were asked to provide input, both for the process and the content of the "new" code of ethics. Those in attendance were strong in their support for the importance of having a code of ethics for the profession that would provide an ethical framework for health educators, regardless of the setting in which health education was practiced.

The Ethics Task Force of the coalition reviewed the two existing codes (SOPHE and AAHE) along with the supporting documents for both and decided that they would enlist the support of a consultant to assist in the unification process. Claire Stiles of Eckerd College was subsequently retained to offer comments about the proposals of the task force, as well as the various drafts that would be developed.

A presentation on behalf of the Ethics Task Force was made in November 1997 at the national APHA meeting in Indianapolis, and the first draft of the Unified Code of Ethics was presented. Attendees were asked to comment about the draft document and were asked to take copies of the draft document to distribute among their constituencies. Comments from professionals in the field were returned to and considered by the task force.

A second (revised) draft of the Unified Code was presented during the March 1998 AAHE meeting in Reno. Comments received from the APHA Indianapolis meeting and field distribution had been incorporated into the document. In addition, the AAHE Ethics Committee had the opportunity to comment about the new document. During the presentation in Reno, participants were put into small groups to discuss and comment on each of the articles included in the draft document. These comments were subsequently incorporated into the document and the stage was set for a series of meetings designed to elicit commentary from professionals in the field, as well as those who attended the meetings of national professional health education organizations.

Following yet another revision of the emerging code, presentations on behalf of the task force were made in San Antonio in May 1998 at the joint SOPHE/Association of State and Territorial Directors of Health Promotion and Public Health Education (ASTDHPPHE) meeting; in San Diego in June 1998 at the national meeting of the American College Health Association ACHA; and in Colorado Springs in October 1998 at the national meeting of ASHA. Throughout this process, comments and suggestions about the code were received and examined by the task force. Throughout this process of revision and refinement, care was taken to retain the context and concepts present in the original SOPHE and AAHE documents.

The first final draft of the Unified Code of Ethics was presented in Washington, D.C., at the November 1998 meeting of the APHA. The coalition also met in conjunction with APHA, and it was decided that the final draft of the Unified Code would be prepared for presentation to the field in 1999.

In April 1999 the Unified Code of Ethics was presented in Boston at the national AAHE meeting. During that meeting the coalition also met and it was decided that all delegates to the coalition, as well as the task force members, would examine closely the work that had been done and offer comments and suggestions. It was further decided that coalition delegates would be sent a copy of the entire document (both the long and short forms), so that the documents could be discussed during the coalition's May 1999 conference call. During that conference call, the delegates voted to present the Code of Ethics to their respective organizations, for ratification during the remainder of 1999.

On November 8, 1999, the coalition delegates met in Chicago in conjunction with the APHA's annual meeting. At that meeting, the Code of Ethics was a topic of discussion. Letters had been received from all the delegate organizations indicating that they had approved the document. It was moved and seconded that the Code of Ethics be approved and distributed to the profession. There being no further comments by the CNHEO delegates, the Code of Ethics was approved unanimously as a Code of Ethics for the profession of Health Education.

The Code of Ethics that has evolved from this long and arduous process is not seen as a completed project. Rather, it is envisioned as a living document that will continue to evolve as the practice of Health Education changes to meet the challenges of the new millennium.

References

Association for the Advancement of Health Education (AAHE). (1994). Code of ethics for health educators. *Journal of Health Education, 25* (4), 197–200.

Bloom, F. K. (1999). The Society for Public Health Education: Its development and contributions: 1976–1996. Unpublished doctoral dissertation, Columbia University.

Brown, K. M., Cissell, W., DuShaw, M., Goodhart, F., McDermott, R., Middleton, K., Tappe, M., & Welsh, V. (1996). The health education profession in the twenty-first century: Setting the stage. *Journal of Health Education, 27* (6), 357–364.

Taub, A., Kreuter, M., Parcel, G., & Vitello, E. (1987). Report from the AAHE/SOPHE Joint Committee on Ethics. *Health Education Quarterly, 14* (1), 79–90.

Members of the Ethics Task Force

Mal Goldsmith (ASHA)

Alyson Taub (SHES Section, APHA)

June Gorski (SOPHE)

Ken McLeroy (PHEHP Section, APHA)

Larry K. Olsen (ASHA), Committee Chair

Wanda Jubb (SSDHPER)

CODE OF ETHICS FOR THE HEALTH EDUCATION PROFESSION

Long Version[2]

Preamble

The health education profession is dedicated to excellence in the practice of promoting individual, family, organizational, and community health. Guided by common ideals, health educators are responsible for upholding the integrity and ethics of the profession as they face the daily challenges of making decisions. By acknowledging the value of diversity in society and embracing a cross-cultural approach, health educators support the worth, dignity, potential, and uniqueness of all people.

The Code of Ethics provides a framework of shared values within which health education is practiced. The Code of Ethics is grounded in fundamental ethical principles that underlie all health care services: respect for autonomy, promotion of social justice, active promotion of good, and avoidance of harm. The responsibility of each health educator is to aspire to the highest possible standards of conduct and to encourage the ethical behavior of all those with whom they work.

Regardless of job title, professional affiliation, work setting, or population served, health educators abide by these guidelines when making professional decisions.

Article I: Responsibility to the Public

A health educator's ultimate responsibility is to educate people for the purpose of promoting, maintaining, and improving individual, family, and community health. When a conflict of

[2] Used with the permission of the Coalition of National Health Education Organizations.

issues arises among individuals, groups, organizations, agencies, or institutions, health educators must consider all issues and give priority to those that promote wellness and quality of living through principles of self-determination and freedom of choice for the individual.

Section 1
Health educators support the right of individuals to make informed decisions regarding health, as long as such decisions pose no threat to the health of others.

Section 2
Health educators encourage actions and social policies that support and facilitate the best balance of benefits over harm for all affected parties.

Section 3
Health educators accurately communicate the potential benefits and consequences of the services and programs with which they are associated.

Section 4
Health educators accept the responsibility to act on issues that can adversely affect the health of individuals, families, and communities.

Section 5
Health educators are truthful about their qualifications and the limitations of their expertise and provide services consistent with their competencies.

Section 6
Health educators protect the privacy and dignity of individuals.

Section 7
Health educators actively involve individuals, groups, and communities in the entire educational process so that all aspects of the process are clearly understood by those who may be affected.

Section 8
Health educators respect and acknowledge the rights of others to hold diverse values, attitudes, and opinions.

Section 9
Health educators provide services equitably to all people.

Article II: Responsibility to the Profession

Health educators are responsible for their professional behavior, for the reputation of their profession, and for promoting ethical conduct among their colleagues.

Section 1
Health educators maintain, improve, and expand their professional competence through continued study and education; membership, participation, and leadership in professional organizations; and involvement in issues related to the health of the public.

Section 2

Health educators model and encourage nondiscriminatory standards of behavior in their interactions with others.

Section 3

Health educators encourage and accept responsible critical discourse to protect and enhance the profession.

Section 4

Health educators contribute to the development of the profession by sharing the processes and outcomes of their work.

Section 5

Health educators are aware of possible professional conflicts of interest, exercise integrity in conflict situations, and do not manipulate or violate the rights of others.

Section 6

Health educators give appropriate recognition to others for their professional contributions and achievements.

Article III: Responsibility to Employers

Health educators recognize the boundaries of their professional competence and are accountable for their professional activities and actions.

Section 1

Health educators accurately represent their qualifications and the qualifications of others whom they recommend.

Section 2

Health educators use appropriate standards, theories, and guidelines as criteria when carrying out their professional responsibilities.

Section 3

Health educators accurately represent potential service and program outcomes to employers.

Section 4

Health educators anticipate and disclose competing commitments, conflicts of interest, and endorsement of products.

Section 5

Health educators openly communicate to employers expectations of job-related assignments that conflict with their professional ethics.

Section 6

Health educators maintain competence in their areas of professional practice.

Article IV: Responsibility in the Delivery of Health Education

Health educators promote integrity in the delivery of health education. They respect the rights, dignity, confidentiality, and worth of all people by adapting strategies and methods to meet the needs of diverse populations and communities.

Section 1

Health educators are sensitive to social and cultural diversity and are in accord with the law when planning and implementing programs.

Section 2

Health educators are informed of the latest advances in theory, research, and practice, and use strategies and methods that are grounded in and contribute to development of professional standards, theories, guidelines, statistics, and experience.

Section 3

Health educators are committed to rigorous evaluation of both program effectiveness and the methods used to achieve results.

Section 4

Health educators empower individuals to adopt healthy lifestyles through informed choice rather than by coercion or intimidation.

Section 5

Health educators communicate the potential outcomes of proposed services, strategies, and pending decisions to all individuals who will be affected.

Article V: Responsibility in Research and Evaluation

Health educators contribute to the health of the population and to the profession through research and evaluation activities. When planning and conducting research or evaluation, health educators do so in accordance with federal and state laws and regulations, organizational and institutional policies, and professional standards.

Section 1

Health educators support principles and practices of research and evaluation that do no harm to individuals, groups, society, or the environment.

Section 2

Health educators ensure that participation in research is voluntary and is based upon the informed consent of the participants.

Section 3

Health educators respect the privacy, rights, and dignity of research participants, and honor commitments made to those participants.

Section 4

Health educators treat all information obtained from participants as confidential unless otherwise required by law.

Section 5

Health educators take credit, including authorship, only for work they have actually performed and give credit to the contributions of others.

Section 6

Health educators who serve as research or evaluation consultants discuss their results only with those to whom they are providing service, unless maintaining such confidentiality would jeopardize the health or safety of others.

Section 7

Health educators report the results of their research and evaluation objectively, accurately, and in a timely fashion.

Article VI: Responsibility in Professional Preparation

Those involved in the preparation and training of health educators have an obligation to accord learners the same respect and treatment given other groups by providing quality education that benefits the profession and the public.

Section 1

Health educators select students for professional preparation programs based upon equal opportunity for all, and the individual's academic performance, abilities, and potential contribution to the profession and the public's health.

Section 2

Health educators strive to make the educational environment and culture conducive to the health of all involved, and free from sexual harassment and all forms of discrimination.

Section 3

Health educators involved in professional preparation and professional development engage in careful preparation; present material that is accurate, up-to-date, and timely; provide reasonable and timely feedback; state clear and reasonable expectations; and conduct fair assessments and evaluations of learners.

Section 4

Health educators provide objective and accurate counseling to learners about career opportunities, development, and advancement, and assist learners to secure professional employment.

Section 5

Health educators provide adequate supervision and meaningful opportunities for the professional development of learners.

CODE OF ETHICS FOR THE HEALTH EDUCATION PROFESSION

Short Version[3]

Preamble

The health education profession is dedicated to excellence in the practice of promoting individual, family, organizational, and community health. The Code of Ethics provides a framework of shared values within which health education is practiced. The responsibility of each health educator is to aspire to the highest possible standards of conduct and to encourage the ethical behavior of all those with whom they work.

Article I: Responsibility to the Public

A health educator's ultimate responsibility is to educate people for the purpose of promoting, maintaining, and improving individual, family, and community health. When a conflict of issues arises among individuals, groups, organizations, agencies, or institutions, health educators must consider all issues and give priority to those that promote wellness and quality of living through principles of self-determination and freedom of choice for the individual.

Article II: Responsibility to the Profession

Health educators are responsible for their professional behavior, for the reputation of their profession, and for promoting ethical conduct among their colleagues.

Article III: Responsibility to Employers

Health educators recognize the boundaries of their professional competence and are accountable for their professional activities and actions.

Article IV: Responsibility in the Delivery of Health Education

Health educators promote integrity in the delivery of health education. They respect the rights, dignity, confidentiality, and worth of all people by adapting strategies and methods to meet the needs of diverse populations and communities.

Article V: Responsibility in Research and Evaluation

Health educators contribute to the health of the population and to the profession through research and evaluation activities. When planning and conducting research or evaluation, health educators do so in accordance with federal and state laws and regulations, organizational and institutional policies, and professional standards.

Article VI: Responsibility in Professional Preparation

Those involved in the preparation and training of health educators have an obligation to accord learners the same respect and treatment given other groups by providing quality education that benefits the profession and the public.

---

[3] Used with the permission of the Coalition of National Health Education Organizations.

HEALTH EDUCATION SPECIALIST
PRACTICE ANALYSIS (HESPA)
2015 COMPETENCIES AND
SUB-COMPETENCIES

The Seven Areas of Responsibility contain a comprehensive set of Competencies and Sub-competencies defining the role of the health education specialist. These Responsibilities were verified by the 2015 Health Education Specialist Practice Analysis (HESPA) project and serve as the basis of the CHES exam beginning in October 2016 and the MCHES exam in April 2016.

The shaded Sub-competencies entries indicate Advanced – 1 level; <u>underlined entries</u> indicate Advanced – 2 level. These will not be included in the entry-level, CHES examination. However, the advanced-level Sub-competencies will be included in the MCHES examination.

AREA I: ASSESS NEEDS, RESOURCES, AND CAPACITY FOR HEALTH EDUCATION/PROMOTION

1.1 Plan assessment process for health education/promotion

1.1.1 Define the priority population to be assessed

1.1.2 Identify existing and necessary resources to conduct assessments

1.1.3 Engage priority populations, partners, and stakeholders to participate in the assessment process

1.1.4 Apply theories and/or models to assessment process

1.1.5 Apply ethical principles to the assessment process

1.2 Access existing information and data related to health

1.2.1 Identify sources of secondary data related to health

1.2.2 Establish collaborative relationships and agreements that facilitate access to data

1.2.3 Review related literature

1.2.4 Identify gaps in the secondary data

1.2.5 Extract data from existing databases

1.2.6 Determine the validity of existing data

1.3 Collect primary data to determine needs

1.3.1 Identify data collection instruments

1.3.2 Select data collection methods for use in assessment

1.3.3 Develop data collection procedures

1.3.4 Train personnel assisting with data collection

1.3.5 Implement quantitative and/or qualitative data collection

1.4 **Analyze relationships among behavioral, environmental, and other factors that influence health**

1.4.1 Identify and analyze factors that influence health behaviors

1.4.2 Identify and analyze factors that impact health

1.4.3 Identify the impact of emerging social, economic, and other trends on health

1.5 **Examine factors that influence the process by which people learn**

1.5.1 Identify and analyze factors that foster or hinder the learning process

1.5.2 Identify and analyze factors that foster or hinder knowledge acquisition

1.5.3 Identify and analyze factors that influence attitudes and beliefs

1.5.4 Identify and analyze factors that foster or hinder acquisition of skills

1.6 **Examine factors that enhance or impede the process of health education/ promotion**

1.6.1 Determine the extent of available health education/promotion programs and interventions

1.6.2 Identify policies related to health education/promotion

1.6.3 Assess the effectiveness of existing health education/promotion programs and interventions

1.6.4 Assess social, environmental, political, and other factors that may impact health education/promotion

1.6.5 Analyze the capacity for providing necessary health education/promotion

1.7 **Determine needs for health education/promotion based on assessment findings**

1.7.1 Synthesize assessment findings

1.7.2 Identify current needs, resources, and capacity

1.7.3 Prioritize health education/promotion needs

1.7.4 Develop recommendations for health education/promotion based on assessment findings

1.7.5 Report assessment findings

AREA II: PLAN HEALTH EDUCATION/PROMOTION

2.1 **Involve priority populations, partners, and other stakeholders in the planning process**

2.1.1 Identify priority populations, partners, and other stakeholders

2.1.2 Use strategies to convene priority populations, partners, and other stakeholders

2.1.3   Facilitate collaborative efforts among priority populations, partners, and other stakeholders

2.1.4   Elicit input about the plan

2.1.5   Obtain commitments to participate in health education/promotion

2.2   Develop goals and objectives

2.2.1   Identify desired outcomes using the needs assessment results

2.2.2   Develop vision statement

2.2.3   Develop mission statement

2.2.4   Develop goal statements

2.2.5   Develop specific, measurable, attainable, realistic, and time-sensitive objectives

2.3   Select or design strategies/interventions

2.3.1   Select planning model(s) for health education/promotion

2.3.2   Assess efficacy of various strategies/interventions to ensure consistency with objectives

2.3.3   Apply principles of evidence-based practice in selecting and/or designing strategies/ interventions

2.3.4   Apply principles of cultural competence in selecting and/or designing strategies/ interventions

2.3.5   Address diversity within priority populations in selecting and/or designing strategies/interventions

2.3.6   Identify delivery methods and settings to facilitate learning

2.3.7   Tailor strategies/interventions for priority populations

2.3.8   Adapt existing strategies/interventions as needed

2.3.9   Conduct pilot test of strategies/interventions

2.3.10 Refine strategies/interventions based on pilot feedback

2.3.11 Apply ethical principles in selecting strategies and designing interventions

2.3.12 Comply with legal standards in selecting strategies and designing interventions

2.4   Develop a plan for the delivery of health education/promotion

2.4.1   Use theories and/or models to guide the delivery plan

2.4.2   Identify the resources involved in the delivery of health education/promotion

2.4.3   Organize health education/promotion into a logical sequence

2.4.4   Develop a timeline for the delivery of health education/promotion

2.4.5   Develop marketing plan to deliver health program

2.4.6   Select methods and/or channels for reaching priority populations

2.4.7   Analyze the opportunity for integrating health education/promotion into other programs

2.4.8   Develop a process for integrating health education/promotion into other programs when needed

2.4.9 Assess the sustainability of the delivery plan

2.4.10 Design and conduct pilot study of health education/promotion plan

2.5 **Address factors that influence implementation of health education/ promotion**

2.5.1 Identify and analyze factors that foster or hinder implementation

2.5.2 Develop plans and processes to overcome potential barriers to implementation

AREA III: IMPLEMENT HEALTH EDUCATION/PROMOTION

3.1 **Coordinate logistics necessary to implement plan**

3.1.1 Create an environment conducive to learning

3.1.2 Develop materials to implement plan

3.1.3 Secure resources to implement plan

3.1.4 Arrange for needed services to implement plan

3.1.5 Apply ethical principles to the implementation process

3.1.6 Comply with legal standards that apply to implementation

3.2 **Train staff members and volunteers involved in implementation of health education/promotion**

3.2.1 Develop training objectives

3.2.2 Recruit individuals needed for implementation

3.2.3 Identify training needs of individuals involved in implementation

3.2.4 Develop training using best practices

3.2.5 Implement training

3.2.6 Provide support and technical assistance to those implementing the plan

3.2.7 Evaluate training

3.2.8 Use evaluation findings to plan/modify future training

3.3 **Implement health education/promotion plan**

3.3.1 Collect baseline data

3.3.2 Apply theories and/or models of implementation

3.3.3 Assess readiness for implementation

3.3.4 Apply principles of diversity and cultural competence in implementing health education/promotion plan

3.3.5 Implement marketing plan

3.3.6 Deliver health education/promotion as designed

3.3.7 Use a variety of strategies to deliver plan

3.4 **Monitor implementation of health education/promotion**

3.4.1 Monitor progress in accordance with timeline

3.4.2 Assess progress in achieving objectives

3.4.3 Ensure plan is implemented consistently

3.4.4 Modify plan when needed

3.4.5 Monitor use of resources

3.4.6 Evaluate sustainability of implementation

3.4.7 Ensure compliance with legal standards

3.4.8 Monitor adherence to ethical principles in the implementation of health education/ promotion

AREA IV: CONDUCT EVALUATION AND RESEARCH RELATED TO HEALTH EDUCATION/ PROMOTION

4.1 **Develop evaluation plan for health education/promotion**

4.1.1 Determine the purpose and goals of evaluation

4.1.2 Develop questions to be answered by the evaluation

4.1.3 Create a logic model to guide the evaluation process

4.1.4 Adapt/modify a logic model to guide the evaluation process

4.1.5 Assess needed and available resources to conduct evaluation

4.1.6 Determine the types of data (for example, qualitative, quantitative) to be collected

4.1.7 Select a model for evaluation

4.1.8 Develop data collection procedures for evaluation

4.1.9 Develop data analysis plan for evaluation

4.1.10 Apply ethical principles to the evaluation process

4.2 **Develop a research plan for health education/promotion**

4.2.1 Create statement of purpose

4.2.2 Assess feasibility of conducting research

4.2.3 Conduct search for related literature

4.2.4 Analyze and synthesize information found in the literature

4.2.5 Develop research questions and/or hypotheses

4.2.6 Assess the merits and limitations of qualitative and quantitative data collection

4.2.7 Select research design to address the research questions

4.2.8 Determine suitability of existing data collection instruments

4.2.9 Identify research participants

4.2.10 Develop sampling plan to select participants

4.2.11 Develop data collection procedures for research

4.2.12 Develop data analysis plan for research

4.2.13 Develop a plan for non-respondent follow-up

4.2.14 Apply ethical principles to the research process

4.3   Select, adapt, and/or create instruments to collect data

4.3.1   Identify existing data collection instruments

4.3.2   Adapt/modify existing data collection instruments

4.3.3   Create new data collection instruments

4.3.4   Identify useable items from existing instruments

4.3.5   Adapt/modify existing items

4.3.6   Create new items to be used in data collection

4.3.7   Pilot test data collection instrument

4.3.8   Establish validity of data collection instruments

4.3.9   Ensure that data collection instruments generate reliable data

4.3.10 Ensure fairness of data collection instruments (for example, reduce bias, use language appropriate to priority population)

4.4   Collect and manage data

4.4.1   Train data collectors involved in evaluation and/or research

4.4.2   Collect data based on the evaluation or research plan

4.4.3   Monitor and manage data collection

4.4.4   Use available technology to collect, monitor, and manage data

4.4.5   Comply with laws and regulations when collecting, storing, and protecting participant data

4.5   Analyze data

4.5.1   Prepare data for analysis

4.5.2   Analyze data using qualitative methods

4.5.3   Analyze data using descriptive statistical methods

4.5.4   Analyze data using inferential statistical methods

4.5.5   Use technology to analyze data

4.6   Interpret results

4.6.1   Synthesize the analyzed data

4.6.2   Explain how the results address the questions and/or hypotheses

4.6.3   Compare findings to results from other studies or evaluations

4.6.4   Propose possible explanations of findings

4.6.5   Identify limitations of findings

4.6.6   Address delimitations as they relate to findings

4.6.7   Draw conclusions based on findings

4.6.8   Develop recommendations based on findings

4.7   Apply findings

4.7.1   Communicate findings to priority populations, partners, and stakeholders

4.7.2 Solicit feedback from priority populations, partners, and stakeholders

4.7.3 Evaluate feasibility of implementing recommendations

4.7.4 Incorporate findings into program improvement and refinement

4.7.5 <u>Disseminate findings using a variety of methods</u>

AREA V: ADMINISTER AND MANAGE HEALTH EDUCATION/PROMOTION

5.1 **Manage financial resources for health education/promotion programs**

5.1.1 Develop financial plan

5.1.2 Evaluate financial needs and resources

5.1.3 Identify internal and/or external funding sources

5.1.4 Prepare budget requests

5.1.5 Develop program budgets

5.1.6 Manage program budgets

5.1.7 Conduct cost analysis for programs

5.1.8 Prepare budget reports

5.1.9 Monitor financial plan

5.1.10 Create requests for funding proposals

5.1.11 Write grant proposals

5.1.12 Conduct reviews of funding proposals

5.1.13 Apply ethical principles when managing financial resources

5.2 **Manage technology resources**

5.2.1 Assess technology needs to support health education/promotion

5.2.2 Use technology to collect, store, and retrieve program management data

5.2.3 Apply ethical principles in managing technology resources

5.2.4 Evaluate emerging technologies for applicability to health education/promotion

5.3 **Manage relationships with partners and other stakeholders**

5.3.1 Assess capacity of partners and other stakeholders to meet program goals

5.3.2 Facilitate discussions with partners and other stakeholders regarding program resource needs

5.3.3 Create agreements (for example, memoranda of understanding) with partners and other stakeholders

5.3.4 Monitor relationships with partners and other stakeholders

5.3.5 Elicit feedback from partners and other stakeholders

5.3.6 Evaluate relationships with partners and other stakeholders

5.4 **Gain acceptance and support for health education/promotion programs**

5.4.1 Demonstrate how programs align with organizational structure, mission, and goals

5.4.2 Identify evidence to justify programs

5.4.3 Create a rationale to gain or maintain program support

5.4.4 Use various communication strategies to present rationale

5.5 Demonstrate leadership

5.5.1 Facilitate efforts to achieve organizational mission

5.5.2 Analyze an organization's culture to determine the extent to which it supports health education/promotion

5.5.3 Develop strategies to reinforce or change organizational culture to support health education/promotion

5.5.4 Facilitate needed changes to organizational culture

5.5.5 Conduct strategic planning

5.5.6 Implement strategic plan

5.5.7 Monitor strategic plan

5.5.8 Conduct program quality assurance/process improvement

5.5.9 Comply with existing laws and regulations

5.5.10 Adhere to ethical principles of the profession

5.6 Manage human resources for health education/promotion programs

5.6.1 Assess staffing needs

5.6.2 Develop job descriptions

5.6.3 Apply human resource policies consistent with laws and regulations

5.6.4 Evaluate qualifications of staff members and volunteers needed for programs

5.6.5 Recruit staff members and volunteers for programs

5.6.6 Determine staff member and volunteer professional development needs

5.6.7 Develop strategies to enhance staff member and volunteer professional development

5.6.8 Implement strategies to enhance the professional development of staff members and volunteers

5.6.9 Develop and implement strategies to retain staff members and volunteers

5.6.10 Employ conflict resolution techniques

5.6.11 Facilitate team development

5.6.12 Evaluate performance of staff members and volunteers

5.6.13 Monitor performance and/or compliance of funding recipients

5.6.14 Apply ethical principles when managing human resources

AREA VI: SERVE AS A HEALTH EDUCATION/PROMOTION RESOURCE PERSON

6.1 Obtain and disseminate health-related information

6.1.1 Assess needs for health-related information

6.1.2 Identify valid information resources

6.1.3 Evaluate resource materials for accuracy, relevance, and timeliness

6.1.4   Adapt information for consumer

6.1.5   Convey health-related information to consumer

6.2   **Train others to use health education/promotion skills**

6.2.1   Assess training needs of potential participants

6.2.2   Develop a plan for conducting training

6.2.3   Identify resources needed to conduct training

6.2.4   Implement planned training

6.2.5   Conduct formative and summative evaluations of training

6.2.6   Use evaluative feedback to create future trainings

6.3   **Provide advice and consultation on health education/promotion issues**

6.3.1   Assess and prioritize requests for advice/consultation

6.3.2   Establish advisory/consultative relationships

6.3.3   Provide expert assistance and guidance

6.3.4   Evaluate the effectiveness of the expert assistance provided

6.3.5   Apply ethical principles in consultative relationships

AREA VII: COMMUNICATE, PROMOTE, AND ADVOCATE FOR HEALTH, HEALTH EDUCATION/PROMOTION, AND THE PROFESSION

7.1   **Identify, develop, and deliver messages using a variety of communication strategies, methods, and techniques**

7.1.1   Create messages using communication theories and/or models

7.1.2   Identify level of literacy of intended audience

7.1.3   Tailor messages for intended audience

7.1.4   Pilot test messages and delivery methods

7.1.5   Revise messages based on pilot feedback

7.1.6   Assess and select methods and technologies used to deliver messages

7.1.7   Deliver messages using media and communication strategies

7.1.8   Evaluate the impact of the delivered messages

7.2   **Engage in advocacy for health and health education/promotion**

7.2.1   Identify current and emerging issues requiring advocacy

7.2.2   Engage stakeholders in advocacy initiatives

7.2.3   Access resources (for example, financial, personnel, information, data) related to identified advocacy needs

7.2.4   Develop advocacy plans in compliance with local, state, and/or federal policies and procedures

7.2.5   Use strategies that advance advocacy goals

7.2.6   Implement advocacy plans

7.2.7 Evaluate advocacy efforts

7.2.8 Comply with organizational policies related to participating in advocacy

7.2.9 Lead advocacy initiatives related to health

7.3 **Influence policy and/or systems change to promote health and health education**

7.3.1 Assess the impact of existing and proposed policies on health

7.3.2 Assess the impact of existing and proposed policies on health education

7.3.3 Assess the impact of existing systems on health

7.3.4 Project the impact of proposed systems changes on health education

7.3.5 Use evidence-based findings in policy analysis

7.3.6 Develop policies to promote health using evidence-based findings

7.3.7 Identify factors that influence decision makers

7.3.8 Use policy advocacy techniques to influence decision makers

7.3.9 Use media advocacy techniques to influence decision makers

7.3.10 Engage in legislative advocacy

7.4 **Promote the health education profession**

7.4.1 Explain the major responsibilities of the health education specialist

7.4.2 Explain the role of professional organizations in advancing the profession

7.4.3 Explain the benefits of participating in professional organizations

7.4.4 Advocate for professional development of health education specialists

7.4.5 Advocate for the profession

7.4.6 Explain the history of the profession and its current and future implications for professional practice

7.4.7 Explain the role of credentialing (for example, individual, program) in the promotion of the profession

7.4.8 Develop and implement a professional development plan

7.4.9 Serve as a mentor to others in the profession

7.4.10 Develop materials that contribute to the professional literature

7.4.11 Engage in service to advance the profession

A New Perspective on the Health of Canadians
the Canadian publication that presented the epidemiological evidence supporting the importance of lifestyle and environmental factors on health and sickness and called for numerous national health promotion strategies to encourage Canadians to become more responsible for their own health.

abstracts short summaries of research studies that have appeared in selected journals.

accreditation the status of public recognition that an accrediting agency grants to an education institution or program that meets the agency's standards or "requirements" (National Transition Task Force on Accreditation in Health Education, 2013) (Chapter 6).

action stage a stage of the Transtheoretical Model in which a person is overtly making changes.

actual behavioral control having the "the skills, resources, and other prerequisites needed to perform a given behavior" (Ajzen, 2006) (Chapter 4).

adjusted rate a rate that is statistically adjusted for a certain characteristic, such as age, expressed for a total population.

administrative and policy assessment is "an analysis of the policies, resources, and circumstances prevailing in an organizational situation to facilitate or hinder the development of the health program" (Green & Kreuter, 2005, p. G-1) (Chapter 4).

advocacy "the actions or endeavors individuals or groups engage in in order to alter public opinion in favor or in opposition to a certain policy" (Pinzon-Perez & Perez, 1999, p. 29) (Chapter 1).

Affordable Care Act (ACA) the official title of healthcare reform legislation that was passed by Congress in March 2010. All of the provisions of the ACA will be fully implemented by 2020.

American Academy of Health Behavior (AAHB) society of researchers and scholars in the areas of human behavior, health education, and health promotion.

American Alliance for Health, Physical Education, Recreation and Dance (AAHPERD) was the largest organization of professionals involved in physical education, physical activity, dance, school health, and sport—all specialties related to achieving an active, healthy lifestyle. This organization evolved into SHAPE.

American Association for Health Education (AAHE) was a professional association within AAHPERD. As of May 1, 2013, the AAHE was formally retired.

American College Health Association (ACHA) a professional association comprising mostly individuals who work in colleges and universities.

American Public Health Association (APHA) a professional association for those individuals working in all fields of public health.

American Red Cross (ARC) a quasi-governmental organization.

American School Health Association (ASHA) a professional association comprising individuals interested in coordinated school health.

anonymity exists when no one, including those conducting the program, can relate a participant's identity to any information pertaining to the program.

Asclepiads a brotherhood of men associated with the Asclepian temples who first began the practice of medicine based on a more rational basis.

Asclepius the Greek god of medicine, for whom many temples were built.

assessment the estimation of the relative magnitude, importance, or value of objects observed.

attitude toward the behavior an attitude about a certain behavior; a construct of the theory of planned behavior.

bacteriological period of public health the period of 1875 to 1900, during which great advancements in the study of bacteria occurred.

behavioral capability the knowledge and skills necessary to perform a behavior.

behavior change philosophy involves a health education specialist using behavioral contracts, goal setting, and self-monitoring to help foster and motivate the modification of an unhealthy habit in an individual with whom the health education specialist is working.

beneficence "simply doing good" (Balog et al., 1985, p. 91) (Chapter 5).

benevolence see *beneficence*.

caduceus the serpent and staff symbol of medicine, which was the symbol of the Asclepian temples.

capacity "refers to both individual and collective resources that can be brought to bear for health enhancement" (Gilmore & Campbell, 2005, p. 7) (Chapter 6).

CDCynergy (or Cynergy) a health communication planning model developed by the Office of Communication at the Centers for Disease Control and Prevention.

certification "a process by which a professional organization grants recognition to an individual who, upon completion of a competency-based curriculum, can demonstrate a predetermined standard of performance" (Cleary, 1995, p. 39) (Chapter 6).

Certified Health Education Specialist (CHES) a health education specialist who has met all necessary requirements and has been certified by the National Commission for Health Education Credentialing, Inc.

chain of infection a model used to help explain the spread of a communicable disease from one host to another.

Coalition of National Health Education Organizations, USA (CNHEO) a coalition made up of representatives from eight professional associations, of which health education specialists are members.

code of ethics "document that maps the dimensions of the profession's collective social responsibility and acknowledges the obligations individual practitioners share in meeting the profession's responsibilities" (Feeney & Freeman, 1999, p. 6) (Chapter 5).

Code of Hammurabi the earliest known written record concerning public health.

cognitive-based philosophy a philosophy that focuses on the acquisition of content and factual information to increase knowledge so a person is better equipped to make health-related decisions.

communicable disease model a model used to help explain the spread of a communicable disease from one host to another via the elements of agent, host, and environment.

communicable diseases those diseases for which biological agents or their products are the cause and that are transmissible from one individual to another (McKenzie et al., 2012) (Chapter 1).

community empowerment "the process by which people gain control over the factors and decisions that shape their lives. It is the process by which they increase their assets and attributes and build capacities to gain access, partners, networks and/or a voice, in order to gain control" (World Health Organization, 2013) (Chapter 6).

community health "the health status of a defined group of people and the actions and conditions to promote, protect and preserve their health" (Joint Committee, 2012, p. 15) (Chapter 1).

community health education health education/promotion programs conducted in departments of health, voluntary agencies, hospitals, religious organizations, and so on.

competencies "reflects the ability of the student to understand, know, etc." (National Commission for Health Education Credentialing, Inc., 1996, p. 12) (Chapter 6).

Competencies Update Project (CUP) a project to review and update both entry-level and advanced-level health education/promotion competencies.

comprehensive school health instruction the development, delivery, and evaluation of a planned curriculum, preschool through grade 12, with goals, objectives, content sequence, and specific classroom lessons that include, but are not limited to, the following major content areas: community health, consumer health, environmental health, family life, mental and emotional health, injury prevention and safety, nutrition, personal health, prevention and control of disease, and substance use and abuse (Joint Committee on Health Education Terminology, 1991a, p. 102) (Chapter 2).

concepts the primary elements, building blocks, or major components of theories.

confidentiality exists when only those responsible for conducting a program can link information about a participant with that person and have promised not to reveal such to others.

consequentialism see *teleological theories*.

conservative a person who generally distrusts governmental regulations and tax-supported programs for addressing social or economic problems.

construct a concept that has been developed, created, or adopted for use with a specific theory.

contemplation stage a stage of the Transtheoretical Model in which a person is seriously thinking about change in the next six months.

continuum theories those behavior change theories that identify variables that influence actions and combine them into a single equation that predicts the likelihood of action (Weinstein, Rothman, & Sutton, 1998; Weinstein, Sandman, & Blalock, 2008) (Chapter 4).

credentialing a process whereby an individual or a professional preparation program meets the specified standards established by the credentialing body and is thus recognized for having done so.

crude rate the rate expressed for a total population.

cue to action a construct of the health belief model that motivates a person to act.

cultural competence "a developmental process defined as a set of values, principles, behaviors, attitudes, and policies that enable health professionals to work effectively across racial, ethnic, and linguistically diverse populations." (Joint Committee, 2012, p. 16) (Chapter 1).

death rates the number of deaths per 100,000 resident population, sometimes referred to as mortality or fatality rates.

decision-making philosophy the belief that the use of scenarios, case studies, and simulated problems is the best method to motivate persons to adopt positive health behaviors.

demographic profile a statistical breakdown of the population of a country, region, state, or city by age group, sex, race, and ethnicity.

deontological theories (or formalism or nonconsequentialism) "are those that claim that certain actions are inherently right or wrong, or good or bad, without regard for their consequences" (Reamer, 2006, p. 65) (Chapter 5).

determinants of health include genetics, health behaviors, social circumstances, environmental conditions, and access to health services.

Diffusion Theory a theory that provides an explanation for the movement of an innovation through a population.

Directors of Health Promotion and Education (DHPE) a professional association composed of individuals who, by position, head their state or territory public health education/promotion efforts.

disability-adjusted life years (DALYs) a measure of health that takes into account the severity of the health condition, age, and impact on the future.

disease prevention "the process of reducing risks and alleviating disease to promote, preserve, and restore health and minimize suffering and distress" (Joint Terminology Committee, 2001, p. 99) (Chapter 1).

distributive justice deals with the allocation of resources (Summers, 2009) (Chapter 5).

early adopters a group of people who are interested in innovation but do not want to be the first involved.

early majority a group of people who may be interested in an innovation but will need some external motivation to get involved.

eclectic health education/promotion philosophy a philosophical approach held by health education specialists that no one philosophy is "right" for all situations and circumstances and that the best philosophy involves blending the various philosophical approaches or using different approaches depending on the setting (school, community, worksite).

ecological approaches see *socio-ecological approach*.

ecological assessment is "a systematic assessment of factors in the social and physical environment that interact with behavior to produce health effects or quality-of-life outcomes" (Green & Kreuter, 2005, p. G-3) (Chapter 4).

ecological perspective see *socio-ecological approach*.

educational assessment is "the delineation of factors that predispose, enable, and reinforce a specific behavior, or through behavior, environmental changes" (Green & Kreuter, 2005, p. G-3) (Chapter 4).

elaboration the amount of cognitive processing (i.e., thought) that a person puts into receiving messages (Petty, Barden, & Wheeler, 2009) (Chapter 4).

electronic database computerized storage disks containing a large compilation of references; each database is specific to a general subject area (e.g., education, medicine) and provides access to the cumulative information found in several index or abstract sources on that subject area.

emotional-coping response to learn, a person must be able to deal with the sources of anxiety that surround a behavior.

empowerment "social action process for people to gain mastery over their lives and the lives of their communities" (Minkler, Wallerstein, & Wilson, 2008, p. 294) (Chapter 1).

enabling factor "any characteristic of the environment that facilitates action and any skill or resource required to attain a specific behavior" (Green & Kreuter, 1999, p. 505) (Chapter 4).

endemic occurs regularly in a population as a matter of course.

environment "all those matters related to health which are external to the human body and over which the individual has little or no control" (Lalonde, 1974, p. 32) (Chapter 1).

environmental assessment "a systematic assessment of factors in the social and physical environment that interact with behavior to produce health effects or quality-of-life outcomes. Also referred to as *ecological assessment*" (Green & Kreuter, 1999, p. 505) (Chapter 4).

epidemic an unexpectedly large number of cases of an illness, specific health-related behavior, or health-related event in a population.

epidemiological assessment "the delineation of the extent, distribution, and causes of a health problem in a defined population" (Green & Kreuter, 2005, p. G-3) (Chapter 4).

epidemiological data information gathered when measuring health and ill health.

epidemiology "the study of the distribution and determinants of health-related states or events in specific populations, and the application of this study to control health problems" (Dictionary of Epidemiology as cited in Last, 2007, p. iii) (Chapter 1).

epistemology the study of knowledge (Thiroux, 1995) (Chapter 5).

Eta Sigma Gamma (ESG) the national health education honorary.

ethical good/bad and right/wrong.

ethical dilemma "a situation that forces a decision that involves breaking some ethical norm or contradicting some ethical value" (Pozgar, 2013, p. 534) (Chapter 5).

ethics "the study of morality, one of the three major areas of philosophy, also referred to as moral philosophy" (Thiroux, 1995) (Chapter 5).

evidence a body of data that can be used to make decisions about planning.

evidence-based practice the process of systematically finding, appraising, and using evidence as the basis for decision making when planning health education/promotion programs (Cottrell & McKenzie, 2011) (Chapter 1).

expectancies values people place on expected outcomes.

expectations beliefs about the likely outcomes of certain behaviors.

formalism see *deontological theories*.

freeing or functioning philosophy proponents of this philosophy help the person make the best health choices possible for that person, based on the individual's needs and interests, not on societal expectations.

generalized model a planning model that includes the five major steps in developing a program.

global health "health problems, issues, and concerns that transcend national boundaries and are beyond the control of individual nations, and are best addressed by cooperative actions and solutions" (Joint Committee, 2012, p. 17) (Chapter 1).

goodness (rightness) a state or quality of being good; one of the five principles of common moral ground.

government documents unclassified publications authored and disseminated by federal, state, or local agencies intended for public use.

governmental health agencies agencies designated as having authority for certain specific duties or tasks outlined by the governmental bodies that oversee them.

graduate research assistantship an award given to a graduate student who works closely with one or more faculty members on a research project; the student is usually granted tuition assistance and a stipend in return for the work.

graduate teaching assistantship an award given to a graduate student who teaches for the program and in return is usually granted tuition assistance and a stipend.

hard money funds used to support health education/promotion positions and programs that are part of the regular budget of an employer.

health "is a dynamic state or condition that is multidimensional (i.e., physical, emotional, social, intellectual, spiritual, and occupational), a resource for living, and results from a person's interactions with and adaptation to the environment" (Joint Committee, 2012, p. 10) (Chapter 1).

health advocacy "the processes by which the actions of individuals or groups attempt to bring about social, environmental, and/or organizational change on behalf of a particular health goal, program, interest, or population" (Joint Committee, 2012, p. 17) (Chapter 1).

health behavior see *lifestyle*.

Health Belief Model an intrapersonal theory that "addresses a person's perceptions of the threat of a health problem and the accompanying appraisal of a recommended behavior for preventing or managing the problem" (Glanz & Rimer, 1995, p. 17) (Chapter 4).

healthcare organization "consists of the quantity, quality, arrangement, nature and relationships of people and resources in the provision of health care" (Lalonde, 1974, p. 32), also referred to as the healthcare system.

healthcare settings locations for health education/promotion programs, including public and for-profit hospitals, free-standing medical care clinics, home health agencies, and physician organizations such as health maintenance organizations (HMOs) and preferred provider organizations (PPOs).

health disparity the difference in health between different populations often caused by two health inequities—lack of access to care and lack of quality care (McKenzie et al., 2012) (Chapter 1).

health education "any combination of planned learning experiences using evidence based practices and/or sound theories that provide the opportunity to acquire knowledge, attitudes, and skills needed to adopt and maintain healthy behaviors" (Joint Committee, 2012, p. 17) (Chapter 1).

health education research "a systematic investigation involving the analysis of collected information or data that ultimately is used to enhance health education knowledge or practice, and answers one or more questions about a health-related theory, behavior or phenomenon" (Cottrell & McKenzie, 2011, p. 2) (Chapter 6).

health education specialist "an individual who has met, at a minimum, baccalaureate-level required health education academic preparation qualifications, who serves in a variety of settings, and is able to use appropriate educational strategies and methods to facilitate the development of policies, procedures, interventions, and systems conducive to the health of individuals, groups, and communities" (Joint Committee, 2012, p. 18) (Chapter 1).

health field a term that includes all matters that affect health; far more encompassing than the healthcare system.

Health Field Concept a framework that was developed in Canada to study health; it has four elements: human biology, environment, lifestyle, and healthcare organization.

health literacy the capacity of individuals to access, interpret, and understand basic health information and services and the skills to use the information and services to promote health.

health promotion "any planned combination of educational, political, environmental, regulatory, or organizational mechanisms that support actions and conditions of living conducive to the health of individuals, groups, and communities" (Joint Committee, 2012, p. 17) (Chapter 1).

health-related quality of life (HRQOL) "those aspects of overall quality of life that can be clearly shown to affect health—either physical or mental" (CDC, 2011b, ¶ 3) (Chapter 1).

Healthy People the first major U.S. government document recognizing the importance of lifestyle in promoting health and well-being.

Healthy People 2000: National Health Promotion and Disease Prevention Objectives a document that contains the health objectives for the United States during the 1990s.

Healthy People 2010: Understanding and Improving Health a document that contains the health objectives for the United States during the first decade of the 2000s.

Healthy People 2020 the latest listing of National Health Objectives for the United States through the year 2020.

Hippocrates a Greek physician from the Asclepian tradition who eventually became known as the father of medicine.

holistic philosophy the philosophy that the mind and body blend into a single unit; the person is a unified being.

human biology "all those aspects of health, both physical and mental, which are developed within the human body as a consequence of the basic biology of man [sic] and the organic make-up of an individual" (Lalonde, 1974, p. 31) (Chapter 1).

Hygeia the daughter of Asclepius granted the power to prevent disease.

impact evaluation "the assessment of program effects on intermediate objectives including changes in predisposing, enabling, and reinforcing factors, behavioral and environmental changes, and possibly health and social outcomes" (Green & Kreuter, 2005, p. G-5) (Chapter 4).

implementation "the act of converting program objectives into actions through policy changes, regulation and organization" (Green & Kreuter, 2005, G-5) (Chapter 4).

indexes reference books that provide links to articles from many refereed journals, books, and selected reports; each index is written to target specific subject headings, so one index is not all-encompassing for all subjects.

individual freedom (equality principle, or principle of autonomy) people, being individuals with individual differences, must have the freedom to choose their own ways and means of being moral within the framework of value of life, goodness, justice, and truth-telling (Thiroux, 1995) (Chapter 5).

informed consent requires (a) disclosure of relevant information to prospective participants about the program; (b) their comprehension of the information; and (c) their voluntary agreement, free from coercion and undue influence, to participate (OHSR, 2006) (Chapter 5).

innovators the first people to adopt an innovation.

intention "is an indication of a person's readiness to perform a given behavior, and it is considered to be the immediate antecedent of behavior" (Ajzen, 2006) (Chapter 4).

International Union for Health Promotion and Education (IUHPE) a professional association open to individuals who are interested in health education/promotion on a global basis.

intervention alignment matching appropriate strategies and interventions with projected changes and outcomes.

intervention mapping a six-phase program planning model guided by diagrams and matrices that incorporate outputs of the assessment process with relevant theory to help develop appropriate interventions for priority populations.

justice (fairness) "human beings should treat other human beings fairly and justly in distributing goodness and badness among them" (Thiroux, 1995, p. 184) (Chapter 5); a basic principle of ethics.

laggards the last group of people to get involved in an innovation, if they get involved at all.

late majority a group of people who are skeptical and will not adopt an innovation until most people in the social system have done so.

liberal generally, a person who favors governmental programs to address perceived social and economic inequities between segments of society.

licensure "a process by which an agency or government (usually a state) grants permission to individuals to practice a given profession by certifying that those licensed have attained specific standards of competence" (Cleary, 1995, p. 39) (Chapter 6).

life expectancy "the average number of years of life remaining to a person at a particular age and based on a given set of age-specific death rates—generally the mortality conditions existing in the period mentioned. Life expectancy may be determined by race, sex, or other characteristics using age-specific death rates for the population with that characteristic" (NCHS, 2013, p. 452) (Chapter 1).

lifestyle "an aggregation of decisions by individuals which affect their health and over which they more or less have control" (Lalonde, 1974, p. 32) (Chapter 1).

likelihood of taking action chances that a person will behave in a particular way; a construct of the health belief model.

local health department (LHD) a governmental organization that is located in a city or county.

locus of control one's perception of the center of control over reinforcement.

logic model used in program planning and evaluation. Researcher creates a visual to indicate the relationship between program resources, program activities, and desired program outcomes (Chapter 4).

macrolevel having health education/promotion interventions targeted to the community as a whole, instead of to individuals.

maintenance stage the stage of the Transtheoretical Model in which a person is taking steps to sustain a behavior change and resist temptation to relapse.

Master Certified Health Education Specialist (MCHES) an advanced level of certification available for certified health education specialists (CHES) who have 5 continuous years as a certified health education specialist or for those with a master's degree in health education or a master's degree in another field with at least 25 semester hours of health education classes The MCHES exam must be taken and passed to receive this credential.

MAPP is the acronym for the planning model titled Mobilizing for Action through Planning and Partnerships created by the National Association of County and City Health Officials.

MATCH an acronym for Multilevel Approach To Community Health.

M.A., M.Ed., M.H.S., M.P.H., M.S., M.S.P.H. degree designations available to master's-level health education/promotion students, depending on the institution they attend and their area of emphasis.

Medicaid government health insurance for the poor.

Medicare government health insurance for the elderly and disabled.

metaphysics the study of the nature of reality (Thiroux, 1995) (Chapter 5).

miasmas theory a belief that vapors, or miasmas, rising from rotting refuse could travel through the air for great distances and result in disease when inhaled.

microlevel targeting health education/promotion interventions to individuals.

model "is a composite, a mixture of ideas or concepts taken from any number of theories and used together" (Hayden, 2009, p. 1) (Chapter 4).

moderate a person who acts in a more situationally specific manner in regard to using tax-supported programs to solve social problems.

modifiable risk factors changeable or controllable risk factors.

moral good/bad and right/wrong.

moral philosophy see *ethics*.

moral sensitivity being aware that an ethical problem exists and having an understanding of what impact different courses of action may have on the people involved (Rest et al., 1999) (Chapter 5).

multicausation disease model a model that explains the onset of disease caused by more than one factor.

multitasking the skill of coordinating and completing multiple health education/promotion projects at the same time.

National Commission for Health Education Credentialing, Inc. (NCHEC) the organization that oversees the health education certification process.

National Task Force on the Preparation and Practice of Health Educators the group that oversaw development of the roles and responsibilities of health education specialists and ultimately the CHES credentialing system.

National Wellness Institute, Inc. (NWI) a professional association for those interested in wellness programs.

needs assessment a process that helps program planners determine what health problems might exist in any given group of people, what assets are available in the community to address the health problems, and the overall capacity of the community to address the health issues (McKenzie et al., 2009) (Chapter 6).

networking establishing and maintaining a wide range of contacts in the profession that may be of help when looking for a job and in carrying out one's job responsibilities once hired.

noncommunicable diseases those that cannot be transmitted from an infected person to a susceptible, healthy one (McKenzie et al., 2012) (Chapter 1).

nonconsequential see *deontological theories*.

nongovernmental health agencies those that operate, for the most part, free from governmental interference as long as they comply with the Internal Revenue Service's guidelines for their tax status (McKenzie et al., 2012) (Chapter 8).

nonmaleficence "the non-infliction of harm to others" (Balog et al., 1985, p. 91) (Chapter 5).

nonmodifiable risk factors unchangeable or uncontrollable risk factors.

objective statement describing specific, measurable cognitive or affective changes in the learner. An objective establishes a performance standard for the learner.

open access journals are journals that are available to the reader online without restriction to cost, membership, or legal barriers with the exception that the reader must be able to access the Internet.

outcome evaluation "assessment of the effects of a program on its ultimate objectives, including changes in health and social benefits or quality of life" (Green & Kreuter, 2005, p. G-6) (Chapter 4).

ownership a feeling of responsibility for program outcomes.

Panacea the daughter of Asclepius granted the power to treat disease.

pandemic an outbreak over a wide geographical area, such as a continent.

participation the active involvement of those in the priority population in helping identify, plan, and implement programs to address the health problems they face.

peer-reviewed journal a journal that publishes original manuscripts only after they have been read and critiqued by a panel of experts (peers) in the field.

perceived barriers the cost of engaging in a health behavior; a construct of the Health Belief Model.

perceived behavioral control a belief held by people that they have control over a behavior; a construct of the theory of planned behavior.

perceived benefits a belief that a particular health recommendation would be beneficial in reducing a perceived threat; a construct of the Health Belief Model.

perceived seriousness/severity a belief that a health problem is serious; a construct of the Health Belief Model.

perceived susceptibility a belief that one is vulnerable to a health problem; a construct of the Health Belief Model.

perceived threat a belief that one is vulnerable to a serious health problem or to the sequelae of that illness or condition; a construct of the Health Belief Model.

philanthropic foundation "endowed institution that donates money for the good of humankind" (McKenzie et al., 2012, p. 57) (Chapter 8).

philodoxy literally means "the love of opinion" but often is used in the context of letting opinion define reality.

philosophy a statement summarizing the attitudes, principles, beliefs, values, and concepts held by an individual or a group.

philosophy of symmetry a philosophy of health with physical, emotional, spiritual, and social components of health.

popular press publications publications ranging from weekly summary magazines (e.g., *Newsweek*) to monthly magazines (e.g., *Better Homes and Gardens*); articles often include editorials. Information from these sources should be heavily scrutinized before using.

population-based approaches community health methods that are used to help change behavior in groups of people. Examples include policy development, policy advocacy, organizational change, community development, empowerment of individuals, and economic supports.

population health "a cohesive, integrated, and comprehensive approach to health care that considers the distribution of health outcomes within a population, the health determinants that influence distribution of care, and the policies and interventions that affect and are affected by the determinants" (Nash, Fabius, Skoufalos, Clarke, & Horowitz, 2016, p. 448) (Chapter 1).

portfolio a collection of evidence that enables students to demonstrate mastery of desired course or program outcomes.

postsecondary institution in the United States, an institution that provides further education after high school.

PRECEDE-PROCEED an acronym for a theory of implementation that stands for Predisposing, Reinforcing, and Enabling Constructs in Educational/Environmental Diagnosis and Evaluation and Policy, Regulatory, and Organizational Constructs in Educational and Environmental Development.

precontemplation stage the stage of the Transtheoretical Model in which a person is not thinking about change in the next six months.

predisposing factor "any characteristic of a person or population that motivates behavior prior to the occurrence of the behavior" (Green & Kreuter, 2005, p. G-6) (Chapter 4).

preparation stage the stage of the Transtheoretical Model in which a person is actively planning change.

prevention the planning for and measures taken to forestall the onset of, limit the spread of, and rehabilitate after pathogenesis or other health problems.

primary data original data gathered by the health education specialist as part of a needs assessment; this includes data gathered from telephone surveys, focus groups, and interviews.

primary prevention preventive measures that forestall the onset of illness or injury during the prepathogenesis period.

primary sources published studies or eyewitness accounts written by the person(s) who actually conducted the study or observed the event.

privacy "the claim of individuals, groups, or institutions to determine for themselves when, how, and to what extent information about them is communicated to others" (Westin, 1968, p. 7) (Chapter 5).

procedural justice deals with whether or not fair procedures were in place and whether those procedures were followed (Summers, 2009) (Chapter 5).

process evaluation "the assessment of policies, materials, personnel, performance, quality of practice or services, and other inputs and implementation experiences" (Green & Kreuter, 2005, p. G-6) (Chapter 4).

professional ethics "actions that are right and wrong in the workplace and are of public matter. Professional moral principles are not statements of taste or preference; they tell practitioners what they ought to do and what they ought not to do" (Feeney & Freeman, 1999, p. 6) (Chapter 5).

professional health associations/organizations organizations that promote the high standards of professional practice for their respective professions, thereby improving the health of society by improving the people in the professions (McKenzie et al., 2012) (Chapter 8).

Promoting Health/Preventing Disease: Objectives for the Nation a document containing 226 health objectives for the United States to be accomplished during the 1980s.

public health "an organized effort by society, primarily through its public institutions, to improve, promote, protect and restore the health of the population through collective action. It includes services such as health situation analysis, health surveillance, health promotion, prevention, infectious disease control, environmental protection and sanitation, disaster and health emergency preparedness and response, and occupational health, among others" (from WHO, 2016, available at http://www.who.int/healthsystems/hss_glossary/en/index8.html) (Chapter 1).

public health agencies also called "official governmental health agencies"; agencies usually financed through public tax monies and typically offering health promotion and education programs.

quality assurance "The planned and systematic activities necessary to provide adequate confidence that the product or service will meet given requirements" (Quality Assurance Solutions, 2010) (Chapter 6).

quasi-governmental health agencies agencies that possess some of the characteristics of a governmental health agency but also possess some of the characteristics of nongovernmental agencies.

rate "a measure of some event, disease, or condition in relation to a unit of population, along with some specification of time" (NCHS, 2013, p. 468) (Chapter 1).

reciprocal determinism "Environmental factors influence individuals and groups, but individuals and groups can also influence their environments and regulate their own behavior" (McAlister, Perry, & Parcel, 2008, p. 171) (Chapter 4).

reduction of threat a belief that a particular health recommendation would be beneficial in reducing a threat at a subjectively acceptable cost; a construct of the health belief model.

reform phase of public health the period from 1900 to 1920 during which many federal regulations were passed to protect and improve the public's health.

reinforcement a response to behavior that increases the chance of recurrence.

reinforcing factor "any reward or punishment following or anticipated as a consequence of a behavior, serving to strengthen the motivation for the behavior after it occurs" (Green & Kreuter, 2005, G-7) (Chapter 4).

research ethics "comprises principles and standards that, along with underlying values, guide appropriate conduct relevant to research decisions" (Kimmel, 2007, p. 6) (Chapter 5).

responsibilities the seven major responsibilities of all entry-level health education specialists.

risk factors those inherited, environmental, and behavioral influences "which are known (or thought) to increase the likelihood of physical or mental problems" (Slee et al., 2008, p. 510) (Chapter 1).

role delineation the process of identifying the specific responsibilities, competencies, and subcompetencies associated with the practice of health education/promotion.

Rule of Sufficiency the programs, strategies, initiatives, and methods implemented must be sufficiently robust, or effective enough, that the stated objectives will have a reasonable chance of being met.

School Health Advisory Council (SHAC) community members such as parents; medical, health, and safety professionals; and political, religious, and corporate or business leaders who assist with the planning and promotion of school health initiatives.

School Health Education Evaluation Study a landmark study that examined the entire health program of selected schools in the Los Angeles area.

school health education/promotion instruction health education programs that instruct school-age children/youth about health and health-related behaviors.

School Health Education Study a nationwide study that examined the status of health education and resulted in the development of an important curriculum.

search engine site on the World Wide Web specifically designed to search for all links associated with a word or phrase that the user wants information on; the search engines greatly decrease the time it takes to search for information on the Web; examples are Google, Yahoo®, and Bing.

secondary data preexisting data used by a health education specialist in a needs assessment.

secondary prevention preventive measures that lead to early diagnosis and prompt treatment of a disease or an injury to limit disability, impairment, or dependency and to prevent more severe pathogenesis.

secondary sources articles that often provide an overview or a summary of several related studies or that chronicle the history of several related events, written by someone who did not conduct the study or observe firsthand the event that is written about.

self-control (self-regulation) gaining control over one's own behavior by monitoring and adjusting it.

self-efficacy people's confidence in their ability to perform a certain desired task or function.

service learning course credit for students to work with a community agency to meet an identified community need.

SHAPE America (Society of Health and Physical Educators) membership organization of health and physical education professionals—preK-12 educators to university professors.

situational analysis is "the combination of social and epidemiological assessments of conditions, trends, and priorities with a preliminary scan of determinants, relevant policies, resources, organizational support, and regulations that might anticipate or permit action in advance of a more complete assessment of behavioral, environmental, educational, ecological, and administrative factors" (Green & Kreuter, 2005, pp. G-7 & G-8) (Chapter 4).

SMART is an acronym for a social marketing planning model titled the Social Marketing Assessment and Response Tool.

Smith Papyri the oldest written document related to health, which describes various surgical techniques and dates back to 1600 B.C.E.

social assessment "the assessment in both objective and subjective terms of high-priority problems or aspirations for the common good, defined for a population by economic and social indicators and by individuals in terms of their quality of life" (Green & Kreuter, 2005, p. 492) (Chapter 4).

social capital "the relationships and structures within a community, such as civic participation, networks, norms of reciprocity, and trust, that promote cooperation of mutual benefit" (Putnam, 1995, p. 66) (Chapter 4).

social change philosophy a philosophy emphasizing the role of health education/promotion in creating social, economic, and political change that benefits the health of individuals and groups.

social determinants of health "conditions in the environments in which people are born, live, learn, work, play, worship, and age that affect a wide range of health, functioning, and quality-of-life outcomes and risk" (USDHHS, 2013, ¶ 4) (Chapter 1).

social ecology an approach to health education/promotion that goes beyond individual behavior change to examine and modify the social, political, and economic factors impacting health behavior decisions.

social marketing "the application of commercial marketing technologies to the analysis, planning, execution, and evaluation of programs designed to influence the voluntary behavior of target audiences in order to improve their personal welfare and that of their society" (Andreasen, 1995, p. 7) (Chapter 4).

social media "media that uses the Internet and other technologies to allow for social interaction" (McKenzie et al., 2012, p. 448) (Chapter 1).

social network "web of social relationships that surround people" (Heaney & Israel, 2008, p. 190) (Chapter 4).

social networking connecting to other individuals (or organizations) that are tied (connected) by one or more specific types of interdependency, such as friendship, kinship, common interest, financial exchange, occupational or professional interests, or beliefs. Facebook, Myspace, LinkedIn, Twitter, YouTube, and Instagram are just a few examples of social networking sites that may be of value to health education specialists.

social norms "what are perceived to be true and acceptable" (Simons-Morton et al., 2012, p. 158) (Chapter 4).

Society for Public Health Education, Inc. (SOPHE) a professional association for health education specialists.

Society of State Leaders of Health and Physical Education a professional association composed of individuals who, by position in a state or territorial department of education, represent their state or territory.

socio-ecological approach behavior has multiple levels of influences.

soft money funds to support health education/promotion positions and programs secured through grants or contracts, which may be discontinued at the end of a designated period.

specific rate a rate for a particular population subgroup, such as for a particular disease (i.e., disease-specific) or for a particular age of people.

stage theories those behavior change theories that comprise an ordered set of categories into which people can be classified (staged) and for which factors could be identified that could induce movement from one category to the next (Weinstein & Sandman, 2002) (Chapter 4).

sub-competencies A "cluster of simpler but essential related skills or abilities within a competency" (NCHEC & SOPHE, 2015, p. 90) (Chapter 6).

subjective norm a belief held by people that others (individuals or groups) think they should do something and that they care about what others think; a construct of the theory of planned behavior.

technology any device used by society to increase access to or opportunity for people to be exposed to that device—for example, computers and television have increased educational access and opportunities for many people; thus, they are examples of technology.

teleological theories (or **consequentialism**) evaluate the moral status of an act by the goodness of the consequences (Reamer, 2006) (Chapter 5).

termination zero chance of relapsing after a behavior change.

tertiary prevention preventive measures aimed at rehabilitation following significant pathogenesis.

tertiary sources publications such as pamphlets, handbooks, or brochures containing information collected from primary or secondary sources.

theories/models of implementation theories and models used in planning, implementing, and evaluating health education/promotion programs.

theory "a set of interrelated concepts, definitions, and propositions that presents a systematic view of events or situations by specifying relations among variables in order to explain and predict the events of the situations" (Glanz et al., 2008b, p. 25) (Chapter 4).

Theory of Planned Behavior an intrapersonal theory that addresses individuals' intentions to perform a given behavior as a function of their attitude toward performing the behavior, their beliefs about what is relevant, what others think they should do, and their perception of the ease or difficulty in performing the behavior.

traditional family a family having two parents and their children.

Transtheoretical Model of Change also known as the stages of change model, it is an intrapersonal theory that addresses an "individual's readiness to change or attempt to change toward healthy behaviors" (Glanz & Rimer, 1995, p. 17) (Chapter 4).

truth telling (honesty) to tell the truth; one of the five principles of common moral ground.

value of life a basic principle of ethics: no life should be ended without strong justification.

variable the operational form (practical use) of a construct.

voluntary health agencies "organizations that are created by concerned citizens to deal with health needs not met by governmental agencies"

(McKenzie et al., 2012) (Chapters 7 and 8); these organizations rely heavily on volunteer help and donations to function.

wellness "an approach to health that focuses on balancing the many aspects, or dimensions, of a person's life through increasing the adoption of health enhancing conditions and behaviors rather than attempting to minimize conditions of illness" (Joint Committee, 2012, p. 10) (Chapter 1).

Whole School, Whole Community, Whole Child (WSCC) Model an ecological approach for improving student learning and health in our nation's schools by focusing on the whole school with the school in turn drawing resources and influences from the whole community to address the needs of the whole child (Association for Supervision and Curriculum Development, available at http://www.ascd.org/programs/learning-and-health/wscc-model.aspx).

worksite health promotion health education/promotion programs offered by business and industry entities for their employees.

years of potential life lost (YPLL) a measure of premature mortality calculated by subtracting a person's age at death from 75 years (NCHS, 2013) (Chapter 1).

Chapter 1
P.7,8: Jaime Harding

Chapter 2
P. 35: The Metropolitan Museum of Art/Image Resource, NY; p. 37: Richard Ashworth/ Robert Harding Picture Library Lts/Alamy Stock Photo; p. 38: Alinari/Art Resource, New York; p. 39 (top): Garry Gay/Alamy Stock Photo; p. 39 (bottom): Mrakor/Fotolia; p. 41: Stevanzz/Fotolia; p. 46: Robert Harding World Imagery; p. 49: Library of Congress; p. 50: U.S. Department of Health and Human Services; p. 52: PVDE/Bridgeman Images; p. 53: James Gathany/Centers for Disease Control and Prevention; p. 58: Library of Congress Prints and Photographs Division Washington [LC-DIG-nclc-02986]

Chapter 3
P.77: James Girvan; p. 79: Mark Boster/Los Angeles Times/Getty Images

Chapter 4
P. 103: Oleg Baliuk/Shutterstock; pp. 116–117, Trevor Newby

Chapter 5
P. 142 (left): Underwood Archives/Getty Images; p. 142 (right): Kenneth Benjamin Reed/ Shutterstock; p. 145: Mohammed Zaatari/AP Images; p. 149: Kevork Djansezian/Getty Images

Chapter 6
P. 166: Helen P. Cleary; pp. 169–170: Angela Adams; p. 173: Gary Gilmore; p. 181: Lucky winner/Alamy Stock Photo; pp. 191–192: Jovanni Reyes

Chapter 7
P.205: David Buffington/Photodisc/Getty Images; pp. 208–209: Carolyn Conley; p. 210: Raymond Boyd/Getty Images; pp. 211–213: Jennifer O'Donnell; pp. 216–217: Ashton Putnam; pp. 222–223: Nicole Gaudette;p. 227: Robert Clay/Alamy; pp. 228–229: Heather Rhodes; pp. 233–234: Elizabeth Peeler; pp.235–237: Emily Miller; pp. 239–241: Patricia Stewart; pp. 243–244: Jeremy Herzberg; pp. 247–249: Louise Villejo

Chapter 8

P. 256: James F. McKenzie; p. 262: XiXinXing/Alamy Stock Photo; p. 263: Klaus-Dietmar Gabbert/picture-alliance/dpa/AP Images; pp. 265–267: Melissa E. Shelton; pp. 270–271: Sheridan Stanley

Chapter 9

P. 283: ACE Stock Limited/Alamy Stock Photo; pp. 284–285: Janet Kamiri; p. 294: U.S. National Library of Medicine; p. 296: Centers for Disease Control and Prevention

Chapter 10

P. 309: Robert Kneschke/Fotolia; 313,(top) Siberia/Fotolia; (bottom: Richard Lord/The Image Works;